Domination & Submission:

The BDSM Relationship Handbook

MICHAEL MAKAI

ISBN: 1492775975
ISBN-13: 978-1492775973

DEDICATION

This book is for the people
who are simply tired of pretending to be
something or someone they are not,
and are ready for a change.

CONTENTS

All people dream, but not equally. Those
who dream by night in the dusty recesses of their mind,
wake in the morning to find that it was vanity.
But the dreamers of the day are dangerous people,
for they dream their dreams with open eyes,
and make them come true.

-- *D. H. Lawrence*

Preface

Don't read this book.

By that, I mean don't *just* read this book. Please ponder it. Question it. Study it. Get mad about it. Laugh *at* it. Laugh *with* it. Use it. Abuse it. Talk about it. Recommend it. Criticize it. Burn it. Gift it. Pass it along to a friend. *Do something* with it.

This book is for those who may be either curious about the Domination/submission lifestyle, or find themselves suddenly a part of it, and needful of information to fill the gaps in their knowledge and experience. Though written from the admittedly highly subjective perspective of a male heterosexual Dominant with over thirty years of real-life experience in D/s relationships, great pains have been taken to apply a modicum of objectivity to the endeavor.

It's probably important to state up-front that there is, always has been, and always will be a great deal of controversy both in and outside of the D/s lifestyle about many of the topics discussed in this book. Frankly, there is *barely* any consensus even on the question of whether Domination/submission constitutes a "lifestyle" *at all.* Opinions on that particular question range from the one extreme of classifying it as a *mental disorder and aberration*, to the other of elevating it to the status of a faux religion or divine truth. The reality can be found somewhere in the mushy middle, where this lifestyle is simply a choice between consenting adults on one of the most important aspects of *any* relationship dynamic. We're talking, of course, about the essential question: *who is really in charge and what, exactly, does that mean?*

Note the very specific wording. When we say "*really*" in charge, we're acknowledging a dirty little secret about human relationships in general. Quite often – perhaps more often than we care to admit – the person who *thinks* he or she is in charge, *really isn't.* We will discuss that and similar topics at length later in the book. Many of these questions will open a large can of worms that, frankly, many people would prefer to keep closed and tucked away somewhere cool and dark.

We will also be exploring in depth a question that I consider to be the core issue that is at the heart of the Domination/submission lifestyle. That question is: Is D/s *who you are*, or is it *something that you do?* If you have not yet asked yourself that question, and come up with an acceptable answer, you may be getting just a little ahead of yourself in your quest for knowledge about the lifestyle. For the purposes of this book, we will treat Domination/submission as a *mindset and relationship dynamic*; certainly an important aspect of *who you are*. As we explore further the mechanics of *what one does* in this lifestyle, we will attempt to consistently refer to that as BDSM, or *Bondage Discipline Sadism and Masochism.*

Why should it be important to make the distinction? Consider the fact that most people who are D/s at their core do not want to spend the rest of their lives with someone who considers it a Saturday night kink that can be discarded on a whim at some point in the future. Imagine the horror of a submissive who wakes up one morning to discover that the Dominant she depends upon and worships as Lord and Master has suddenly decided it's *his turn* to be the submissive. Unfortunately such things can, *and do*, happen with annoying regularity in the lifestyle.

I consider Domination/submission to be what happens in your head and heart. It's all about *how you love,* and how you express that love. BDSM is more about what *physically* happens between you and your partner or playmates. It's *something you do.* Is there often a certain degree of overlap? Of course there is, all the time. In fact, for most people, the more overlap the better. But there are also relationships where they can be completely separate, and some people happen to *like* it that way. The stereotypical 1950's television sitcom marriage that portrayed the husband as king of his castle, and his spouse as a stay-at-home submissive housewife who fretted about *"ring around the collar"* is probably a good portrayal of how D/s can exist without BDSM.

How do you know whether you're dominant or submissive at your core? The odds are actually pretty good that you are *neither* and, frankly, there's *absolutely nothing wrong with that.* The great majority of human beings that inhabit this planet comprise the 80% or more who have an equitable mixture of *both* dominant and submissive tendencies. Perhaps 10% have inherently dominant personalities, and another 10% submissive personalities. One should always be careful about assuming that a person's career choices or relationship dynamics reflect or define their core personality. Quite often, submissive people are thrust into jobs and relationships that require them to function in a dominant role. That's not to say they find joy or fulfillment in it. Just because someone may be *good* at being dominant doesn't necessarily mean they *have to like it.* The same sort of thing happens to dominant people who are required to function as subordinates at work or in relationships.

We'll discuss various ways to help a person to determine their core D/s personality type elsewhere in this book. As a general rule of thumb, the mere fact that you may be uncertain and questioning about your role probably places you in that not-so-rare category that I like to call "*normal.*" Most people are perfectly comfortable assuming *either* role, depending on the needs and appropriateness of the given situation. A hard-wired or *true* Dominant knows no other way to be, and is often profoundly uncomfortable assuming the role of a submissive, under *any* circumstances. Similarly, a hard-wired or *true* submissive would sooner cut off her right arm than have to take on a dominant role. If neither of those reactions sounds very familiar to you, then you're probably like *most* people, meaning you fall somewhere *between* those two extremes.

If BDSM is a growing sexual fascination for you, or simply an opportunity for you and your partner to try something new and exciting, that's perfectly okay. You can learn a *lot* from this book, and adopting some BDSM interests and techniques can definitely be a healthy and deliciously kinky way to spice up what otherwise might be a pretty routine sex life. It is important, however, to know the difference between a *kink* and a *lifestyle*, and to be honest about that with your potential partners.

The Domination/submission lifestyle, like any other lifestyle choice, can be a complex yet rewarding way to live if you and your potential partner(s) are guided by similar values, follow familiar protocols, and share the same vision. Conversely, your experience with the lifestyle can end up being a train wreck if you fail to take inventory of your own capacity to live in a D/s relationship, as well as your tolerance levels for the great diversity of expression you'll encounter from others in this lifestyle.

A Domination/submission relationship can be as comforting as a warm blanket or as frightening as an unexpected encounter with a knife-wielding stranger in a dark alley. It can be uplifting and empowering, or it can be abusive and dangerous. It can bring great joy into your life, or tremendous sadness. Ultimately, it will be whatever you and your partner make of it. If you fail, it won't be because there is something wrong with the lifestyle. It will be because you were inadequately prepared to live it.

That is why you should fully understand *what* you're getting into, *why* you're doing it, and whether you are *suited* for it. It is only *after* those key questions have been answered, that you should be at all concerned with whether or not you might be any *good* at it.

A final *caveat,* which I feel compelled to make before you read much further, would be to explain my conscious decision to dispense with the practice of footnoting all factoids and their sources. I am a firm believer in the words of financial wizard Bernard Baruch, who once quipped, "Every man has a right to his own opinion, but no man has a right to be wrong in his facts." I have gone to great lengths to be as meticulous as possible in researching and validating the facts, statistics and data that

I've cited in this book. I've also shared many of my personal opinions and anecdotes, which I always attempt to identify as such. The controversial topic and treatment of my *first* book, published in 2012 under a pseudonym, taught me an extremely valuable lesson. That book was painstakingly researched, heavily footnoted, and meticulously researched from the most credible and authoritative sources available. In the end, that simply *didn't matter*.

Readers who were predisposed to agree with my world-view *ignored* the thirty-plus pages of footnotes. Conversely, readers who held *differing* views from mine seemed all too willing and eager to *automatically* dismiss any source of data that supported an opposing point of view as being *non-credible*. Consequently, the notes which were provided as an expression of my earnest desire to be scrupulously accurate and transparent in my research became, instead, nothing more than a distraction and liability.

The lesson I learned from that experience was this: The measure of a book's success isn't found in its footnotes, it can only be found in its *utility*. If you find the information contained in the pages of this book to be *useful* to you, then that is a *very good thing*. In that case, I would recommend that you put that information to work at making your relationships more fulfilling, and your life better. I would also ask you to recommend or give the book to your friends and relatives who might derive some benefit from it.

If, on the other hand, you don't much like the facts and statistics that I've presented in this book, or if you strongly disagree with my admittedly unique lifestyle perspective, *that's* perfectly okay *too*. You are certainly entitled to your own *opinions*, if not your own set of *facts*. I would encourage you, if you're any good at articulating your thoughts and are ready to write a best-selling book, to *give me a call*. Maybe I can help you out.

The bottom line is I hope you will enjoy reading this book as much as I enjoyed writing it, and that you will feel that the price you paid for it was money well-spent.

ACKNOWLEDGMENTS

I want to express my undying gratitude to
the very special people in my life who helped make this
book possible. You believed in me, even when I found
it hard to believe in myself. You encouraged, cajoled, and
cheered me when I needed it most. You put up with my grump.
You are my synergist, muse, and inspiration.
Thank you so very much.

"We are defined by how we use our power."

-- *Gerry Spence, The Rat Hole (2003)*

CHAPTER 1: THE DOMINANT

What is a Dominant?

Just as we might expect any reasonable discussion of the *solar system* to focus first upon our *sun*, we're going to begin our examination of Domination/submission *(D/s)* relationships by taking a look at the self-appointed center of the D/s universe, the *Dominant*. In any relationship, it is always the *interplay* of personalities that helps us to understand the true nature of the relationship dynamic at work. It isn't so much about what happens *inside* of their heads, as it is about what happens *between* the partners in the relationship. This is very much the case in a *D/s relationship*, where the true expression of one's core personality is enhanced by a partner who not only understands it, but encourages it and thrives upon it. After all, it's hard to be a leader without a follower, and vice-versa.

In this chapter, we will explore the part that the Dominant plays in this little waltz. Some of the questions we'll address are: What is a Dominant? What drives a Dominant? How does someone know if he or she is a Dominant? How does one approach, or please a Dominant? What are the risks and drawbacks of being a Dominant, or being involved with one? We'll discuss those, and other relevant questions, because at the risk of appearing to contradict what I've just said in the preceding paragraph, it *is* important to understand what is going on *inside* of a Dominant's head as a precursor to understanding what occurs *between* a Dominant and his or her submissive.

Knowing a Dominant's heart and mind can often be a difficult thing. A Dominant, generally speaking, does not appreciate being psychoanalyzed, categorized, or labeled. The reason can be simply stated thusly: *Scientia potentia est.* Knowledge is power. For a Dominant, life is all about *power*, in one form or another. It needn't always be about power over other people. Sometimes, it can be as simple as the power to control or change his own life circumstances, to alter his environment, or to choose his own path.

If you really want to learn about a person's true character, the part of him that stays safely tucked away from view most of the time, just give him a little *power*. There is no faster, nor more accurate way to see what lies buried beneath the public veneer. You've no doubt seen what happens to petty bureaucrats when they're given just a *little bit* of power. Various university psychological experiments have shown that when individuals are given the power to *anonymously* administer electrical shocks to another individual, they quickly become increasingly and surprisingly cruel in doing so. Just imagine what can happen when someone is handed *absolute power* over another human being. The results are often not very pretty.

How does one avoid that ugly and potentially *dangerous* possibility? One way is to learn the difference between a true Dominant and a pretender. A pretender is someone who is simply infatuated with the notion that having *absolute power* over another human being for the first time in his miserable, powerless life might be *really cool.* If you're a submissive who would prefer to avoid becoming an unwitting part of someone's tragically warped, doomed-from-the-start psycho-social experiment, *avoid the pretenders*.

Before we go any further, let's clarify some terminology.

Throughout this book, I'll often refer to a Dominant as *"he"* and a submissive as *"she"*. Please be assured that this is *not* the result of any gender bias, but simply a way to avoid the awkward and clunky *"he or she"* – or even worse, the grammatically incorrect *"they."* It is also done out of recognition that, in a purely *statistical* sense, Dominants are far more likely to be male, and submissives to be female. Additionally, society generally characterizes dominance and submission as male and female traits, respectively. I really *am* fully aware and appreciative of the many good people both in and out of the lifestyle who defy the stereotypes. I am a *wordsmith*, and my job is to connect with an audience with a predominantly *vanilla* perspective. For those who may not have heard the term used in this context before, *vanilla* is the word used by those in the D/s lifestyle to describe those *outside of it.*

You'll also see me using the terms *"true Dominant"* or *"true submissive."* This will probably infuriate some folks, especially those who may be unsure or insecure about their place on the Dominant-submissive spectrum. Please remember that the great majority of people fall somewhere in the middle, with a rather equitable mix of *both* Dominant and submissive tendencies and character traits. That's *perfectly normal* and acceptable, even in this culture that sometimes views *normalcy* as abhorrent. There's no crime in being a lot like the great majority of humanity.

A very tiny percentage of people will find themselves at either extreme of the scale, feeling not just more comfortable there, but *profoundly uncomfortable* with the mere thought of being anywhere else. That isn't to say that they can't *function* in roles outside of their core D/s orientation; just that doing so brings them no sense of joy or fulfillment. For some, working or living counter to their core D/s orientation brings them a great deal of emotional stress and makes them want to escape to their inner *happy place* all the more. So, how does one spot the *"true Dominant"* in a world where people often change their roles the way we change our socks? The answer lies in that emotional stress and *happy place*.

Everyone experiences stress. It's an integral part of life, and completely unavoidable. In many ways, we are *defined* by how we handle that stress and by how we process it. Imagine the difference between how you might expect an optimist to handle stress, versus how you might expect a pessimist to handle the same stressful situation. Imagine further how surprised you might be if a good friend, who always seemed cheerful and optimistic on the surface, inexplicably shifts into *"doom and gloom"* mode whenever the *crapola* hits the fan. Does that sound like anyone you know? If so, then you've experienced first-hand the phenomenon we're talking about.

Your friend operates one way on the surface, when things are going the way they should, and another way *below* the surface, when things *aren't* going quite so well. While we may sometimes refer to this as seeing someone *"freak out,"* in reality, what you're seeing is simply a case of someone *reverting to type*. At a certain point, under extreme duress, a person no longer *cares* what anyone thinks and they abandon their carefully crafted façade and fall back upon their *core coping strategy*. Sometimes that core personality characteristic is in sync with their public persona and sometimes it isn't. Frankly, being in sync isn't really all that important to our purposes. My sole purpose in calling your attention to it is so you can apply what we'll call the First Commandment of D/s Relationships: **Know Thyself.**

Knowing yourself is the singularly most important thing you must accomplish before even *considering* entering into a D/s relationship or adopting a BDSM lifestyle. Again, let me be clear about this. There is a *huge* difference between the BDSM *activities* that are a casual part of the Saturday night kink that spices up your sex life, versus entering into a D/s relationship or *adopting it as a way of life*. There's nothing wrong with *either*, but you should just be sure never to confuse the two, and ensure that when you transition from one to the other, that you do it with your *eyes open*.

So, how well *do* you know yourself? Are you a *true Dominant?* What makes you *think* so? Are Dominants *born* that way, or can someone be *trained* to become a Dominant? We'll explore those questions and others like them in the remainder of this chapter.

Let's begin by asking a few simple introspective questions.

Introspection

Do you like being told what to do? Practically everyone answers *"no"* to this question, at first blush. After all, *no one* likes to be told what to do, particularly if it's done rudely, or when it's not necessary. But I want you to think very carefully, and ask yourself this: When I am confused, or hurt, or lost... when life seems to be crashing down around my shoulders, do I *then* like being told what to do? If you were to find yourself in a burning building, and an authoritative voice yells, *"Everyone run to the rear exits!"* do you reflexively *do so*, or do you instantly suspect that doing so might be a *fatal mistake*, if for no other reason, than because everyone *else* will be doing so? If your *immediate and visceral reaction* to any directive, no matter how reasonable, polite, or helpful, is generally *negative* then (at the risk of sounding like the punch line from a certain redneck comedy routine) *you just may be a Dominant.*

This is not to say that a Dominant can't take orders. *Of course* they can take orders. A Dominant does what he has to do, but he doesn't necessarily have to *like it.* In my particular case, even though I have been a die-hard Dominant all of my life, I was also able to have a very successful military career. I had two basic strategies for coping with being told what to do. First, I learned how to become *so good* at what I did, that even my superiors consistently came to me for advice and, second, I quickly got promoted to positions where I eventually became the one giving the orders.

Unfortunately, many people are eager to accept the common misconception that Dominants can't or won't take orders, or conversely, that because he does, he must not *really* be a Dominant.

Just because every two-year old child is at the center of his or her own universe and doesn't want to be told what to do doesn't mean that every Dominant must behave like a two-year-old and throw a tantrum when he doesn't get his way. It is, however, why it's always important to be able to differentiate between what a person *does* and who a person *is*.

Are you stubbornly independent, even to a fault? Imagine wandering through an unfamiliar city, looking for the train station. Do you prefer to wander on your own, even if it takes twice as long to get to your destination, rather than ask someone for directions? Does it rub you the wrong way to accept help from someone, even if you sorely need it or are probably entitled to it? Are you the kind of person for whom the three most difficult words in the English language are "I need help?" If so, then you just may be a Dominant.

Pride can be a double-edged sword for the Dominant. It shapes and defines him like no other character trait yet it is simultaneously his greatest weakness. Despite the fact that he necessarily has an extraordinarily healthy ego, the Dominant is always painfully aware that he is *far* from perfect. Nevertheless, he often creates and nurtures for himself and others the illusion that he is *always* in control and rarely in need of assistance. To accept help, even when it is sorely needed, is to allow a chink in the carefully crafted illusion that makes him what and who he is.

If a Dominant allows you to help him, in even the tiniest way, you should probably consider that a great honor. In doing so, he has revealed a part of himself that he would rather not be confronted with, much less have to reveal to others. It is also an integral part of the *power exchange* that occurs between Dominant and submissive, which we'll discuss at greater length elsewhere in this book.

Do people seem all too willing to grant you authority over various aspects of their lives? Examples might range from the serious to the mundane, such as trusting you with the keys to their homes or with access to their online accounts, or something as simple as ordering for them in restaurants. Are you often asked to help make important decisions for others, more because of your decision-making ability than because of your expertise on the subject at hand? When you are a member of a group or organization, are you frequently nominated for or elected to positions of authority, whether you want to be or not? If so, you just may be a Dominant.

Are you energetic and task oriented? Dominants tend to be very focused on accomplishing their goals, even if the goals may be unclear or out of reach at times. You won't typically find a Dominant spending a lot of time soul searching, or second guessing his decisions. He is an unstoppable force until he hits an immovable object, in which case he often simply pivots and shoots off in another direction, until the next immovable object is encountered. When a Dominant is asked *why* he does what he does, the answer is almost invariably, *because he can.* If this sounds like *you*, you just may be a Dominant.

Are you sometimes hard to get along with? *Anyone* can be difficult to get along with at times, but the key in this instance is the *why.* A Dominant is usually more focused on *facts* than *feelings*. This tendency to overlook the feelings of others can sometimes result in the Dominant being characterized as harsh, disrespectful, or lacking compassion. At the same time, one advantage to this character trait in Dominants is the fact that you *always know where you stand* with him. He is not one to tiptoe around an issue in order to spare your feelings. Dominants are often characterized as being brutally honest and unafraid to tell you what they think. If your feelings get bruised by his direct manner, his response will usually be, *"Get over it."* If that sounds all too familiar, you just may be a Dominant.

You've probably noticed that much of what we've said about Dominants thus far has been about *how he feels*, or how *others feel* about him. That's because what sets the Dominant apart from the rest of humanity is his unique world view, and how he *relates* to others. *Anyone* can bark orders or learn to crack a whip. That doesn't necessarily make him a

Dominant. What makes him a Dominant is *how he thinks and feels, how others perceive him, and how he relates.*

Training a Dominant

Can a person be *trained* to be a Dominant? The answer is complicated, and depends entirely upon what kind of Dominant you're referring to, how badly the person in question wants it, and whether he is capable of fundamental change on a core personality level.

The first factor is: *What kind of Dominant* are you trying to produce through training? If the answer to that question is, you're looking to train a person *who can be taught to act in a Dominant role,* well then *of course* you can train someone to be a Dominant. Anyone with even a modicum of *acting ability* will fit the bill nicely. Of course, the issue *then* becomes, to what extent can you expect that person to *"stay in character"* and will he be capable of fulfilling those expectations? One should always remember that a person who is *taught to play the role of a Dominant* and puts on that mantle may eventually grow bored with the role at some point and cast it off. While it is true that such an eventuality may not be too critical in a *mutual role play* environment, it can be completely *devastating* in other situations. When serious relationship commitments are made based upon the reasonable expectation *that your partner is actually a Dominant* and is *supposed to stay that way*, the end of a role play can signal bad times ahead.

But what if you're seeking to produce what we've thus far been referring to as a *true Dominant* through training? Is it at all possible? If it *is* possible, is it something that anyone should attempt to do? As usual, the answers can be complicated, but here they are, in a nutshell: Yes, it is possible. It's very difficult, *but it is possible*. Whether it should be attempted depends entirely on the trainer, the person being trained, his reasons for *wanting* to be trained, how *badly* he wants it, and whether he is *capable* of such a fundamental character changes. Let's briefly examine each of those factors in turn.

Anyone who attempts to train another person to be a true Dominant must first be a true Dominant, himself. If this is not the case, his efforts will be doomed from the start. It would be a lot like a *non-dancer* trying to teach someone to *cha-cha*, or a *negaholic* attempting to teach someone how to be an *optimist.* Anyone who may be contemplating an attempt to turn someone else into a Dominant should first engage in some serious soul searching. It is not a decision that should ever be made lightly. Even when the trainer has all of the right *credentials,* there is also the not-so-insignificant matter of whether he has the *training skills* to be up to the task. I like to think I am a pretty good driver, but whenever I try to teach someone how to drive, there's usually a lot of screaming, choking, and crying involved. Teaching someone *how to be,* as opposed to teaching them *what to do,* is even harder. It is *never* an easy thing. *Ask any shrink.*

Anyone who wants to be trained as a Dominant has some important questions to answer, as well. The question that should be at the very top of that list is this one: *Why do you want to be a Dominant?* There are many possible responses that can be given to that question, but there is really only one that makes any sense at all and should be considered the *only correct answer.* It is: *Because I know that at my core, that is who I am, and I want to learn to express and conduct myself in harmony with that.*

Here are just a *few* of the many *incorrect* answers I've been given in response to this question:

- I hear being dominant is a sure way to get lots of sex. Is that true?
- I'm kinky, being dominant is kinky... *Well, duh!*
- I can't seem to get laid any *other* way, so I'll try being a Dominant.
- That whole *whips and chains thing* just sounds *so cool.*
- I like the idea of being able to tell people what to do.
- I want sex slaves. There's no limit on how many I can have, is there?

- I really hate women. / I think women are inferior. / Revenge is sweet.
- I really hate men. / I think men are inferior. / Revenge is sweet.
- My girlfriend / boyfriend / husband / wife thinks I should be a Dominant.
- I'm bored / I'm crazy / I'm curious / I'm sick / I'm a moron.

As hard as it may be to believe, those are all *real reasons* that real people have given me - in complete earnestness - for wanting to become a Dominant. If any of them sound applicable to *you*, my sincere and heartfelt advice to you is, *please put any thought of becoming a Dominant completely out of your head.* Find another hobby. Learn to dance, or something. Your future submissives will thank you. Your fellow Dominants will thank you. Your girlfriend / boyfriend / husband / wife / significant-other who suggested it to you in the first place will thank you.

If the prospective trainer is credible and capable and the would-be Dominant sincerely wants to be trained for all the right reasons, the next hurdle is to learn whether the Dominant-in-training is capable of changing the way he thinks, feels, and conducts himself accordingly. This task usually falls into the category of *"far easier said than done."* One way to explore this part of the process is to ask deep, thought-provoking questions that are designed to take a person beyond the superficial stereotypes that are generally associated with the D/s lifestyle in general, and with being a Dominant in particular.

One of those questions is: What does it *really mean to you* to have a submissive, or slave? The superficial, stereotypical answer is usually something like: *I get to tell someone what to do, and she has to obey me.* But how many people have really given much thought to anything beyond that point? I always follow that question up with a few more, like the following:

- What if you tell your submissive what to do, and she *doesn't* obey you? What *then?*
- Why in the world should your submissive *want* to obey you?
- What if your directives turn out to be wrong, misguided, or even dangerous?
- What are the limits to your responsibilities to your submissive, or her responsibilities to you?
- Are you required to fulfill any, or all, of *her* needs?
- Where do you *draw the line* at meeting her emotional, physical, intellectual, financial, social or educational needs?
- Would you be prepared to put her through school, pay her bills, or care for her if she were incapacitated?

If some of those questions sound an awful lot like the sort of questions people should be asking before entering into a *marriage*, guess what? It's *no coincidence.* Frankly, a marriage can be a *lot less complicated* than a D/s relationship. A marriage is typically viewed (at least, in the vanilla world) as an *equal partnership* between two people. But a D/s relationship places a disproportionately heavy burden upon a Dominant to be a leader, mentor, teacher, provider, guide, inspiration, planner, problem solver, and *so much more.*

It would certainly be simpler for everyone concerned if the answer to *all* of those questions is: *We have no real responsibilities to each other. We are simply role playing, or enjoying an online-only relationship. Much* simpler. But you should always be mindful of the fact that the *emotions* that are felt in those venues are *quite real* to those involved and can often cause people to blur the lines between role playing and real life. Before that happens to you and/or someone you play with, ask yourself some of the questions above, even - no, *especially* - if you aren't quite sure what your answers will be.

Another important question that any would-be Dominant should ask himself is: *Would you still want to be a Dominant, even if it meant that there would be absolutely no sex involved?* If you honestly can't separate being a Dominant from the *sexual* aspects of the lifestyle, then perhaps your reasons for wanting to be a Dominant are just a *tad* superficial. A Dominant shouldn't be defined by his sexual activities, and sex should never be the primary motivation for wanting to be a Dominant, any more than it should be the primary focus of a meaningful relationship. It's entirely possible to be a Dominant, in or outside of a relationship, without ever expressing that aspect of your personality *sexually.* Obviously, for *most* people, that would not be the *ideal* arrangement, but it *is* possible and it happens more often than you might think.

What Kind of Dominant Would *You* Be?

If you are on the path to becoming a Dominant, ask yourself this question: *What kind of Dominant would you be?* For those of you who *already* consider yourselves Dominants, ask it like this: *What kind of Dominant are you?* There are *many* different kinds of Dominants in this lifestyle and just as many types of D/s relationships, which are defined predominantly (is that a pun? I just never know any more) by the Dominants that *lead* them. Please spend some time pondering the following questions. It's okay if you don't have easy answers to all of them just yet. They are *supposed* to be hard. Ponder them sincerely now, and revisit them occasionally in the future as you progress along your path. Refer to the glossary at the end of this book for definitions of terms with which you may be unfamiliar.

- Are you a *cruel* or *kind* Dominant?
- Are you a *sadist?* If so, *how much* of a sadist?
- Does it matter to you if your partner is a masochist?
- Are you monogamous or polyamorous?
- If you are polyamorous, are you polyfidelous?
- Do you hold your partners to a different loyalty standard than you set for yourself?
- Are there aspects of being a Dominant that appeal to you more than others?

- How important is protocol to you, and what part does it play in your relationships?
- Do you *punish* your submissives? If so, how?
- How do you handle conflict?
- Do you easily become angry? How do you express your anger?
- What is the best way for your partner(s) to manage a conflict with you?
- Do you prefer a submissive who is a masochist? Why or why not?
- How *much* masochism is *too much*?
- Do you prefer your D/s relationship to be public or private?
- What should or shouldn't your *vanilla friends* and family know about your lifestyle?
- Do you prefer your partners to be subs or slaves?
- Do you have lots of rules or very few? Are they *formal* or *informal?* Are they *inviolate,* or *flexible?*
- Is it important for you to connect and socialize with others in the D/s lifestyle?

Types of Dominants

There are many different kinds of Dominants that you'll encounter in the D/s lifestyle and, as you may well imagine, it's rare that anyone will match an archetypal profile exactly. As is the case with *any* stereotype, the more you know about an individual, the less they will seem to match any generalization. As I mentioned earlier, I also think it's important to determine, to the best of your ability, the degree to which being a Dominant is *hardwired* into the person's brain, as opposed to being the product of *role play* behavior. This is one area where *assumptions* can lead to some *reeeeeally* bad decisions.

What follows, in no particular order, is a list of what I consider to be the eight general types of Dominants and a ninth category of *non*-Dominant.

The Sadistic Dom

A Sadistic Dominant is one who enjoys or becomes sexually aroused from inflicting physical or emotional pain or discomfort upon his partners. Whether or not his partner is a masochist *(someone who enjoys pain)* is usually irrelevant to the pleasure that a Sadistic Dominant gets from inflicting it. Within this category of Dominant, there is a wide spectrum of sadism that can range from the *minimally sadistic yet skilled pain-inflictor* on one end, to the abusive or pathologically dangerous *extreme sadist* at the other end of the scale. For a pathological sexual sadist, the mere thought of causing someone permanent or crippling bodily harm *or even death* may actually be a *turn-on*. One should therefore always take great caution, especially when meeting or playing with a sadistic Dominant for the first time, to attempt to learn *what's on his mind*, and to protect yourself in the event that things start down a path that you did not anticipate. How badly *can* things go, if and when they *do* take a turn for the worse? For the answer to *that* question, consider the fact that some of the worst serial killers in our nation's history have been sadistic Dominants. Fortunately, there are quite a few simple steps that you can take to help ensure that your very first encounter with a sadistic Dominant (or for that matter, *anyone* that you may be meeting for the first time) is *safe, sane, and consensual.* Those steps are discussed at great length in Chapter 8: *Meeting for the First Time.*

Clinically speaking, the general consensus of the medical professionals who happen to be in the business of psychoanalyzing and categorizing sexual deviancy is that there are four general classes of *sexual sadists.* They are:

- The Class I Sexual Sadist is a person who has sexually sadistic urges, but *doesn't act upon them.* In a nutshell, he's *all about the fantasy.*
- The Class II Sexual Sadist is someone who *acts* upon his sexually sadistic impulses, but only does so with *consenting partners.* As sexual sadists go, *this is good.* This also describes about half of the people in your local BDSM munch group.

- The Class III Sexual Sadist is someone who acts out his sexually sadistic impulses with *non-consenting individuals*, but does not want to seriously injure or kill them. Sure, he's a predator and rapist but, apparently, he's *the Care Bear kind.*
- Class IV Sadist: A person who acts out his sexually sadistic urges with *non-consenting* individuals and *does want to seriously injure or kill them.* So, on the off-chance that you raced through that sentence without observing the caution sign, please allow me to refocus your attention upon it once more: *"does want to seriously injure or kill."* It has a little more *oomph* if you tack the word *"you"* on at the end of it, but if you *really* want the *full effect,* try adding, *"and cook you and feed you to the people he hates at a church barbeque."*

Anyone who may be considering a play date or entering into a relationship with a Sadistic Dominant is *strongly advised* to seek out one of the *first two* varieties, rather than the *latter* two. Consent, in this lifestyle, is *everything*. There is a little word with big ramifications for non-consensual sexual activity - in *or* out of the lifestyle. In most states, it's called *rape*.

The Gorean Slave Master

The Gorean Slave Master is a Dominant who follows the traditions of *Gor,* a fictional planet described and popularized in the pulp erotic science fiction novels published by John Frederick Lange, Jr. under the pen-name *John Norman.* The Gor series of novels, thirty-two of them in all, gained considerable popularity in the 1970s and 80s and were loosely based on the works of Edgar Rice Burroughs, specifically his *John Carter of Mars* novels. John Norman's novels created a robust mythical extraterrestrial cultural framework to fuel the erotic imaginations of millions of mostly-adolescent males at the time, but it was his nonfiction book, *Imaginative Sex,* which was published first in 1974 and republished in 1997 with more of a BDSM focus, that made *Gor* a significant subculture within the D/s lifestyle. It is worth noting that John Norman has *never* advocated for the adoption of the societal customs or sexual practices of the fictional planet Gor by anyone in *real life*. Even so, since the Gor phenomenon seems to have taken on a life of its own that *even its creator* could never have foreseen, it might be helpful to know something about it. For a more in-depth discussion of Gor, including its real life applications, be sure to check out Chapter 7: *The Gorean Way.*

A Gorean Slave Master, almost by definition, is a male Dominant who prefers *slaves* to submissives and subscribes to a highly stylized, authoritarian, and ritualistic way of life described in the Gor novels. In John Norman's books, males are predominantly *freeborn*, while some females are born slaves, and others are captured and made slaves. Female slaves are trained in the art of pleasuring, and are often used for sexual purposes with no consideration given to their thoughts on the matter. Slaves, who typically wear *silks and bells* similar to what might be considered traditional middle-eastern *harem* attire, are expected to learn a variety of sexual submission poses, and to accept being routinely loaned out or given to others for sexual favors. Slave girls are often taught to avoid direct eye contact with males, speak of themselves in the third person, and to perform serving rituals and dances. Theoretically, at least, the customs and protocols of a Gorean relationship are enforced by the *sword*. Think: *Conan the Barbarian* meets *I Dream of Jeanie*.

The Daddy or Mommy Dom

The Daddy Dom or Mommy Domme is typically a Dominant whose primary mode of expressing himself in the D/s lifestyle is through a nurturing sort of *paternalism* or *maternalism*. The relationship dynamic *may* involve sexual *or* nonsexual *age play*, erotic or nonsexual spankings, incest role-play, and other forms of role play. It is often erroneously assumed, both by people in *and* outside of the D/s lifestyle, that Daddy or Mommy Doms harbor *pedophilic* thoughts and tendencies. The truth is, Daddy and Mommy Doms are statistically no more likely to be pedophiles than any other random sampling of the general population. Daddy and Mommy Doms are *not* attracted to children; they are attracted to *adults* who embrace their inner child and exhibit childlike *behaviors*, which *may or may* not be sexual in nature. Consider this rather self-evident observation: Daddy and Mommy Doms prefer *adults* who enjoy and are skilled at expressing themselves in this dynamic because, frankly, *actual children would be terrible at it.*

For the sake of simplicity, we'll henceforth dispense with the clunky practice of referring to this category of Dominant as the *Daddy or Mommy Dom*, and just call it *what it is* for the vast majority of the folks who comprise this particular D/s subculture – the *Daddy Dom*. Just remember that anything we say about the Daddy Dom probably applies equally to Mommy Dommes, as well.

Most Daddy Doms find fulfillment in the *relationship dynamic* that exists between the Dominant and his submissive, who is usually referred to as *baby, babygirl, little one,* or other pet name that suggests and reinforces the submissive's child-like status in the relationship. The components of the relationship dynamic that a Daddy Dom seeks – no, *craves* - from his babygirl usually include the ability to *trust* absolutely and without reservation, a spirit of wide-eyed innocence and playfulness, an eagerness for mentoring and guidance, and the kind of gleeful no-holds-barred adoration and worship that only little girls and puppies seem capable of demonstrating.

Lifestyle Daddy Doms should be willing to take their Daddy responsibilities *beyond the bedroom*. That can mean helping their babygirls to make the kinds of decisions that would be difficult for an adult, spending an evening watching her favorite cartoons, reading stories aloud to her, brushing her hair, or just holding her when she is frightened or feeling down. It can also require loads of patience, which may be needed when doing things like shopping, explaining things, disciplining, or dealing with little tantrums. Any Dominant who might be considering the Daddy Dom lifestyle should seriously consider *all* of the aspects of being in this kind of relationship, and *not* just the *pervy* ones.

The FemDom Mistress

The FemDom Mistress is something of an anomaly in the categorization of Dominants, for the simple reason that while practically all of the other categorizations of Doms are *gender-neutral*, the FemDom is *always* a dominant *woman* who makes the most of a unique combination of *force* and sexual *role reversal*. The FemDom, who may prefer either male *or* female submissives, is also sometimes referred to as a *Domme, Domina, Dominatrix, or Mistress*. Traditional FemDom BDSM scene activities include pegging *(anal intercourse utilizing a strap-on dildo)*, face-sitting, forced feminization of male submissives, CBT *(cock and ball torture)*, forced felching *(orally sucking semen out of a person's anus. Yes,* there really *is* a word for that), tie-and-tease play, forced orgasm, orgasm deferral or denial, various forms of physical or verbal humiliation, and sexual sadism in general. Though it isn't necessarily a requisite part of a FemDom's *repertoire*, there is often a significant element of *misandry*, or hatred of men, involved, whether real or role-played.

A sub-category of FemDom is the *FinDom*, which is a contraction of *Financial Dominant*. A FinDom expects her submissives to support her financially by *paying tribute* to her in the form of cold hard cash or lavish gifts. She typically maintains an online *wish list* of items that she hopes someone will purchase for her. Submissives who show their devotion to a FinDom by paying this tribute usually do so without any expectation of receiving anything in return except, perhaps, scorn and continued exploitation. It should come as no surprise to anyone that *some* FinDoms are more authentic than others. How do you recognize the phonies? They're the ones posting photos taken at their trailer park.

The Bear Dom

The *Bear Dom* is typically a burly gay or bisexual male Dominant who prefers diminutive and youthful gay or bisexual male submissives. Some Bear Doms are attracted to *lady-boys* and boyish *females*, as well. They are called Bear Doms mostly for their tendency to exhibit hyper-masculinity and somewhat exaggerated male characteristics such as a muscular or stocky build and abundant body hair. Bear Doms are commonly encountered in the BDSM leather and LGBT subcultures.

The Lesser God Dom

The Lesser God Dom *(sometimes referred to as Lord, Prophet, Pharoah, or Pharoanic Lord)* is a Dominant who expects and thrives on the worship of his submissives. This adoration and worship, which can sometimes take the form of highly ritualistic activities and behaviors, has but one purpose, which is the ego gratification of the Lesser God. It is relatively common for the real-life households of Lesser God Doms to forsake all traditional forms of religion in order to practice their own *home-grown* religion, with the Dominant at its head and submissives as religious acolytes. In such cases, the Dominant is usually regarded by his submissives as a deity, or as a prophet of God.

The Lesser God generally prefers slaves to submissives and, in either case, often considers them simply as expendable vessels to be used for his own pleasure or procreation. He is more likely than not to be polyamorous and/or polygamous. When the Lesser God has a full stable of slaves, whether real-life or role-played, it is relatively common to see a high degree of specialization among the acolytes. Some may be considered *breeders* and used solely for the purpose of bearing and raising children, while others may be considered pleasure slaves, income earners, or recruiters of new slaves. For the Lesser God, being called *"God's gift to mankind"* isn't an insult at *all;* it's a way of life.

The Collector Dom

The *Collector Dom (sometimes referred to as a Farmer Dom)* is a type of Dominant who is far more likely to be encountered *online* than in real life. The Collector is focused on building a stable of submissives, similar to a *harem*. For the Collector, *quantity* always trumps *quality*. In *his* way of thinking, the measure of a Dom's standing is *how many submissives* he can accumulate, without much regard for who, or even what, those submissives may be. It is relatively common for a Collector Dom to attempt to collar a submissive *mere minutes* after meeting her for the first time in an online chat room or on a BDSM social network, which sometimes results in the so-called Dom being comically unaware of his own submissives' ages, genders, or *even their names*.

The Collector is typically an adolescent male in his teens or early twenties who has recently stumbled upon D/s in an online chat room or lifestyle-related website. He is agog and obsessed with the thought that he can *actually acquire slaves* online the same way he shops for *Pokemon* cards. He typically doesn't understand the difference between a submissive and a slave and may, in fact, be completely ignorant of the meaning of the term *submissive.* For the Collector, *it's all about slaves* and *more is always better*. To absolutely no one's surprise but his own, he soon learns that *keeping* them is an entirely a different matter - a matter to which he hasn't given an iota of thought. Luckily for the Collector, there is always an endless supply of naive teens willing to role play *"slave for a day."* The important thing, for the Collector, is to be able to boast, *"You have a slave? Hah! That's nothing! I have twenty-seven of them!"*

There are two *very good reasons* why the Collector Dom phenomenon exists almost exclusively in the *cyber realm*, rather than in the *real world*. First, being a sophomore in high school and having a ten o'clock curfew can be problematic in the accumulation of slaves in *real life*. And second, it's a lot harder in real life to keep twenty-seven angry slaves from beating you to a bloody pulp.

The Ineffable Dom

I'm going to invent a final unique category of Dominant, which I hereby christen the *Ineffable Dom. Ineffable* is a word that essentially means *"impossible to be categorized or adequately described in words."* It's a word that became fashionable during the middle-ages as a way for many philosophers to oxymoronically describe God as *indescribable.* My reason for creating this category out of whole cloth is in recognition of the fact that many lifestyle Dominants just can't be neatly pigeon-holed into any of the other categories. They are, quite simply, *atypical or unique.*

The Ineffable Dom is typically a Dominant who has been in the D/s lifestyle for several years or longer and has, mostly through trial and error, learned what does and doesn't appeal to him and what works best in his D/s relationships. Over this span of time, he has consciously explored and borrowed traits and characteristics from other more traditional Dominant categories. Additionally, the synergy created with each new partner brings new facets to the Ineffable Dom's understanding and interests. The Ineffable Dom steals unashamedly from any D/s lifestyle tradition that strikes his fancy, taking what he considers the best bits and pieces of each and tossing them all into a hodge-podge D/s stew that, surprisingly, can turn out to be quite *delicious.* Never discount or underestimate a Dominant simply because he cannot adequately describe in 25 words or less what *kind* of Dominant he is. He may just be an *Ineffable Dom.*

The Tin Pot Dom

The *Tin Pot Dom* is no more a Dominant than the person who wears a dollar store eye patch on *Talk Like a Pirate Day* (September 19th, by the way) is really a *pirate.* Tin Pot Doms generally fall into two categories.

The first is the *role player.* This Tin Pot Dom doesn't consider what he does as a *deception;* he considers it *role play.* As far as *he* is concerned, D/s isn't a *lifestyle;* it's *entertainment.* He sees what he does - role playing the part of a Dominant - as a perfectly natural and appropriate behavior, mainly because he believes he is interacting with people *who are doing precisely the same thing*. It hasn't quite dawned on him that those people *really may be Dominants and submissives,* and not just *acting out roles.* The role player Tin Pot Dom believes that *everyone* is simply making it up as they go along, so he feels pretty confident doing so *himself*. The ridiculous notion of doing any *homework* on how *real Dominants* might conduct themselves makes about as much sense to him as trying to learn how *real vampires* behave.

Eventually, the role player Tin Pot Dom realizes his mistake but, by then, it's usually too late to recover from it gracefully. The great majority of them will simply drop the role completely, quickly assume another identity, and *then* start doing a little homework on the lifestyle. Some may even go so far as to explore how they might fit into the lifestyle in *reality*, rather than through role play. If they are smart and/or lucky, they will find mentors or friends who will help them navigate the tricky path from *role play* to *reality*.

You probably know more of these folks than you think. They're usually the people who tell you, "I'm a submissive (or switch), *but I used to be a Dom."* Translation: "I used to *role play* being a Dominant until one day, I realized that there really *were* such things, and that *I wasn't one."*

Just because someone *discovers* the D/s lifestyle through *role play* doesn't necessarily mean they can't successfully adopt it as a *way of life* and find happiness in a D/s relationship. All who arrive at this lifestyle come by different paths, and no path is intrinsically better than another. The important thing is that they arrive safe and sound. Such is *not* always the case with the *next* type of Tin Pot Dominant.

The second category of Tin Pot Dom is the *self-delusional* variety. This poor bastard *really believes* in his innate superiority and unrecognized demi-godhood, despite the overwhelming body of evidence to the contrary. He develops his strategies and techniques, not out of any sense of deception, but from a purely pragmatic sense of what has worked for him in the past. He simply plays the odds. He *knows* that if he approaches twenty complete strangers and commands each of them to drop to their knees and submit to him that nineteen of them will *slap him silly*, but the *twentieth* just might do it. He knows that eventually, he will find someone who is willing to *buy into his delusion* and *feed it*, and that's all that matters.

If you happen to be that unlucky person who has bought into his delusion, he also knows that separating you from the D/s community-at-large will insulate you from dissenting voices which might warn you about him. He knows he is shunned by others in the lifestyle but, then again, what else would you expect from such *riff-raff?* He *knows* all of this, because *he's seen it work for him* time and again, and it's *hard to argue with success*. Anyone who steadfastly refuses to recognize his innate superiority is simply a *bit-player or antagonist* in a grand drama that is played out on center-stage in his own little parallel universe.

You might be tempted to *pity* the self-delusional Tin Pot Dom until you realize the full magnitude of the *damage* that his kind does to submissives, to the D/s lifestyle, and to society in general. As a result of this person's delusional and often paranoid behavior, submissives often end up stripped of their dignity, sense of self-worth, self confidence and trust. Others in the lifestyle are forced constantly to defend our way of life because of the widespread stereotypes and misconceptions that result from the actions of these bad apples. Even worse, there are those high-profile, extreme cases where the worst of these self-delusional, criminally insane individuals kidnap people and keep them chained in their basement or bury them in their backyards.

Now, before I am accused of engaging in *fear-mongering,* or the wanton and indiscriminate *slander* of all the poor, innocent, harmlessly self-deluded Tin Pot Doms everywhere, I hope you'll allow me to just say that I did *not* mean to imply that *all* self-deluded Tin Pot Dominants are *psycho loons*. I meant to imply that *most* of them are.

Alrighty, then. Let the accusations *fly.*

My Two Cents

There you have it, my perspective on what I consider to be the eight *major* categories of Dominants and a *ninth* for the TPDs who are role players or self-delusional. My perspectives on this and other D/s lifestyle topics have been shaped and impacted by thirty-five years of D/s relationships, a lifetime of unusual life experiences, and an admittedly eccentric world-view. I suppose the key to getting your money's worth from this book will be your ability to take from it what is useful to your relationships and activities, and to simply disregard the rest. There isn't much in the D/s lifestyle that can be characterized as *right or wrong*. It is either useful to you, or it is not.

Frankly, I fully expect that some of the things I say in this book are going to cause some people to foam at the mouth and perhaps even say *not-nice* things about me. That's *okay.* It's all part of the *process.* I'd be far more concerned if everyone were *agreeing* with me, since that's usually my first clue that I'm dead *wrong* about something.

Speaking of *being wrong,* I am truly fortunate to be able to count among my dearest friends my former collared submissive, a woman who has turned *tactfully telling me that I'm wrong* into a virtual *art form*. She has been an invaluable aide and adviser in the production of this book from concept to completion, and I trust her instincts and opinions without reservation. So, when she *ever-so-tactfully* told me *well into the writing of the book* that I was *doing it wrong,* I listened.

She told me that my readers wanted *more* than an informative or even entertaining book about D/s and BDSM relationships. *Anyone* could write *that* book, she said. What they *wanted,* she assured me, was the chance to be *voyeurs.* They wanted a *peek into my head*. They wanted to know how someone like *me,* a Dominant with over thirty-five years of experience in this lifestyle and in these kinds of relationships, *thinks and feels and acts.*

And, to be brutally honest, I wanted *absolutely no part of that.*

I have always been an exceedingly private person, and *not* without *good reason*. At various times in my life, I have been targeted in one way or another by criminals, enemy soldiers, union thugs, law enforcement officers, political activists, crooked lawyers, newspaper reporters, and even jealous husbands. Some of those people pointed *real guns* loaded with *real bullets,* at me. Others used less obvious, but even more insidious methods that, frankly, made me nostalgic for *gunplay*. I learned some important lessons from all of that, the most valuable being: *Don't make yourself a target.*

And now, I was being asked to do *just that.*

My immediate reaction was to simply dismiss the idea, outright. I really did *not* want to make any part of this book *all about me.* I've spent my entire life playing my cards close to the vest. I wasn't about to suddenly start playing them face up on the table. Paranoia may not be a winning strategy for *everyone*, but it's always worked pretty well for *me*. I promised her that I'd at least *think about it*. And, I did.

After about a *week* of thinking about it, I realized she was *right.* There really *was* only one thing I could offer to my readers that *no one else* could, and that was *me* - or more accurately, my own unique experiences and thoughts. The rest of it, *anyone* could write. I gave it a little more thought, and finally arrived at what I believe is a reasonable *compromise* between *"The BDSM Textbook That Anyone Could Have Written"* and *"Mike Makai's XXX Memoirs."*

At the end of each chapter, I've added a section called *"My Two Cents."* There, you'll find personal anecdotes, opinions or reflections culled from my lifetime accumulation of unique experiences in the D/s and BDSM lifestyles. The stories range from pleasant recollections to painful memories; but they are true, and they are told from the heart.

If you prefer your BDSM relationship handbooks to be more *scholarly* than *memoirish*, feel free to skip merrily past those parts and on to the next chapter. *Seriously*, I won't mind. *Not one teensy-weensy bit.*

My Two Cents on Being a Dominant

What kind of a Dominant am I? My first impulse has always been to categorize myself as an *Ineffable Dom*, but I've recently come to realize that I've always done so *not* so much because my style of dominance *can't be described*, but because *I just don't like having to describe it.*

If I had to categorize myself, I would be very tempted to create a whole *new* classification for myself and the relatively small number of other Dominants who are *like* me. I would designate it the *White Knight Dom*. Yes, I *know* what you're thinking. You're thinking that a person would have to be pretty darn *full of himself* to think he can willy-nilly create a whole new category of Dominant just for himself and, in fact, you would be *absolutely right.* Fortunately, when it comes to being full of myself, *I am eminently qualified*.

The White Knight Dom wants to right wrongs, slay dragons, rescue beautiful women, treat his submissive like a princess, and become King – and he wants to do it all before lunch. He is driven by a deep sense of chivalry and altruism that transcends what he considers to be the sordid and tawdry business of self-gratification. The White Knight *lives* to find solutions to *your* problems. He gets off on learning what makes *you* tick. He truly isn't happy unless *you're* happy. Where other Dominants might seek out submissives for their own gratification, the White Knight seeks them out because that's what a White Knight *does* as he solves riddles, completes quests, and slays monsters. For the White Knight, conduct and protocol count for a lot. This is why a submissive's ability to convincingly pull off the classic transformation from *"princess in public, to whore in the bedroom"* is so important to him. The gallant knight expects – no, *demands* – that anyone he rescues from the clutches of the beast be future *Queen* material. The White Knight aspires to be King of his castle, sovereign of the realm, and to be afforded all the rights and privileges thereof.

There *are* disadvantages of being a White Knight, some of them quite profound, indeed. The first and most obvious is you simply can't save *everyone,* no matter how much you may *want* to, no matter how hard you *try*. Second, there are fewer and fewer princesses to go around, which frankly, is exactly the way princesses *like* it. Even when a princess *can* be found and rescued, the fairy tales rarely mention what happens *next*. The White Knight returns to the castle with his prize in hand, only to be greeted by a royal chorus of crestfallen princesses crying out, *"Geez, Sir Knight! Not another princess!"*

Another disadvantage involves the dirty little secret that White Knights would prefer remain unspoken: *Not all problems have solutions.* When faced with an unsolvable predicament, particularly if someone depends upon his ability to *fix* whatever may be wrong, the White Knight's shortcomings are felt far more intensely.

People can often sense the White Knight's problem-solving abilities and chivalrous aura and, as a result, sometimes even complete strangers will bare their souls and bring their problems to him, hoping and expecting him to make things right.

And sometimes, he actually *does*.

"Surely there is a time to submit to guidance
and a time to take one's own way at all hazards."

- - *Thomas Huxley*

CHAPTER 2: THE SUBMISSIVE

What is a Submissive?

Depending upon whom you ask, a submissive may be described as anything from a *human doormat* to a conspiratorial behind-the-scenes *puppet-master* who controls her Dominant without his knowledge. The *reality*, as usual, can be found somewhere between those two extremes.

For our purposes, we'll simply define a submissive as a person who acts in a compliant or submissive role in life, and *especially in relationships*. A submissive may be what we call a *"true submissive"* in the sense that these traits are firmly *hard-wired* into her psyche and she simply doesn't know any other way to be, or she may be acting out a *submissive role*, whether consciously or unconsciously. A submissive is defined *primarily* by her deep-seated desire to *serve* and *please* another, while feeling loved, cherished and cared for. You might be surprised to learn that even the submissive who is an extreme masochist or who craves degradation and humiliation still wants to feel as appreciated and treasured as any other kind of submissive.

We will also, for the purposes of this book, continue in the habit of referring to submissives with the feminine pronoun *"she."* As we stated previously, this is not being done out of any gender bias on the author's part, nor in the erroneous belief that all submissives are female or, conversely, that all females are or should be submissive. No, nothing of the sort. It is simply a hat-tip to the fact that in our society, submission is typically seen as a *feminine trait*, and statistics have generally supported the notion that the majority of submissives in the D/s lifestyle just *happen* to be female. Besides, having to say *"he or she"* in every other sentence just hurts my brain.

Despite having a handy dictionary-style definition, many readers will still be left with lingering questions regarding whether they, themselves, might be submissives. To assist you with that conundrum, we'll explore a series of probing questions on the subject, just as we did in the previous chapter. As I cautioned you in our earlier discussion on Dominants, much depends upon how well you know yourself, or at the very least, upon your willingness to do some soul-searching as you ponder these questions. Additionally, you should give considerable thought to whether your answers are describing your innate, *hard-wired* core character traits, or *roles* which you are able to assume or cast off as the situation demands. A *true submissive* cannot simply remove her *"submissive hat"* and replace it with a *"Dominant hat."* That's because *her* submission is hard-wired *into her head*, and not her *hat.*

Anyone in the D/s lifestyle who has the ability to shift their behavior from submissive to Dominant and back again at will is appropriately called a *"switch."* Outside of the D/s lifestyle, there's another name for people who can switch back and forth between these roles as appropriate. We call these people *"normal."* There's nothing at *all* unusual about someone who *excels* in her career as an obedient underling to the CEO, a domineering supervisor to those she manages in her department, a submissive partner to her spouse at home, and tyrant to her children. That's what most normal people *do* on a day to day basis. It is only when you add the *whips and chains* aspect that it starts to sound *kinky*. For more on *switches*, see Chapter 3: *The Switch.*

Introspection

If you are someone who is wondering if you are *"hard wired"* to be a submissive, or whether you are suited to assume the *role* of a submissive, some introspection can help you to sort through the issues involved. Take a few moments to ponder the following thought-provoking questions as a way to explore your potential *inner subbiness*:

Does the idea of service, particularly service to someone you love and respect, make you happy? *Service* is a concept that few people give much thought to these days. Obviously, it can mean different things to different people but, generally speaking, it refers to behaving in ways that *benefit others.* Performing service can be one of the most fulfilling things you can do, whether you are a submissive or not. I served my country as a soldier for twenty years, and I know without a doubt that I am a better person for having done so. But not all service has to be quite so difficult or life-changing. Doing a little yard work for the elderly widow who lives next door, or volunteering your time to the local food bank are just a few examples of the types of service that benefit the one who performs the service as much as the recipient. If performing service to help a *complete stranger* can bring you joy and fulfillment, imagine how much happier you might be if you were given the opportunity to do something similar for someone that you love and respect. If the idea of service to the one you love warms the cockles of your heart, then you just might be a submissive.

Do you find yourself instinctively sacrificing your own comfort, well-being, or material things for others? This question is similar to the previous one regarding service, but there is a distinct difference between service and sacrifice. *Service* is cooking dinner for your kids. *Sacrifice* is *going hungry* so your kids can have dinner. Some people have *such* a giving nature, they don't know *how or when to stop* giving, even when it threatens to leave them in dire straits. Feeding the *hungry* is one thing; giving your last crust of bread to someone who owns a grocery store is another thing *entirely*. Unfortunately, our society is full of wolves who prey upon these sacrificial lambs and their loving, generous nature. If you're the sort of person who seems to *attract* the kind of people who take advantage of your sense of sacrifice, then you just might be a submissive.

Do you generally prefer to avoid contention and confrontation at all costs? People typically fall into two categories when it comes to dealing with personal confrontation. There are those who enthusiastically leap into the fray, swinging their sabers and boisterously singing a swashbuckling pirate song, and there are those who would rather have a root canal. An argument or fight with someone who is self-assertive, aggressive, or intimidating can send someone who is non-confrontational into an emotional death spiral of discomfort, self-doubt, and anger. Not *all* submissives react to confrontation in this way, but if *you* do, you just might be one.

Does the idea of having to make important decisions without assistance make you uncomfortable? In each of our lives, there will inevitably be critical decisions that have to be made about our finances, careers, relationships, quality of life, and similar matters. How often do you typically make those decisions *alone?* When you *do*, how *comfortable* are you about doing so? Or, do you seek out the advice and guidance of a trusted family member, friend or colleague? Remember, you're not being asked whether or not you are *capable* of making decisions on your own. The question is *how do you feel about it?* If having the benefit of assistance or guidance from a trusted friend would make you feel much better about in making that critical decision, you just may be a submissive.

In chaotic, confusing, or dangerous situations, do you instinctively look for someone who knows what is going on to tell you what to do or where to go? As I stated previously, most people can perform admirably in *either* a dominant or submissive role as needed in their day-to-day lives. To learn whether you are psychologically *hard-wired* to be a submissive, you need to dig a little deeper than that. One way to do that is to consider where your mind retreats to when it needs to find its *happy place* - the mental sanctuary where you find joy, where your soul can recharge. Another way to accomplish the same thing is to take note of what happens when you are under a great deal of stress or duress, when fear and confusion short-circuit your ability to *act out a role.* It is in those moments of dread and anxiety that the facade is stripped away momentarily and the foundational character traits are laid bare for all to see. The question *isn't* whether or not you are *fearful*. The question is: *When experiencing terrible fear, do you instinctively become a leader or a follower?* If you find more comfort as a follower than as a leader in times of great stress or danger, then you just may be a submissive.

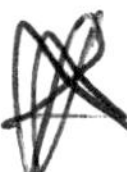

Does it give you a thrill when the person you love takes charge in the bedroom? Once again, let me caution you about misinterpreting the question. This is *not* a question about whether you *can* or *do* take charge sexually in the bedroom. This question is about *how you feel when someone else does*. Remember, D/s isn't necessarily about *what you do.* It's about *who you are, how you relate,* and *how you feel.* Some people find this difficult to believe, but your *competency* at demonstrating dominant behaviors in your sex life has *nothing to do* with whether or not you may be a submissive. But whether or not having your *hair pulled* during rough sex sends *tingles* to your crotch *just might*. If the mere *thought* of your partner showing you who's boss in the bedroom causes your heart to go *all aflutter*, then you just may be a submissive.

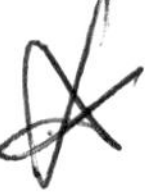

Do you seem inexplicably attracted to highly assertive, self-confident people? Have you developed a sort of intuitive radar for spotting the alpha individual in any room? If so, you are definitely not alone. Many natural submissives have, over the course of their lifetimes, developed and honed this ability, often without even realizing it. Similarly, many gays and lesbians are able to utilize a finely tuned *"gaydar"* sense that helps them to spot subtle body language and other nonverbal cues that can help to identify potential partners. When you walk into a room full of strangers, do your *"spidey senses"* immediately home in on that *alpha person?* Is your curiosity naturally drawn to the person telling a funny story in the center of a cluster of laughing people? Or perhaps you can simply feel his or her direct gaze upon you from clear across the room. If any, or all, of these scenarios sound familiar to you, you just might be a submissive.

Do you feel good about changing your appearance, behavior, or habits in order to please your partner? People generally tend to fall into three categories, when it comes to altering how they look or act in order to please someone else. Just for fun, I sometimes like to characterize the three categories as *salmon, cats, and dogs.*

Salmon *swim against the current*. The salmon folks are those who are fiercely independent and completely uncompromising when it comes to their appearance and behavior. A person in this category not only enjoys blazing her own path, but often seeks out and enjoys the opportunity to swim against the tide of opinion, even if it is the opinion of the person whose opinion she values the most. She's the one who says, *"Honey, I love you, but if you try to tell me what to wear, how to look, or how much I should weigh, I will rip your balls off and feed them to the dog."*

Cats are *aloof*. A cat person is one who is ambivalent or even apathetic about this issue. If her appearance or behavior pleases her mate *great,* but his opinion carries no more weight - *and often less* - than anyone else's does. She worries about what people think, just not so much about what her *partner* thinks.

Dogs are *eager to please*. They are not only *willing* to alter their appearance and behavior to please their partners, *they live for it.* The dog person derives a tremendous amount of joy and fulfillment from the approval that comes from her mate as the result of any change in her wardrobe or hair color, the success of her diet, or progress in overcoming bad habits. If you fit into this *latter* category; if you've ever found yourself asking your partner what you should wear, how you should eat, or whether you should quit smoking, then there's a very good chance that you might be a submissive.

Pencils down! Pass your papers to the front of the class. Let's take a moment here to reiterate the point that there are no *right or wrong* answers to any of the preceding questions. They are simply designed to *get you thinking* about what is *really going on* inside of your head and in your heart. It is entirely possible to have answered all of the introspection questions in the *negative*, and yet *still be a submissive*. Conversely, you could have been nodding in complete and utter agreement with every question, and *still not be a submissive*. To say it can be an incredibly *complicated* issue would be a gross understatement.

If only it were as easy as going to the pharmacy, purchasing a test kit, and taking it home to pee on a little plastic stick. Red for Dominant, blue for submissive, purple for switches, and yellow for everyone else. Life really would be *so* much simpler.

The Gift of Submission

Much has been said in D/s circles about the so-called *"Gift of Submission"* that is believed by many to be bestowed upon a Dominant by his submissive. For many, especially those who may be new to the D/s lifestyle, it can be a concept with a great deal of utility. After all, it sometimes needs to be said that one's submission is not something that can be taken from you by force. It is something that you *give willingly* to someone who deserves it. So, in the sense that it is willingly *given*, submission is most definitely a *gift*.

There are also some people who may not fully appreciate the very real and intrinsic *value* of one's submission to her Dominant. If a submissive is plagued with serious self-esteem issues, she may view *herself* as worthless and, therefore, her *submission* as equally worthless. In such a case, it becomes necessary and appropriate to teach her that not only does *she* have value, but her *submission* is a gift of great value which should not be wasted on the unworthy. In such a case, the metaphor of submission as a *gift* can be very useful.

One occasionally hears discussion of the *gift of submission* as something which must be *earned.* I, for one, am not entirely comfortable with that notion, but am certainly willing to take a closer look at it. Can you think of any other situation or scenario in our society where *gifts* must be *earned?* We have words for the things we *earn* in our culture; words like *wages, paychecks, tips and bonuses.* I will certainly admit that a Dominant *should* earn a submissive's trust, respect and love as their relationship evolves but, at the beginning of any relationship, there is often going to be a significant *leap of faith* involved. At that point, a Dominant may have demonstrated certain traits that make him attractive and potentially *worthy* of such a *leap of faith*, but it is doubtful he has *earned* much.

A gift, *by definition*, is something that is given with no strings attached and no expectation of getting anything in return. When something is bestowed upon another with the expectation of getting something else in return, that is what the *legal beagles* like to call *quid pro quo*, which is Latin for trading *"this for that."* This begs the question, is a person's submission to her Dominant a *gift*, or is it *quid pro quo?* Most people would respond that *every* submissive expects *something in return* for her submission. That *something* may include love, respect, guidance, leadership, mentoring or affection, to name just a few of the infinite possibilities. So, yes, *there usually are strings attached.* But that isn't necessarily a bad thing.

By the way, one rarely - *if ever* - hears mention of a *"gift of domination."* And no, I'm *not* just looking for a crass opportunity to toot my own *Dommy horn*. If a person's submission has intrinsic value then doesn't a person's domination? Since we've already firmly established the *quid pro quo* nature of most D/s relationships, then perhaps the most *useful* and descriptive metaphor would be the notion of a *gift exchange.* The only explanation I have been able to come up with for this apparent lack of any mention of the *gift of domination* is the fact that Dominants – *with their big honkin' egos* - rarely have to be convinced of the value of their contribution to a relationship.

Total Power Exchange

Domination/submission relationships are often referred to as a form of *power exchange* or sometimes, *total power exchange (TPE)*. As we've mentioned previously, there is obviously *something* being mutually exchanged in these relationships, but what is it, *exactly*? For many, it's difficult to understand the notion that *power* is somehow being exchanged in *both* directions between a submissive and a Dominant. One of the reasons it can be unclear is the fact that quite often, we are talking about *two completely different relationship dynamics*. On one hand, the *D/s dynamic* governs the emotions and interactions in a long-term, committed, and loving D/s relationship. On the other hand, the *BDSM dynamic* governs play activity and physical interactions with our mates *and* play partners.

Another reason for the general lack of clarity on this issue may be that there are many different ways we can define *power*. There is even some controversy over the question of whether something can be considered *real* power if it isn't *exercised or exploited*. Some people believe that it isn't so much *power* that is exchanged in TPE, as it is *authority*. The intrinsic difference between power and authority can best be explained thusly: If we were talking about a *car*, then *power* would be what was under the hood. *Exercising* that power would mean taking the car out for a spin. Having the *authority* to do so might involve a driver's license, possessing the keys, or having the title and registration.

In a long-term, committed D/s relationship, *both* power and authority are exchanged to an exponentially greater degree than in any short-term, uncommitted BDSM *play scenario*. The reasons for this should be fairly obvious but, to the casual observer, the true nature of the two way exchange may not be. It may be easy to see the *authority* that a submissive grants to her Dominant to *exercise power* over her life. It's also easy to see that, even though her Dominant may be *exercising* that power, the submissive always retains the power and authority to *revoke* it at will, at any time. Additionally, she typically retains the power or *ability* to do for herself what she has granted her Dominant the *authority* to do; she simply chooses not to *exercise* that power.

Consider the submissive who may be perfectly *capable* of managing her own household budget, but has ceded the *authority* to do so to her Dominant. Another example is the submissive who may be required to get *permission* from her Dominant to have an orgasm – *any orgasm* – even though the *power* to bring herself to orgasm has always been there, and always will be. In these two examples, the *power is retained* even as the *authority is given*.

Let's take a look at the kinds of power and authority a Dominant in a long-term committed D/s relationship might give to his submissive. Any power that is derived from *consent*, such as the power to choose or reject a Dominant or to leave a dysfunctional D/s relationship, isn't something that is granted to the submissive by the Dominant. Those powers are considered by many to be *god-given, cultural, and legal* in nature, and universal to *everyone*. So, if the power to say *no* to a Dominant shouldn't be considered part of this so-called power exchange, then *what should?*

I believe the answer lies in asking the question in a different way. Every Dominant should make it a point to ask his submissive some variation of the following: *"Have I empowered you? If so, how?"* The responses you get just might surprise you. Here are just a few of the real responses that I have received when I have posed that question to a submissive:

- You empowered me by forcing me to be independent at times, even when I wanted nothing more than for you to handle certain things for me. By directing me to carry out tasks that I would normally have avoided, you taught me that I am smarter, stronger and far more resourceful than I ever thought possible.

- You empowered me with the power to let go. Before, I would worry myself sick over certain things, but *now*, I know that if I've put a problem into your hands, I can just let go of it, and trust that you will do what is right.

- You empowered me with self-confidence and the sure knowledge that I am loved and cherished. Knowing that you treasure my submission gives me strength and a real sense of worth.

- You empowered me by *trusting* me with your flaws, weaknesses, and secrets. I know you don't share these things with just anyone, and the fact that you share them with *me* makes me feel very special. This knowledge could hurt you, even destroy you, and yet you trust me with it.

- You empowered me with the authority to act and speak for you in certain situations. When I am weak or indecisive, I am able to draw on your judgment and guidance and say, "My Master would not be pleased if I were to do what you've asked of me."

- You empowered me with the ability to learn and grow, and to reach my full potential – whether it is in my education, career, personal goals, or as a submissive. You make me want to be a better person, not just a better submissive, because I want you to be proud of me.

- You empowered me to be a synergist and gave me the ability to be a catalyst in your life. You gave me a chance to work side-by-side with you to inspire you, motivate you, nudge you, or challenge your assumptions.

- You empowered me by showing me those little things that make a difference in your life and bring you joy. Others may *think* they know you, but they don't know you like I do.

It would be difficult for anyone to hear or read these responses and not know for a fact that the phenomenon of *power exchange* is a very *real* one. There is no question that *both* a Dominant and his submissive can be *empowered* by their relationship dynamic. The degree to which that empowerment is fulfilling, significant, meaningful, or symmetrical is *entirely up to you.*

Types of Submissives

If you are in the BDSM lifestyle or involved in a D/s relationship, you *may* know some of the following categories of submissives by different names. You may even know of additional categories or traits that are not fully represented here, and that's *okay*. No book on this subject is going to be able to capture every aspect of the lifestyle or its many subcultures. Even so, I'm sure you'll recognize many of the character traits and behaviors we're about to explore, and perhaps even learn a little about yourself and others you may know.

As we go through these categories, you may find yourself wondering why there is no category designated for the *"sex slave."* The reason is simply that, in my humble opinion, *there is no such category* of submissive. A submissive in *any* of the following categories could accurately be referred to as a *sex slave,* particularly by those with a limited understanding of the D/s or BDSM lifestyles. I believe that sex is something that a person *does*; it is *not* a very good description of *who someone is*. Frankly, *anyone* can have sex or role-play the part of a sex slave. That doesn't really tell us anything useful about who they are, how they love, or how we can love them.

The Acolyte

The Acolyte is a submissive who is usually in a D/s relationship with a Lesser God Dom. There is a very real distinction between *being in a relationship* with the Lesser God Dom, versus *being attracted to* a Lesser God Dom. The reason for this distinction is actually quite simple. The Acolyte is a member of an intense D/s personality cult. She rarely enters into any relationship with a Dominant as an Acolyte; she is invariably *converted* to it.

The Acolyte may be referred to as a *disciple, follower, worshipper or priestess,* and considers herself not only her Dominant's *number one fan,* but also as a holder of *sacred knowledge,* a gatekeeper with the keys to her Dominant's inner sanctum, and a part of a relationship that will endure through eternity, transcending even death. The reason for that belief is rooted in the quasi-religious foundations of this sort of D/s relationship. The Lesser God and his Acolytes are part of their own private *religion*, where sin and redemption are redefined and the Dominant sits at the center of his worshippers' universe as a god or prophet. They don't expect or need the rest of us to understand, as long as it continues to work *for them*.

Of all the submissive types, the Acolyte usually is in the greatest danger of *potential* abuse, even more so than the Novice *(see below).* A Lesser God Dom considers himself unbound by any rules other than those me makes for himself, and the Acolyte typically exists in a detached, isolated and sometimes *amoral* reality in the presence of her own personal god. When things are going *well* in this kind of relationship, they tend to go *very* well. But when things begin to go *badly* – and they *often* do - it can be a disaster of *biblical* proportions. Within their quasi-religious paradigm, *death* is often viewed as a mere *illusion* or as a *graduation* from one level of awareness to the next. This can become problematic when the Lesser God Dom is revealed to his Acolytes to be a mere mortal, or when the group feels threatened by outsiders.

The relationship between the Acolyte and her Dominant always reminds me of the movie *Ghostbusters.* In that movie, an immense and horrifying demon peers at the diminutive Dr. Ray Stantz *(brilliantly played by Bill Murray)* and asks in a booming voice, *"Are you a God?"* Dr. Stantz tentatively replies, "No." His response triggers an incredible, demonic display of lightning, destruction, and chaos from the demon. In the midst of it all, fellow ghostbuster Winston Zeddemore grabs Stantz by the collar and screams, *"Ray,* when someone asks you if you're a god, *you say yes!"*

The Brat

No category of submissive has been more misunderstood, mischaracterized, nor been made the brunt of as many jokes, as *the*

Brat submissive. A Brat is a submissive who is *generally* well-behaved, but has made misbehavior, teasing, and limited kinds of defiance or disobedience an *integral* part of her Dominant-submissive dynamic. Preferably, this occurs with the full awareness and at least the *implied approval* of her Dominant. When such is *not* the case, problems will invariably arise. There is term for submissives who conduct themselves as Brats without the approval of their Dominants. We call them *phony submissives.*

There is a widespread misconception in the D/s lifestyle that Brats are always well-behaved with their Dominants, and that it is only with *other* Dominants and submissives that they exhibit their inner brat. This ridiculous notion completely ignores the fact that it is the dynamic between the submissive and her Dominant that defines her. No submissive (nor Dominant, for that matter) is defined by *how they treat everyone outside her relationship.* If such *were* the case, categorizations would not only be impossible, but meaningless. This silly notion also requires us to believe that we can truly see what happens behind closed doors in *someone else's* relationship dynamic, in order to say, *"She behaves perfectly with her Dom, it is only with others that she is a brat."* Frankly, it defies credibility to believe that anyone could be challenging, rude, or disrespectful to everyone in the world *except* her Dominant. It is *far* more likely that the submissive's bratty behavior is *universal* and *whitewashed* by a Dominant is complicit in it because prefers to keep his own inability to deal with it a secret. The internet abounds with web site tutorials for frustrated Dominants on *"How to Train Your Bratty Submissive."* Unfortunately, most of them miss the point entirely and should, instead, be tutorials on *"How to Spot and Avoid a Phony Submissive."*

On the other hand, if a Brat's behavior is an integral *and approved* part of the relationship dynamic, then it becomes a delicate balancing act that must continually be tweaked and reevaluated by both the submissive and her Dominant. The very serious question of *how much* disobedience or disrespect is *too much* can only be answered by the individuals in that relationship, and will almost always raise questions about whether or not the submissive is *"topping from the bottom."* Topping from the bottom is a technique used by *some* submissives to manipulate, control, or influence a Dominant's decision-making process. It is quite often accomplished without the Dominant even being aware of it and, *sometimes,* without the *submissive* being conscious of it, *either.* It is my humble opinion that any submissive who routinely tops from the bottom should not be considered a true submissive. That isn't to say she isn't a *good person*. It just means she isn't a *submissive*.

The Cow/Pig

The Cow or Pig submissive is one who enjoys being treated like a domesticated farm animal. Unlike the Pet submissive *(see below),* the Cow/Pig submissive thrives on humiliation, degradation, and abuse from her Dominant. For this reason, the Cow/Pig is usually most compatible with a Sadistic Dom. Often, the relationship dynamic between the two focuses on the *real or imagined* unattractiveness of the submissive, and frequent or extreme body modifications such as *branding or scarification* are fairly common for the Cow/Pig submissive. Cages, crates or pens are typically where the Cow/Pig submissive feels most comfortable. She may spend time in these enclosures for play-time only, or during select portions of the day, or even to sleep in. Cow/Pig submissives are rarely allowed to sit or lie on household furniture, and they are sometimes expected to eat table scraps or slop from a bowl or trough placed on the floor. Curiously enough, in spite of all the hoopla about the Cow/Pig submissive being *unworthy, subhuman and ugly*, her Dominant almost *always* somehow finds the intestinal fortitude to *have sex with her.* Go figure.

The Domestic

The Domestic submissive, sometimes referred to as a *service submissive,* is one who is expected to perform domestic duties in the

Dominant's household such as cooking, cleaning, childcare, chauffeuring, and yard work. More often than not, the Domestic sub is expected to be available sexually to the Dominant, his other submissives, or guests. In some relationships, *humiliation* role play is quite often a significant part of the dynamic. It is entirely possible, but relatively rare, for a Domestic submissive to be in a completely *nonsexual* D/s relationship. The Domestic sub may be involved with virtually *any* kind of Dominant; however, the most *likely* scenario is a relationship with a Sadistic Dom, FemDom, or Lesser God Dom.

The Kajira

A female *Gorean slave* is referred to as a *kajira (plural: kajirae)* which, in the fictional language of John Norman's novels about the planet *Gor,* means "slave-girl." While the great majority of Gorean slaves are female, there are some males who consider themselves to be Gorean slaves, and they are called *kajirus (plural: kajiri).* Another term that is sometimes used synonymously for *kajira* is *sa-fora*, which is said to mean *"daughter of the chain."* (For an more in-depth examination of Gorean traditions, see Chapter 7: *The Gorean Way.*)

Kajirae, almost *by definition*, are typically involved in relationships with Gorean Masters, however it is fairly common to find submissives who consider themselves kajirae *(or at the very least, trained as one)* involved with *other types* of Dominants. The reason for this is actually quite simple. The Gorean D/s lifestyle is based on a work of science fiction, and can be difficult to implement in any *practical* way in a *real-life* setting. Consequently, there are many submissives who are initially attracted to the Gorean traditions because of the rich back-story, the many opportunities for fascinating role play, and its highly-stylized and erotic customs, only to find themselves seeking other facets of the D/s lifestyle once it becomes apparent that a *real-life* Gorean relationship can be hard – *really hard.*

Theoretically, kajirae do not have any rights, nor are they allowed to own any property. They are expected to render absolute obedience to their Masters, whether or not they harbor any affection or love for him. The penalties for disobedience are quite harsh and, at least in the *novels*, include the penalty of *death*. Kajirae may be sold, given away, or loaned out to others for sexual favors, and they may not refuse nor even voice disapproval of it. Kajirae are often expected to wear highly-stylized silks, bells and jewelry, and to learn a variety of dances, serving rituals, poses, and sexual positions. It is relatively common for kajirae to speak of themselves in the third person and to avoid direct eye contact with free persons, though there is some controversy regarding whether this is prescribed in the fiction or simply a custom that has become attached to the subculture.

Gorean philosophy teaches that there is a *natural order* of things, and that natural order includes the subordination of women by men. The role and status of women in the Gorean tradition can best be summed up by this proverb from John Norman's writings: *"There are only two sorts of women – slaves, and slaves."* If feminism and the empowerment of women are among your primary guiding principles, it's a pretty fair bet that *kajira training* is just going to *piss you off*.

The Little

The Little, sometimes referred to as a *Baby, Babygirl, Babyboy, Lolita, Loli, Lolly, Little Girl, Little One, or Tot*, is a submissive who finds great joy in embracing her inner child. This sort of *age play* often involves behaving, speaking, dressing in a child-like manner, or engaging in typical child-appropriate activities, and *may or may* not involve sex or other adult-appropriate themes. While *most* Littles and their Daddy Doms find age play to be sexually stimulating, there are also many who simply find comfort in the simulated adult-child dynamic and do *not* associate it in *any way* with sex. As we stated in the previous chapter and reiterate here, anyone who associates the Daddy Dom/Little relationship dynamic with pedophilia in any form is buying into an erroneous and potentially harmful stereotype.

The degree to which a Little can actually be *hard-wired* in this way, as opposed to *role-playing*, is often the source of debate. The salient issue is rarely whether such a thing is possible, but whether or not it would be *ethical* to be involved in a relationship with a Little, *if it is.* Fortunately, for almost everyone involved, the overwhelming majority of Littles are perfectly capable of slipping in and out of the role of *innocent waif* as needed and appropriate, both in and out of the bedroom. It is not at all unusual to see a lifestyle babygirl who, at the end of a long workday as a high-powered executive and an evening of helping her teenage kids with their homework, wants nothing more than to watch her favorite cartoons with her Daddy and to have a bedtime story read aloud to her as she drifts off to sleep.

It would be easy to assume that all Littles eventually end up in relationships with Daddy Doms or, at the very least, *potential* Daddy Doms, but such is not always the case. Since age play is typically frowned upon and shunned by the general population, Littles and Daddy Doms often learn to suppress or conceal their true orientation, which makes their quest for suitable life-partners who share their way of thinking far more complicated and difficult than it ought to be. It certainly doesn't help that when most people *outside* of this lifestyle hear the words *lolita* or *babygirl,* their first thought is usually of a sexually abused under-aged girl, rather than a kinky middle-aged housewife with a pacifier in her mouth. Their practical need to stay *under the radar* has led to the exponential growth of online venues where real-life Littles and Daddy Doms are able to meet, mingle and develop relationships.

One of the down-sides of Daddy Dom/Little relationships is the unfortunate fact that they reward childish behavior. Because the dynamic can mask naiveté and places more emphasis on *cuteness* than *common sense*, these online venues also tend to attract people who are *actually* mind-numbingly immature or under-aged. Imagine how you might feel to learn that your exciting new online friend, who just happens to be *awfully good* at playing the role of a naughty twelve-year-old, *isn't acting*. This, my friend, is what *nightmares* are made of.

The Novice

The category of *Novice* covers a *lot* of ground, but it should suffice to say that the Novice submissive is typically a person who has very recently discovered and become excited about the D/s or BDSM lifestyle, and has decided that she badly wants to be a part of it. The problem is, it usually isn't simply a matter of badly *wanting* to be a part of it, but of badly *going about it*, as well. This often involves a frenzied quest to find a Master - *any Master* - and to have that accomplished by *dinner time*. This condition is often referred to as *sub frenzy,* which we discuss at greater length elsewhere in this book. As one might expect, the Novice submissive's efforts usually end in miserable failure but, *occasionally*, she is unexpectedly presented with the worst possible outcome: *success*.

When *that* happens, the Novice is usually hastily collared by an inexperienced or phony Dominant, used and abused physically, emotionally, and sexually, and then unceremoniously dumped like yesterday's Chinese take-out. The Novice's first collar typically lasts about as long as it takes the so-called Dominant to reach an orgasm or, conversely, to learn that it isn't going to happen. Sometimes, the collar will just fade away in a muddled fog of uncertainly over the following days or weeks as the hapless Novice struggles to figure out what went wrong and whether or not she still has a Dominant. Nevertheless, the undeterred Novice usually sets out again to do it all over again, *ad nauseum,* again and again, and again.

It should come as no surprise that the Novice submissive has a very high likelihood of eventually becoming someone who passionately believes that *BDSM is for losers*. After all, she has nothing but her own pathetic experiences upon which to base her judgment. This makes me sad. So, how does someone successfully navigate the treacherous path from Novice to *true submissive?* There is no clear and definitive road map that is guaranteed to help you find your way, but there *are* three principles which I believe can make that journey safer, quicker, and tremendously more fulfilling.

The first is quite simply this: *Time is your friend.* Don't be in such a hurry to find, submit, or commit to a Dominant. He isn't a carton of milk. There's no expiration date stamped on his ass. He'll still be there tomorrow, or next week, or even next month. If it is *meant to be*, then a few days or weeks won't make much difference in the grand scheme of things. It's often tempting - *even irresistible* - to leap into a relationship while your endorphins are pumping and your heart is racing. But it is also almost always going to be a *mistake*. *Take your time.*

The second principle would be: Consider a collar, if one is involved, as *symbolic of your mutual commitment*. (We'll discuss collars in greater depth in Chapter 5: *The Collar*.) At the very least, before entering into any D/s relationship, ask yourself and/or the prospective Dominant the following questions: What, *exactly,* is the nature of the commitment I am making here? What are your obligations to *me*? Am I an equal partner, unequal partner, or *property?* What happens if either of us fails to live up to these commitments? How have you handled these issues in the past? Are you any *good* at this? There's nothing disrespectful or inappropriate about any of these question. *Don't* be afraid to ask. Trust me on this. The time to learn the answers to these questions is *before* you wear the collar, *not after.*

The third principle is *crucial*, and often much more difficult than the first two. Here it is, in a nutshell: *If you have serious trust issues, don't bother.* Don't even *think* about jumping into a D/s relationship. The bedrock and foundation of every D/s relationship is *trust.* Entering into or even considering a D/s relationship knowing that you *cannot trust* is a little like skydiving without a parachute. It may start out great, but it *doesn't end well.*

The Painslut

The Painslut is typically an *extreme masochist*, which is someone who enjoys or is aroused by sensations of intense or extreme pain. While *masochists* can and do exist in every other major category of submissive, Painsluts rate their own category in the pantheon of submission for one simple reason. The Painslut's *primary* interest, attraction, and fetish is *pain* – pure and simple, completely unadulterated, and in *heaping quantities.* Many of the masochists in the other categories view *pain* as a *wonderful thing*, but they typically value pain on a par with the *other* good things in a relationship. The Painslut goes well beyond seeing pain as a *good* thing. For the Painslut, it is usually the *best* thing and, sometimes, the *only* thing. The inclusion of the suffix *slut* is not incidental, by the way. Painsluts are often known as much for their sexual *promiscuity* as they are for their extreme brand of masochism.

The Pet

A Pet submissive is one who assumes the role of a cherished animal companion to her Dominant, who typically role plays the part of *owner, caretaker, trainer, breeder, or rider.* Pet submissives typically are able to slip in and out of character as needed in order to deal with the mundane aspects of their *vanilla* lives. In some cases, Pet submissives attempt to stay in character 24/7, which is what takes their role play from being a mere kink to being a full-blown *lifestyle*.

The animal roles chosen by Pet submissives *generally* fall into three major categories: *kittens, puppies, and ponies.* Kitten play allows the submissive to demonstrate feline characteristics, seductive mannerisms, and perhaps even a streak of independence. Puppy play is more often than not characterized by eager devotion, playfulness, mischievousness, collars and leashes. Pony submissives typically fall into three categories themselves: *cart ponies, riding ponies, and show ponies.* Cart ponies pull a small cart called a sulky, which carries her owner. Riding ponies prefer to be ridden directly, either while on all fours, or standing with the rider on her back or shoulders. Since this can be problematic due to the rider's weight, it is often *simulated.* Show ponies are all about the *dressage*, and often wear very elaborate plumes, braids, harnesses, bridles, and other decorative items.

A Pet submissive who assumes the roles of *multiple* types of pets is sometimes known as a *hybrid.* It should also be noted that pet play is also sometimes used by submissive-leaning *switches* to try out roles where disobedience is *expected* and *tolerated*, such as the role of a disobedient puppy. Another point worth noting is the fact that Pet play is frequently a Novice submissive's first real exposure to the D/s dynamic due to its low level of complexity and the relative ease with which one can keep things on a *non-sexual* level. It is relatively common among teenagers in online chat venues to be involved in pet play, either as *furries,* or in other forms of role play. Parents of *very* young teens who are *furries* just might want to ask themselves, *"Who's stroking that kitty?"*

The Pseudo-sub

We mercilessly skewered the poor *Tin Pot Dominant* in the previous chapter, so I suppose it is only fair that we devote equal time and disparagement to *pseudo-submissives.* Frankly, I am often seriously conflicted on this particular topic. After all, I truly do believe that it is ultimately the responsibility of the *Dominant* to recognize these traits in any potential partner *who may honestly and naively believe that she really is a submissive.* If he is sufficiently skilled or at least *lucky* enough to recognize the warning signs, he can then make *informed decisions* about their options and any potential relationship. His options may include abandoning any attempt to forge a relationship, accepting her as she is in a *non-D/s* relationship dynamic, or attempting to train her as a submissive.

Learning that your potential partner is a *pseudo-submissive* can be a rather messy and incredibly painful process for *everyone concerned.*

Typically, the pseudo-sub is someone who may be fairly new to the lifestyle and doesn't quite understand that just because she is a *rope-bunny, spankophile, masochist,* or *bottom,* that this doesn't *necessarily* make her a *submissive.* She usually isn't trying to *deceive* anyone; it's all simply the unfortunate but *predictable* result of erroneously assuming that *because she is a bottom*, she must *also* be a *submissive.*

It really is an honest and easy mistake to make, which makes it very hard to fault someone for making it. On the other hand, these very same sweet yet naively deluded pseudo-submissives have sometimes been known *to go just a little bit postal* when their Dominants suggest that perhaps some *training* might be in order. I'm guessing that it's probably that whole *enraged-psychotic-subbie-with-a-kitchen-knife* reaction that is the source of my mixed emotions on this topic.

Frankly, I can be simultaneously sympathetic *and* cruelly contemptuous of pseudo-submissives. Perhaps that explains why I briefly considered coining a fun new *acronym* for the folks who fall into this category. The acronym would stand for:

Deluded **U**ndisciplined **M**asochists & **B**ottoms **E**arnestly **L**iving the **L**ifestyle in **E**rror as **S**ubmissives

It would be abbreviated as DUMBELLES. But, *no*. I am *not* going to do it, because that would be mean-spirited and wrong on so many levels. Then *again*, you've got to admit, it *is* kind of funny in a *"just-kidding-but-you-know-I'm-really-not"* sort of way.

I'll probably just sneakily *say it* by saying that I am *not* going to say it. After all, being a Dominant is all about having your cake and eating it, too.

Here are some of the tell-tale signs that may indicate that someone may, indeed, be a *pseudo-submissive:*

- A pseudo-sub just *loves* following her Dominant's instructions, just as long as those instructions happen to coincide with what she really wanted to do in the *first place.*

- A pseudo-sub thinks it's critical to get her Dominant's opinion on what color *panties* to wear, but neglects to mention that she bought a car today.

- A pseudo-sub is ever-ready to offer her Dominant advice on how to be a better partner. This usually consists of recognizing her bad moods and just not bugging her at those times.

- A pseudo-sub is never *wrong*. She's just learning life lessons on her own, the *hard* way.

- A pseudo-sub asks her Dominant if he likes what she is wearing, *not* because she wants his opinion, but because she is fishing for a compliment. If she doesn't get one, she sulks or gets angry.

- A pseudo-sub often cares less about her *actual* relationship with her Dominant than she does about what *others think* about her relationship.

- A pseudo-sub uses the word *"why"* as a way to *top from the bottom*. Why don't you like my hairstyle? Why won't you let me do this? Why can't you be more flexible? Why don't you want to have sex right now?

- A pseudo-sub trusts her Dominant, except when it comes to making actual, *important* decision.

- A pseudo-sub thinks the rules only apply to all those *other* submissives. She's *special.*

- A pseudo-sub tells other submissives, "My Master is the best Master in the whole wide world!" At the same time, she asks *him*, "Why can't you be like *other* Dominants?"

- A pseudo-sub thinks that having a Dom will magically fix whatever is wrong with her.
- A pseudo-sub knows the *one true way.* It was on *Tumblr*, so it *must* be true.
- A pseudo-sub has been tied up a hundred different ways and in sixteen different languages. This makes her a *pro*, since everyone knows being tied up takes real skill.
- A pseudo-sub has years of experience at being told what to do by her former Dominant. The fact that she didn't actually *do* any of those things is completely irrelevant.
- A pseudo-sub describes her former Dom as *abusive*, her future Dom as *perfect*, and her current Dom as a *work-in-progress*.

Now, before you go and get your panties in a bunch, let me just say that this laundry list of pseudo-sub warning signs *isn't* meant to be taken completely seriously. Then again, if you *are* going to get your panties in a bunch, please get photographs and send them my way. I think that's kind of *hot*.

This list was actually intended as a tongue-in-cheek commentary on the incredible complexity of D/s relationship and of how *fragile* that dynamic can sometimes be. If any of it seems to hit just a little too close to home, if you recognize yourself or someone you know on this list, I can only hope that you are able to laugh about it and perhaps find a way to use it to improve your relationship. On the other hand, if you have actually known and been involved with me *personally* in the past and think you recognize yourself on that list, I would just like to say:

Ha ha ha! Just kidding! (Does this building have a fire-escape?)

# # #

My Two Cents on Submission

Jade simply couldn't *believe* what she was hearing, and had to ask me to clarify what I'd just said. "Master, did you just say Joanne is going to be *moving here?* To *be with us?"*

I nodded, and replied, "Well, of course! Remember? The three of us talked about it when she visited us last Christmas. At the time, we all thought it was a good idea. Afterward, you even told me privately that you were really looking forward to her moving here from Colorado."

Jade closed her eyes momentarily, and took a series of deep breaths. It was obvious she was struggling to keep her raw emotions in check as she searched for the right words to express exactly how she felt about what I'd just told her. *"Master,"* she confessed haltingly, with downcast eyes, "I only said that because *I didn't think you two were serious!* I honestly, never in a million years, thought she would *actually* quit her job, take her son out of school, pack up a rental truck, and *move here to Texas!"* She was on the verge of tears as she continued, "I love Joanne, but she is *easy to love,* as long as *she* is in Colorado and *we're* in Texas! But *now*, with her coming *here*... I... I just don't *know!* Master, what am I going to do? How am I going to be able to deal with this?"

I replied, "My *love*, you'll welcome her and her son here the way she *expects* to be welcomed and, to the best of your ability, you'll be a good sister-sub to her until things either work out or they don't. And please let this be a lesson to remember *always*. I can't make *good* decisions, if they're based on *bad* information. Please don't *ever* tell me something just because you think that's what I want to hear. There's no way that can ever end well."

Jade hung her head and nodded, uttering an almost-whispered, *"Yes, Master."*

The coming months were about to get very interesting, indeed.

# # #

This sad but true personal story from the dusty archives of my somewhat eccentric life illustrates just one of the *many* reasons why it is *absolutely necessary* for a Dominant to *always* know what is going on inside of his submissive's head. A Dominant may be called upon to make life-changing decisions that affect not only *his* life, but the lives of his submissives *and* their families, both immediate and extended. It is hard *enough* to make good decisions based on timely, factual, and relevant information.

Imagine how difficult the decision-making process becomes when it is based upon information that turns out to be outdated, irrelevant or flat-out *wrong.* Not only does it become infinitely more *difficult*, but the *quality* of any decision arrived at will suffer.

The process becomes a classic case of *junk in, junk out.*

"Tell me what you're thinking" is a question that every submissive should look forward to hearing from her Dominant. Unfortunately, many submissives *dread* it, perhaps for lack of confidence or fear of being inarticulate. That is always a shame, because it is the submissive's *golden opportunity* to influence her Master's decisions and opinions *the right way*.

Charlotte, the Spider: I'm versatile.
Wilbur, the Pig: Does versatile mean full of eggs?
Charlotte: No, it means I can change with ease
from one thing to the next.

- *Charlotte's Web, E.B. White (1973)*

CHAPTER 3: THE SWITCH

What is a Switch?

There are two groups of people in the D/s and BDSM lifestyles who are quite often misunderstood and occasionally even the targets of lingering prejudice even from others in the fetish culture: *Switches* and *Primals*. We'll discuss *Primals* at length in the next chapter. Switches fall into two general categories: BDSM Switches and D/s Switches.

BDSM Switches are individuals who enjoy *performing* in either the role of a *Top* or a *Bottom,* depending upon the circumstances, their moods, or their partners. D/s Switches are people who *feel and relate* to their partners as *Dominants* or *submissives,* for essentially the same reasons. Because the D/s and BDSM cultures are overwhelmingly focused on issues relating to domination and submission, Switches are sometimes regarded by others in the lifestyle with a certain degree of suspicion, condescension or bemusement. The primary source of this prejudicial attitude tends to be the widespread misconception that Switches are simply *confused* or *unaware* of their true orientation. This erroneous belief is founded upon the naive assumption that *everyone* must either be a Dominant or a submissive. The truth of the matter is most people are *neither.* Most people have *both* dominant and submissive characteristics and are able to draw upon them as necessary and appropriate in both their day-to-day lives and their *kink lives*.

As I've mentioned earlier in this book, I firmly believe that most people can be found somewhere on a spectrum between the two extremes of Dominant and submissive. I would venture to guess that only about ten percent of the general population can truly count themselves as Dominants, and another ten percent as submissives. The other eighty percent of the human race falls somewhere in the middle; they exhibit characteristics of either, or both, depending on a variety of factors. These individuals should never feel pressured to *decide* whether they are Dominants or submissives because in truth, *they may be neither,* and there's absolutely nothing wrong with that. Among the *vanilla* population, these folks are simply thought of as being *normal*. Unfortunately, in the BDSM culture, they are often considered *confused*, *just experimenting*, or *still learning* when, *ironically*, it is often the case that an individual has realized that he or she is a Switch only *after* a great deal of soul searching, experimentation and learning.

Decades ago, being a *Switch* generally meant something else, *entirely*. The *classical* definition of *Switch* used to refer to a person (usually a female) who was always submissive to one person, and Dominant towards another. Historically, this manifested itself typically in poly relationships consisting of a male Dominant head of household living under the same roof with two submissive females, one of which was the more dominant. In such a scenario, the more dominant of the two females is *always* submissive to the male Dominant, and yet simultaneously *always* Dominant towards the other submissive female. The meaning of the word has evolved over the past thirty years or so to better serve the purposes of a post-modern BDSM culture that embraces experimentation, self-determination and kink-tolerance. Even so, even today, there are still many people who consider themselves Switches who categorize themselves as such on the basis of the *classical* definition of the word.

In some ways, perceptions of Switches in the BDSM community may be similar to how *bisexuals* are sometimes viewed by straights and gays. Many heterosexuals have an unfortunate tendency to view bisexuals as *gay.* Conversely, there are members of the gay community who demonstrate a bias against bisexuals by characterizing them as *straight people playing at being gay.* Perhaps this is all due to the fact that we all have a very *human* need to interpret our environments in *simple terms*. We want to see things as being black or white. We really don't like all those pesky shades of grey *in-between*. It messes with our sense of balance; we want things *uncomplicated.* You try *one kind* of sushi, discover that you don't care for it, and you say, *"I don't like sushi."* Never mind that there are *literally thousands* of different kinds of sushi out there that you *haven't* tried. *That* would be far too difficult to contemplate.

This tendency to oversimplify things can lead people to believe that certain things are *opposites* and mutually exclusive when, in fact, they are nothing of the sort. Domination and submission are *not* opposites, nor are they mutually exclusive *in any way*. A person can be *both simultaneously,* as in the poly household with the "Dominant submissive" who is always sub to the male head of the household, and always dominant with the other female sub. Many people also erroneously consider *sadism and masochism* to be opposites and mutually exclusive. They are *not*. A person can *easily* be simultaneously a sadist and a masochist and, in fact, it's *extremely common* in the fetish lifestyle. If you're still having a difficult time wrapping your head around this concept, consider this analogy: when a thirty-year-old woman takes her ten-year-old daughter to visit grandma, she is *simultaneously a mother and a daughter.* For the most part, no one thinks there's anything weird about that.

Introspection

How do you know if you're a Switch? It may be overly simplistic to assume that just because you are neither a Dominant nor a submissive, that this automatically makes you a Switch. After all, millions upon millions of *vanilla folk* are neither Doms nor subs *as well*, yet that doesn't make them *Switches*, either. I believe that there are a few definitive traits and characteristics that are common to most Switches. Let's examine them.

The first characteristic would necessarily have to be an involvement in the D/s or BDSM lifestyle. Without *some degree* of involvement in the lifestyle, virtually anyone (kinky *or* vanilla) who doesn't *consider* himself a Dominant or submissive would have to be categorized as a *Switch*. There are at least three good reasons why this would be neither smart nor effective.

First, the mere fact that someone doesn't *consider* himself a Dominant or a submissive doesn't necessarily mean that he *isn't one.* There are a *lot* of people out there who simply haven't yet learned that there are *other people* like them, and that there is a *name* for what they are. Lumping *those* individuals into the category of Switch by *default* would *not* be helpful to them in *any* conceivable way, and could actually *hinder* their journey of self-discovery. Second, any categorization that gives *a member of the vanilla community* a BDSM label, *regardless* of the character traits that he or she exhibits, does a disservice to *both* communities. Finally, the mere application of such a label to a group so large that it applies to eighty percent of the world's population would have the undesired effect of watering down its meaning to the point of not really meaning anything *at all.*

The second characteristic which is common to most Switches is the *enjoyment* of performing in both Dominant and submissive roles, depending upon the circumstances, mood or partner. Please note my very deliberate use of the word *enjoyment.* It isn't enough to simply be *capable* of performing in either role. After all, practically everyone is *capable* of exhibiting both dominant and submissive *behaviors.* I personally know several die-hard submissives who happen to be *quite capable* of functioning very competently in a dominant role, despite the fact that they *dread* it and it literally makes them *nauseous* to do so. What we *should* be asking is: *Do they seek out such opportunities and do they enjoy it?* Do they find *fulfillment* in it? Is *this* where they go to find their *happy place?* If so, they just *may* be Switches.

The third characteristic is tangentially related to the first, and tends to be more a *matter of degree* than it is a *yes or no* proposition. *True* Switches tend to be individuals who have accumulated a great deal of *experience* both in and outside of the lifestyle, had *more than just a few* relationship partners, and should be on the *downhill side* of the self-awareness learning curve. This statement may offend some readers and confound others. In fact, I'd bet the rent money that there's probably someone reading this paragraph *right now* who is thinking, "How *dare* he suggest that just because I'm *relatively new* to the lifestyle, that I might not be a *true* Switch?" Hear me out. I *dare say it* because telling the truth may be a dirty job, but *somebody's* got to do it, and it *might as well be me.*

Why might we expect a true Switch to be on the *experienced* end of the BDSM lifestyle spectrum? The obvious reason would be that *most* Switches tailor their *dominance-orientation* to different situations, circumstances and partners. It stands to reason, then, that if someone has had an *extremely limited number* of experiences and partners, it is likely that he has not had many opportunities to fully explore and plumb the depths of his *switchiness.* It's entirely possible that he has yet to meet that one individual who can help bring forth his *inner Dominant* or his *inner submissive.* Perhaps that crucial *pivotal experience or event* that decides the question for this individual is *still in his future.* At best, anyone who has had very little lifestyle experience to speak of and just a *few* serious D/s relationships might be more accurately described as a *provisional* Switch. In other words, he or she may be a Switch, *subject to change.*

Types of Switches

As complicated as it can be deciding whether or not you *are* a Switch, the issue can become even more convoluted when we progress to the *next* logical question, which is: *What kind of Switch are you?* For our purposes, we will be categorizing them primarily by whether they are predominantly D/s or BDSM, and by their *dominance-orientation*. One should also keep in mind that there is often a significant amount of overlap between a person's D/s *mindset* and his or her BDSM *activities.* I assign Switches to eight categories. They are the Provisional Switch, the Dominant-leaning D/s Switch, the Submissive-leaning D/s Switch, the Balanced D/s Switch, the Top-leaning BDSM Switch, the Bottom-leaning BDSM Switch, the Balanced BDSM Switch, and the D/s-BDSM Switch.

As we cover each of the following categories of Switches, keep in mind that D/s is all about the *relationship dynamic,* while BDSM is about the *kink activities.* For many people, there is a great deal of overlap that occurs between the two but, for others, *there may not be any at all.* It's very much analogous to love and sex. For some people, it's all about *love*. For others, it's all about *sex*. Ideally, *for most people*, it's nice to have *both*, and *preferably* with the same person. At the risk of beating a dead horse, we can take this analogy even further: Being a Switch could, as we mentioned earlier in this chapter, easily be compared to being a bisexual. A man could be madly in *love* with his wife, yet *sexually attracted* to both men *and* women. In such a scenario, his *relationship dynamic* may be purely *heterosexual*, but his *sexual turn-on* is *bisexual.* The same sort of thing often happens when it comes to D/s relationships and BDSM turn-ons.

Provisional Switch

The Provisional Switch, as we explained earlier in this chapter, is a Switch who is relatively new to the BDSM lifestyle and has had comparatively few real-life D/s relationships. His orientation *may* change as he gains experience and becomes involved in more relationships over time. This should carry no stigma or negative connotations, as everyone has to start somewhere, and acknowledging the inevitability of *change* simply makes good sense. Example: Miranda has been in the lifestyle for about a year. She was introduced to it by a friend, and has become active in attending the local group's get-togethers and events, where she has been eagerly learning all that she can. Thus far, she has enjoyed practically everything she has tried, from *both* the Top *and* Bottom perspectives, and hasn't really developed a preference yet. The one thing she *hasn't* done yet is *become involved in a serious relationship* with someone in the lifestyle. She isn't sure how that will change how she feels about the kink stuff that she's learned, and isn't even sure if she should be seeking a *dominant or submissive* partner, or even whether it should be a *guy, a girl or a couple.* In other words, *stay tuned for further developments.*

Dominant-leaning D/s Switch

The Dominant-leaning D/s Switch finds joy and fulfillment in *both* the Dominant *and* submissive roles in a relationship dynamic, with a preference to the Dominant role. Example: Kylie has been a submissive all her life and has been collared to Master James, for three years. Recently, James and Kylie have taken in two other subs who have moved into their home. The new girls were fairly new to the lifestyle, and since James' work often took him out of town for days at a time, he assigned the task of mentoring the girls to Kylie. She was apprehensive about the task at first, but quickly grew to love it. Kylie was surprised to learn that she was naturally submissive to males, but around *other females*, a dominant side of her personality emerged. Over time, this dynamic became the most treasured part of her poly relationship.

Submissive-leaning D/s Switch

The submissive-leaning D/s Switch finds joy and fulfillment in *both* the Dominant *and* submissive roles in a relationship dynamic, with a preference to the submissive role. Example: Jacquelyn is a Switch who is in a committed relationship with Kenneth, who is *also* a Switch. Their relationship is often complicated, and can even get pretty *rocky* at times, *particularly* when the two of them are out of synch, and each vying for dominance in the relationship. Luckily, Kenneth is a Top-leaning D/s Switch, and Jacquelyn is a Bottom-leaning D/s Switch, so when things come to a *draw* between the two of them, Kenneth usually holds the *trump card.*

Balanced D/s Switch

The Balanced D/s Switch is one for whom *both* the Dominant role and the submissive role in a relationship hold *equal appeal.* This is relatively rare, as the overwhelming majority of D/s Switches *do* have a *preference* when it comes to their relationship dynamics. Example: Chuck is a polyfidelous D/s Switch who has two wives, named Julie and Ginger, who live in separate households. Julie is his submissive, and their relationship dynamic never changes. Ginger is his Domme, and their relationship dynamic also never changes. Chuck claims to love both women equally, and expresses no preference for either his dominant or submissive role in the relationships. Interestingly enough, Chuck and his partners keep it relatively *vanilla* in the bedroom, and none of them are active in or seek out others in the lifestyle.

Top-leaning BDSM Switch

The Top-leaning BDSM Switch enjoys *both* topping and bottoming but *prefers* topping, *regardless* of his other emotional and relationship dynamic preferences. Example: Kirk is a Dominant in his primary relationship, and that never changes. However, when he and his submissive Kim attend BDSM play parties, he has been known to enjoy bottoming to some extent. His preference, however, is and always will be topping.

Bottom-leaning BDSM Switch

The Bottom-leaning BDSM Switch enjoys both topping and bottoming but prefers bottoming, regardless of his other emotional and relationship dynamic preferences. Example: William considers himself a monogamous slave to his poly Mistress Victoria, who also has other slaves. Occasionally, his Mistress hosts play parties for the entire clan, and even though William has no significant emotional connection with her other slaves, he does sometimes engage in BDSM play with them, and often switches with a preference for bottoming.

Balanced BDSM Switch

The Balanced BDSM Switch is *equally* attracted to and finds fulfillment in the role of a Top or a Bottom in his kink activities. Example: Sierra is a submissive in her primary relationship with her Dominant Joseph, and that never changes. However, at BDSM play parties, Sierra equally enjoys giving *and* getting spankings, paddlings, floggings and other forms of impact-play.

D/s-BDSM Switch

The D/s-BDSM Switch is able to change his *dominance-orientation* in both his relationship dynamic *and* his kink activities, though the switching may *not* be synchronized by timing, direction or intensity. Example: Bob is a D/s BDSM Switch who is the hinge in a poly "V" relationship, where he is Dominant to Sue, but submissive to Diane. His kink activities with each of his partners stays aligned with his relationship role, but when he attends his local BDSM group play parties, he is equally likely to assume the role of a Top *or* a Bottom.

I am fairly certain that, as a result of what I have written here, I will be deluged with countless letters, messages and emails asking me to divulge the *"authoritative source"* that has served as the wellspring for this unique method of categorizing Switches. To those folks, I can only point to the nearest bottle of tequila. As far as I know, I am the only one crazy enough to have made such an attempt and, frankly, I'm beginning to think that maybe there was a darn good reason why people *way* smarter than me didn't try it.

If You Are a Switch

If you are a Switch, or if you are beginning to suspect that you might be one, my advice to you would be to *embrace who you are*, and refuse to be pressured into having to *decide* between the two ends of the dominance-spectrum, *especially* if you are perfectly comfortable sliding back and forth along its length. On a completely unrelated side note, I probably shouldn't get too comfortable saying *"sliding back and forth along its length."*

For *most* people, their *dominance orientation* is no more a *choice* than their *sexual orientation.* It is simply a matter of *who they are.* It develops and sometimes changes as they mature, just like every other aspect of their personality. It is hardly the set-in-concrete, black-and-white proposition that some people seem to think it is.

Virtually no one would feel justified in demanding that a *bisexual* pick a *heterosexual or homosexual* preference and *just stick to it*, yet there has never been a shortage of people who think it's perfectly acceptable to make similar demands of *Switches.*

If you happen to *be* one of those people, perhaps now would be a good time to rethink your approach.

# # #

My Two Cents on Switches

I've spent much of my life completely *mystified* by Switches, on a *number* of levels. When I was much younger, I was simply *baffled* by their seemingly natural ability to *do what they do*. For someone like *me*, hard-wired since birth as a Dominant and tempered by twenty years of military leadership training and experience, it was a *completely* foreign concept. It might have been easier to convince me that a person could just grow *different sex organs at will*, than to convince me that they could *willy-nilly* change their dominance-orientation.

I've also gotten frustrated at times because *some* Switches seemed unable or unwilling to understand that *not everyone can (or should) do what they do.* Whenever I read or hear someone repeat the mantra that it is impossible to be a good Dominant unless you have first experienced what it is like to be a submissive, my head threatens to undergo what Douglas Adams likes to call a serious case of *nonlinear, catastrophic structural exasperation.* To me, that makes about as much sense as asserting that you can't possibly understand what it is like to be *heterosexual,* unless you've spent some time as a *homosexual,* or vice versa.

Want to know what makes a "good Dominant?" It is someone who finds *joy and fulfillment* in guiding, teaching, caring for and protecting *the right person.* Want to know what makes a "good submissive?" It is someone who finds joy and fulfillment in pleasing, service to, caring for and taking direction from *the right person.* A Switch finds joy and fulfillment in *either, or both,* depending on the circumstances. It really isn't any more complicated than *that.* Things may not be quite so cut and dry when it comes to *Tops and bottoms,* however. If we're talking about the *physical and psychological effects* of certain kinds of *BDSM play,* then I think it makes perfect sense that you should be familiar with *both ends of the equipment.* I certainly would *never* expect a bottom to allow me to use a TENS unit on her if I have never experienced for myself the sensations that it is capable of producing. To *expect* her to consent to such a thing would be arrogant and irresponsible on my part and that stupidity could only be surpassed by her *acceptance* of such a proposition.

To close out this chapter, I'm going to tell you a little story that beautifully illustrates just how *utterly confounded* I have sometimes been, when it comes to Switches.

I have a very good friend named Annie, whom I've known for many years. She's always been an extremely knowledgeable and competent Domme who always impressed me with her wisdom, compassion, and ability to guide and teach submissives of both genders. We would sometimes get together for a few cold beers and share funny stories about the trials and tribulations of being Dominants in an insanely vanilla world.

On one of these occasions, after about four rounds of drinks, Annie asked me, "Why haven't you ever considered taking me on as one of your submissives?" I practically *spit out my beer* and, for a moment, was completely and utterly *dumbfounded.* Anyone who knows me knows that when *I* am at a loss for words, I'm *seriously flummoxed.* I finally stammered, *"Geez, Annie!* I never considered it *because you're a Dominant!* Are you *serious?* This is a *joke*, right?"

She frowned and said, "I'm a Switch. *I thought you knew that."*

"Be a good animal, true to your animal instincts."
- - *D.H. Lawrence*

"Who speaks to the instincts speaks to the deepest in mankind, and finds the readiest response."
- - *Amos Bronson Alcott*

CHAPTER 4: THE PRIMAL

What is a Primal?

The textbook definition (if only there *were* textbooks on such matters) of *Primal,* as it pertains to the D/s lifestyle, might describe it as: 1. a person who trusts and acts upon his or her *animal instincts*; 2. a role that is neither consistently dominant *nor* submissive but can be *either* depending upon the environment, situation and personal dynamic at work; 3. a type of BDSM play that focuses on the *animalistic* aspects of relationships and sexuality.

Primals are a relatively *new* phenomenon in the BDSM culture; one that is still regarded with a great deal of curiosity by those who have long been content to categorize everyone in the D/s lifestyle as a *Dominant, submissive, or switch.* There was just one little problem with that classification method, however. It left an awful lot of people standing on the sidelines, wondering why *they* didn't seem to fit neatly into *any* of those three categories. *Primalism* is often associated with *animal play*, *pet play* or *furries*, and while it may share key characteristics with them, it stands apart from them due to its focus on instincts, perception, disdain for social conventions, and an agonizingly *unpredictable D/s dynamic*. This all may seem a bit confusing to you until you actually *get to know someone* who is a Primal, or suddenly come to the realization that you happen to be one, *yourself.* With that in mind, the best place to start may be by asking yourself the following questions: *Am I a Primal? If I was, how would I know?*

I've come up with just the thing to help you learn the answers to those questions. It's an amusing little quiz, which I've narcissistically entitled "Michael Makai's PRIMAAL Analysis." The PRIMAAL acronym stands for **P**reliminary **R**esearch on **I**nstinctive **M**annerisms & **A**ssessment of **A**nimalistic **L**oving. I created the PRIMAAL Analysis for three reasons. First, I believe it may be able to help a lot of people who may be Primals, and have been struggling to find their *niche* in the D/s culture. Second, I think it does a pretty good job of illustrating many of the common mannerisms and characteristics of Primals to those who may be unclear on the concept. And third, creating it was *a lot of fun*. If you can't have a little *fun* while writing a book, then *what's the point?*

So, at the risk of again sounding like a worn-out Jeff Foxworthy comedy routine, we're going to explore some of the tell-tale signs which *may* indicate that you *just might be a Primal.* To take the quiz, simply use a *pencil* (so you can erase the marks later) to darken the circle next to each statement with which you find yourself in *complete agreement.* If the statement doesn't seem to apply to you, or you are not sure what it means, don't worry too much about it. Just move on to the next statement.

When you're done, tally up the number of marks to get your score, and compare it with the chart that follows the test.

Michael Makai's PRIMAAL Analysis

Preliminary **R**esearch on **I**nstinctive **M**annerisms and **A**ssessment of **A**nimalistic **L**oving

You *could* be a Primal...

- If a battle for dominance is both erotic *and* enraging.
- If you've ever actually growled or snarled at someone, and *meant it.*
- If you've ever *sniffed* someone at your first meeting.
    - Award yourself an extra point if it was below the waist.
- If you've ever *bitten* someone, and *weren't* playing.
    - Award yourself an extra point for drawing blood.
- If you enjoy petting your partner and being petted yourself.
- If you believe that *pouncing* on someone is a perfectly acceptable greeting.
- If you know what the phrase "*heightened senses*" means, because you experience it regularly.
- If you've ever circled another person, evaluating them as prey.
    - Award yourself an extra point if they *were.*
- If you get an incredible thrill from a chase.
    - Award yourself an extra point if it involves tackles and pins.
- If establishing dominance is always unplanned, unscripted, and occurs with each new person.
- If you can *imagine* biting and scratching as being *better than sex.*
    - Award yourself an extra point if it *actually is.*
- If you've ever marked something or someone with your scent as a way of saying, *"Mine!"*
- If the first thing you think of when you hear the word *"pack" isn't* "*suitcase*."
    - Award yourself an extra point if your *pack* takes priority over *family.*
- If you rarely buy band-aids, because you prefer to just *lick* your wounds.

   - Award yourself an extra point if you lick *other people's* wounds, too.
- If your first response to a challenge is usually to *pin, and go for the jugular*.
- If you can always tell when your woman is menstruating by *her scent.*
   - Award yourself an extra point if you can do this with *all* the women you know.
- If you've ever *bitten your itches*, instead of scratching them.
   - Award yourself an extra point if you ever *drew blood* when you did so.
- If you often prefer to use growls, yips, purrs, whines, and barking to actual *words.*
   - Award yourself an extra point for using them in *written format*, as well.
- If you've ever heard a coyote howl, and responded with howling of your own.
- If your fascination with the moon goes *way beyond* thinking it's pretty or romantic.
   - Award yourself an extra point if you actually grow fur or fangs during a full moon.
- If you've ever referred to your children as *cubs, or pups.*
- If you've ever watched a werewolf movie, and rooted for the werewolf.
   - Award yourself an extra point if you cried when the werewolf got whacked.
- If you've ever silenced a barking or growling dog with just a look.
- If you've ever been known to follow a scent to its source, like a bloodhound.
- If you're sometimes obsessed with the thought of *chucking it all* to go live in the woods.
- If you recognize people as much by their scent, as you do by their appearance.
- If your sex partner has ever had to dream up excuses for work to explain bite and scratch marks.
- If animals, both wild and domestic, seem to take an instant and inexplicable *liking* to you.

- If *"puppy pile"* is a good description of your preferred sleeping arrangement.
- If you've ever *licked someone's face* when they were expecting a kiss from you.
    - Award yourself an extra point if they licked you back.
- If you've ever caught yourself thinking, *"the hairier the better"* about *anyone.*
- If you've come to realize you prefer sitting on the floor to sitting in chairs.
    - Award yourself an extra point if you've actually *eaten food* off the floor.
- If you've ever noticed that while your friends were sipping their drinks, you were *lapping yours.*
- If you actually *like* the scents that others usually find awful, such as manure or body odor.
- If you've actually found yourself circling a few times before sitting yourself down.
- If you're still climbing trees past the age of twelve.
    - Award yourself an extra point if you have ever actually *slept or had sex* in a tree.
- If you'd rather spend more time with your friends' pets than with some of your friends.
    - Award yourself an extra point if you actually *do* spend more time with their pets.
- If you've ever thought to yourself, *"Why chase something that doesn't bleed?"*
- If you've ever been asked whether you're a Dom or a sub, and thought, "*How should I know?* I haven't *fought* you yet."

Add 'em up!

Your Score: _____. Compare your score to the chart below. Total Possible Points: 55 Points

How Primal Are You?

0 to 15: You are *way* too civilized for your own good. You not only always use utensils when you eat, but you probably even know what all those different-sized forks at the *hoity-toity* restaurants are used for. You'd rather commune with a *day spa*, than with *nature*. Your pets are secretly plotting to have you for dinner. You seriously need to get out more.

16 to 30: Believe it or not, this makes you pretty normal. *Imagine that!* You *do* share *some* characteristics with Primals but, overall, you scored well within the normative range for most of the other people who take this test. You may be *pervy,* just not *primally pervy.*

31 to 42: You lean *heavily Primal.* You give in to your animalistic impulses and instincts more often than not, but you still maintain a solid foundation of civility and reason which tempers your Primal urges. There's never a dull moment in a relationship with you, and your partners will often have the marks to *prove it. Rawrr!*

43 or higher: You are *definitely* a Primal. You live for the hunt, and thrill to the chase. You can sense weakness or fear from across the room. You evaluate everyone you meet as predator or prey, and you don't mind a bit if the process gets a little messy or bloody. You are guided almost entirely by your instincts and senses, even when they run counter to reason and propriety. You are fiercely loyal to your pack, and to your friends. You're an *animal!*

It's *entirely* possible that some of these characteristics will strike a chord within your psyche even if you're *not* a Primal. *Everyone* has *some* animal instincts, even if they are conveniently tucked out of sight, beneath a civilized veneer. The difference is, while the rest of us are working to deny or conceal those characteristics, *Primals embrace them.*

Semi-legal Mumbo-jumbo Disclaimer: In the unlikely event that you take this test a little too *seriously,* my high-priced attorneys have advised me that I am morally obligated to publicly shame you as a *gullible twit.* This test is provided for *entertainment purposes only.*

Primal Preferences

Now that we've gotten a glimpse of what a Primal *looks like,* it should be significantly easier to draw some conclusions which can help us to more accurately define *what it is that makes a person a Primal* and take a look at what goes on inside of a Primal's head. The psycho-social pieces of the Primal puzzle are important because, for most Primals, this isn't a *role* that they play or a costume that they can put on or take off at will. It is *who they are.* This is not just about *how they act;* it is about *how they think, how they relate, and how they love.*

Let's examine what I've come to call the *Primal preferences.* They are simply a series of generalities, to be sure, but they can be incredibly useful in understanding what makes a Primal *tick.* As always, the use of the male pronoun *"he"* should *not* be interpreted as a bias for one gender over any other. It is a simply a sad acknowledgment of one of the most frustrating limitations of the English language, the aggravating lack of a gender-neutral singular pronoun.

The first *Primal preference,* which cuts right to the heart of the entire Domination/submission culture, is the unique way in which Primals make a determination of dominance. It is a process that invariably occurs *each time* the Primal encounters someone new. In fact, for some Primals it can be an *on-going process,* even with their romantic partners and long-time acquaintances. Establishing dominance is almost always an *ad hoc, unscripted, and unpredictable* thing which can be as simple and innocuous as a momentary glance, or as violent as a *Wrestlemania* cage-match.

This initial and instinctive determination of pecking-order occurs without any conscious thought on the part of the Primal. He doesn't care about whether or not you *want* to be evaluated, nor does he much care about how you evaluate *yourself*. All *he* cares about is how you measure up *in relation to himself.* This fact, alone, can be *quite* disconcerting to those in the D/s lifestyle who have assigned to themselves the traditional role of Dominant or submissive. You may consider yourself a Dominant, but the Primal's instincts may tell him something completely *different* about you, at least in relation to himself. Imagine, for a moment, what thoughts might run through a Dominant's head if a Primal were to tell him, "I know you call yourself a Dominant, but as far as *I* am concerned, *you are a submissive."* Is it any wonder that Primals are widely misunderstood in the lifestyle?

The next *Primal preference* that sets them apart from others in the D/s lifestyle is their instinctive use of, and respect for, *power and strength.* When it comes to demonstrating your worthiness to a Primal, it isn't going to be enough to *talk* about your dominance; you're going to be expected to *demonstrate it.* That demonstration may not *necessarily* involve a physical contest of strength, endurance and tolerance for pain, but you probably shouldn't be too surprised *if it does.*

Another *Primal preference* is their reliance upon predator-prey behaviors. A Primal categorizes all others as either predator or prey, and treats them appropriately. He carefully *observes, stalks, tracks, hunts, chases, and takes down* his prey and relishes every moment of it. If he classifies you as a predator *yourself*, you can expect a Primal to steer a wide path around you, preferring to seek out prey, instead.

The *Primal preference* that is probably most familiar to *non-Primals* is the affinity for the sort of love-play that results in *biting, scratching, nibbling, licking, nuzzling, or a desire to be pet or stroked*. This kind of activity is certainly not *exclusive* to Primals by any stretch of the imagination, but it is far more prevalent among them than it is in the general population. By the way, the technical term for becoming sexually aroused by *biting* is *odaxelagnia.*

Depending upon the situation and his frame of mind, a Primal will often demonstrate a marked reduction, and sometimes even a *complete loss,* of inhibitions. This *situational lack of self-consciousness* may be exhibited in a wide variety of behaviors, to include such things as a general disdain for clothing, the emulation of animal sounds such as barking, howling or growling, and rambunctious play. Quite often, their behavior is mischaracterized by others as *childlike*, when in actuality, it is far more accurate to describe it as *animalistic.*

Another of the *Primal preferences* which often confounds and frustrates their non-Primal partners is what is sometimes characterized as a general *apathy* about sexual skills and techniques. A Primal trusts and embraces his *instincts* in most things, and typically does so in his *sexual technique* as well. Expect your lovemaking with a Primal to be driven by stream-of-consciousness desires and raw, animal impulses. We're talking *on-the-front-lawn* or *on-the-kitchen-table-covered-in-birthday-cake* kind of sex, here. In a nutshell, sex with a Primal may not always be pretty, but it's definitely never *boring.*

Primals, like many of our four-footed friends, endeavor to process the world through all five of their senses *equally*. Where the average human relies primarily on sight and sound, a Primal will often call upon his other senses to distinguish a scent, differentiate a taste, or pinpoint a texture. *Sniffing* or *tasting* a person, place, or thing to learn more about it is a perfectly normal mode of investigation for a Primal. Once a Primal has *codified* you in this fashion, any change in your body chemistry is readily apparent to him. A person's monthly hormonal cycles, menstruation, sexual pheromones, medications, hydration levels, hygiene, diet, and even diseases may be an open book for a Primal to read. In additional to receiving and processing information to a greater extent through scent, taste and touch, a Primal is also far more likely to *transmit* information through those same senses. It is relatively common, for example, for a Primal to mark his or her home, property, and even friends and partners with a distinctive *scent.*

Another preference particular to Primals would be their attachment to the notion of *feeding*, rather than simply *eating and drinking*. The connotations attached to *feeding* suggest a more primitive and instinctive activity that can be applied to more than just *food*. In the modern pop culture parlance of *vampire lore, feeding* takes on a sensuously daring and primal ambience all its own which incorporates itself nicely into the Primal subculture.

Primals typically form tight-knit social groups which they refer to as *packs*, and they often place their allegiance to the *pack* higher than their loyalty to even their biological *families*. Not all Primals are quite so pack oriented; it often depends upon what sort of *animal* they identify with, and which of those animal characteristics they emulate. Even when they *are* members of a pack, different animal characteristics can lead to different sorts of behaviors. Canines, for example, often *hunt* as a pack. Felines, on the other hand, may belong to a *pride*, but prefer to hunt *alone*. Within a pack, hierarchies of dominance and submission are typically more-or-less fixed, with an *alpha individual* (or sometimes an *alpha couple*) leading the pack. Other members of the pack are sometimes referred to as *betas* or *omegas*.

When it comes to mating strategies, it's difficult to predict what a Primal's preference may be. He may show a preference for monogamy, polyamory, strategies based on specific animal species, or *no strategy at all.* Primals certainly *appear* to have a higher likelihood of being *polyamorous* than *monogamous*, but there is little hard data to support that notion. Some identify so strongly with their specific animals, that they will adopt that animal's mating strategies, as well. A *wolf* would therefore employ a strategy of *monogamy*, whereas a *lion* might feel compelled to build a pride of *five or six* mates. It's also entirely possible that for *some* Primals, surrendering to their animal instincts means not really having a strategy *at all*, but simply doing what instinctively feels right at the moment.

What comes as a surprise to many who may not be familiar with Primals is the fact that they typically do *not* identify or connect themselves with the *Furry* subculture. *Furries,* for the benefit of anyone who may have been living in a cave for the past few decades, are people who role-play anthropomorphic *animal characters* with *human characteristics.* A furry may *look* like a dog, or cat, or fox, or skunk, *but he walks and talks and acts just like a human being* in most respects. In other words, a furry is, in practically every way that counts, *the exact opposite* of a Primal. A Primal is a *human* who instinctively thinks, acts, and perceives the word in an *animalistic way.* He considers his *Primalism* a core personality trait, rather than a *role,* and will often view himself as a human-animal hybrid, or *humanimal.* A furry, by contrast, is a *role-player* who is part of a *fandom,* rather than a *lifestyle. His* fascination is with *looking the part* of an animal, while maintaining most or all of the characteristics of humanity.

Another subtle distinction between Primals and Furries concerns the social circles, events and gatherings that are typical to each. Primals are generally considered to be part of the D/s lifestyle, primarily due to their preoccupation with Dominance and submission, even if their expression of it is considered *non-traditional.* Their involvement in the BDSM lifestyle is generally dependent upon the degree to which they *also* subscribe to BDSM related kinks and fetishes. When Primals meet it is, almost by necessity, a *face-to-face* meeting. When they gather in large numbers, it is usually at *fetish events* and *BDSM conventions.*

Conversely, *Furries* are generally considered to be a subset of the *science fiction, fantasy, gaming and comic book fandoms.* Since it is *far* more practical to be a giant, walking, talking kitty-cat wearing human clothes in an *online virtual environment,* the internet is the most common venue for personal encounters. When Furries gather in large numbers, it is usually at *cosplay events* and *comic book conventions.*

One might be tempted to assume that Primals, with their fascination for biting, scratching, and fighting for dominance are, at their core, *sadomasochistic.* That would probably be a mistake. A true *sadist* enjoys inflicting pain upon others, *regardless* of *their* feelings on the matter. A true *masochist* enjoys the sensations of pain, regardless of whom or what the source of that pain might be. There are, of course, an infinite number of gradations between an extremely hard-core sadist or masochist versus someone who is *nominally one.* But the common denominator for *all* sadists and masochists alike is simply the *enjoyment of pain for pain's sake.*

Sadomasochism is *not* a phenomenon that occurs naturally in the animal world with any real frequency. Animals typically hunt, kill, or fight for purely *utilitarian* purposes. True, a *cat* may toy with a mouse before killing it, but that behavior is probably a lot more like *playing with your food* before eating it, than it is an expression of *sadism.* Primals, too, see pain as a necessary and utilitarian part of their mating rituals and for determining dominance. This is *not* to say that Primals can't also be *sadists or masochists*. We're simply saying that Primals shouldn't be considered sadomasochistic *just because they enjoy biting and scratching during sex.*

Each of these so-called *Primal preferences* is a gross generalization which may or may not necessarily apply to any *specific* Primal you may know. Whenever we are dealing with animalistic *instincts*, we have to be prepared to acknowledge that the instincts of a *cat* are going to differ *significantly* from those of a *dog, or a monkey, or a penguin.* And yes, a Primal may identify with just about *any kind of animal imaginable.*

There are a *lot* of questions about Primals which defy any attempt to make generalizations or come to any useful conclusions. Those questions must be answered by each Primal individually, and I would venture to guess that no two answers would be alike. Questions like these, perhaps:

- Are you, as a result of your *instinctive* way of evaluating the world, inherently *amoral?*

- If there were *no limits* to what you could do, how far would you go to alter your physical appearance to resemble your inner animal?
- Do you, as a Primal, prefer other Primals or non-Primals as your potential mates, and why?
- Is the *credibility* or authenticity of another Primal ever in question to you, and if so, why?

Perhaps my readers can, post-publication, provide some inspired answers to these and the countless other unspoken questions that naturally come to mind when pondering the many mysteries of *humanimal* relationships.

In the meantime, let's shift our focus to *another* practical aspect of interacting with a Primal. Before entering into an actual *relationship* with a Primal, you might get the idea that you want to *play with one.* In *this* lifestyle, that usually means a *scene.* A scene with a *Primal...* Now, *there's* a scary thought.

Primal Scenes

A primal scene is not something you see every day. That has a lot to do with the fact that there's very little that a primal does that is *preplanned.* A scene, *almost by definition,* is something that is planned *ahead of time.* There *will,* of course, occasionally be those times when Primals have made plans to do a scene completely unrelated to their *primalism* and serendipity nudges them *off-script.* When it *does* happen, it is rarely predictable, and may even be as alarming to spectators as it is fascinating to them. By the way, the phrase *"primal scene"* can mean very different things to different people. Among psychologists, it is a term which refers to witnessing or imagining *your parents having sex*; something you just might want to keep in mind if you ever decide to discuss this topic with your *shrink.*

Typically, in the BDSM world, a Primal scene simply *happens* without a lot of forethought. What may start as a bit of cautious sniffing and circling can quickly escalate to a scenario where instinct supersedes reason and judgment, and life leaps from mundane to *extraordinarily interesting* in about 2.6 seconds flat.

Mellissa W., a twenty-six-year-old woman from Kansas, considered herself a traditional submissive before she became involved with a Dominant who seemed to play a lot rougher than she had been accustomed to with her previous lovers. That, *in itself* wasn't too unusual. What *surprised* her was her immediate and instinctive reaction to it; a reaction that opened up a part of herself that she had never suspected was there.

> *"We had always been playful and even a little rough at times, but I always figured it was just fun and games. One night I was walking past him and Derek surprised me by grabbing my boob, and I don't know why, but I snatched his hand and bit into the meaty part at the base of his thumb really, really hard. He screamed bloody murder, grabbed me and picked me up, and literally threw me like a sack of potatoes across the room onto the bed. As soon as I realized I wasn't going to die, I was just completely filled with this primal all-consuming rage. I just sprang off the bed like some kind of wild animal, throwing my entire weight on him and knocking him to the floor, while hitting and biting and scratching.*
>
> *We fought and wrestled and rolled around on the floor snarling at each other like pit bulls until we were completely spent. Even then, he somehow managed to pin me down until I stopped struggling. Then we just looked at each other silently for a minute, and suddenly we couldn't stop laughing. Then we had what I can only describe as the most incredible sex, ever. We should have done this a long, long time ago."*

Sometimes, a person may be fully aware of their primal nature, yet still be unsure about how it can be expressed as part of a public scene. After all, it is something that is often misunderstood, even within the BDSM lifestyle, and can sometimes lead to potentially embarrassing or even dangerous situations.

Kevin P., a thirty-year-old living in Florida, described to me the first time he'd allowed his primal side to come out at a public gathering:

> *"I was at one of our group's monthly play parties, held at the spacious home of one of our group members, watching a couple of friends do a knife play scene. Across from me, I noticed Nora, one of the newer members of the group staring directly at me. Once I noticed her, I just couldn't take my eyes off of her. We had chatted briefly at the last get-together, but it was just your typical small-talk. This was something completely different. We probably said more in those few minutes of silently staring at each other than any conversation, no matter how deep, ever could.*
>
> *I walked around the group of people gathered to watch another couple doing a scene. Her gaze never left me as I slowly circled around the group and around her as well. I stopped between the kitchen and the living room. Then it was her turn to circle me, I guess. She started to move past me, and as she did, she put her face right up to my shirt and sniffed me, then moved on past me a few steps and stopped, as if she were daring me to follow her. I moved past her towards the door that led outside to the patio, and opened it. She stepped thru, and I followed out onto the patio, where a few people were enjoying their cigarettes.*
>
> *There, in the back yard, we both started silently circling each other, the way boxers or MMA fighters do in the ring, completely oblivious to the other people on the patio watching us. Our circling got tighter, and turned into touches, pokes, and her raking her fingernails across my*

bare skin. I finally pulled her close to kiss her, but when I did, she turned away from my kiss and sank her teeth so hard into my jawline that it broke the skin! I was surprised, bleeding and angry, and without even thinking, I just slapped her hard across the face. She drew back for a split second, and then clocked me hard right on the nose with her fist. I staggered and almost went down, but figured I'd take her down with me, so I tackled her to the grass, where we wrestled and I bled all over her until the other people on the patio pried us apart and positioned themselves between us.

I stood there, bleeding from my jaw and my nose while she, covered in my blood, paced like an angry feral cat that had been swung around by its tail. Someone mentioned calling the police, and we both instantly and simultaneously said, "No!" She assured them further, saying, "It wasn't a fight... it was..." She paused, and I jumped in to finish her sentence. "Foreplay," I said. They laughed. We laughed. And then we went to my place for sex."

It isn't always simply the unpredictability of a primal scene that can sometimes make it problematic. When I asked my friend *ShadowCat*, a twenty-two-year-old Primal switch who leans heavily dominant, whether she usually sought out other Primals as potential partners, she surprised me with an unexpected response. She said that she typically did *not* prefer other Primals, and explained why:

"Being with other Primals can actually be kind of dangerous for someone like me. I'm a woman, a Primal, and I'm usually a Dominant. But Primals don't care about what you usually are; they make up their own minds about your position in the pecking order. Many just automatically assume that if you're a woman, that there must be a submissive buried deep down inside there, somewhere. They figure all they have to do is beat me into submission to bring it out. Don't get me wrong - I like my sex rough, but I

> *don't want to end up in the hospital, either. Some of these guys just can't get it into their heads that I'm very dominant. Their instincts keep telling them that if they just try a little harder, take the violence up just one more notch, that I'll submit. But I don't and, sometimes, they just don't know when to quit. That usually doesn't end well."*

Primal scenes and other intimate primal encounters always have the potential to be simultaneously exciting *and* terrifying; erotic *and* dangerous. A Primal's instincts can typically do a wonderful job of telling him *who* to play with and *how* to play, but may not always be adequate at telling them *how far is too far, and when to stop.*

Even Primals playing with other Primals would be well-advised to keep that in mind.

Primal Instincts

In the final analysis, primalism is simply a matter of surrendering matters of attraction, love, sex and kink to our most basic instincts. William Bernbach, a prolific advertising executive who had an exceptionally keen insight into how people think and relate once said, "Nothing is so powerful as an insight into human nature... what compulsions drive a man, what *instincts* dominate his action... If you know these things about a man you can touch him at the core of his being."

Trusting and following your primal instincts can not only help you to connect, touch and be touched at your *very core*, but it can sometimes actually help you to make better decisions. *Good instincts* can very often convey hidden truths and guide your actions long before your *intellect* figures things out rationally.

Perhaps an exploration of your *own* primal side is something you should consider.

"For all the talk you hear about *knowledge* being such a wonderful thing, *instinct* is worth forty of it for real unerringness."

Mark Twain

# # #

My Two Cents on Primals

There really wasn't a *word* for what Nicole was, at the time. She was, in my mind, quite simply a *difficult submissive.* On the one hand, she had a truly beautiful spirit and an intense, focused loyalty – not only to me, but to the other members of my house – that was simply amazing. On the other hand, she would often do odd and inexplicable things that would perplex or infuriate me. I didn't know it *then*, but Nicole was a *Primal.*

When she first walked into my life, I was sitting at my desk, working in the front office of a technology business that I'd founded some years previously. The door chimed, and I looked up from my work to see a petite young woman with straight blonde hair to the small of her back and penetrating blue eyes that were focused intently on mine. She seated herself in the chair in front of my desk and we chatted amiably about the services my business had to offer. As we spoke, I noticed an unusual tattoo which covered her entire forearm from wrist to elbow. The tat consisted of orange and black *tiger stripes* that encompassed her arm like a sleeve. I noticed also that her aggressive, penetrating eyes never – *ever* – strayed from their laser-like focus on *mine.* We quickly arrived at a business agreement, and when it came time to finalize the paperwork, she leaned over the desk to sign the contract and did something very odd, something which I found simultaneously fascinating *and* arousing. *She sniffed me.*

A few days later, I received a phone call from my mysterious new client; she was having a little problem with our software. Would I be available to discuss it with her? Incredibly, I heard myself responding, "Sure! Actually, I was just about to break for lunch. It's such a gorgeous day out, I was thinking of having a sandwich in the park. Would you care to join me?" She gave me her address, and told me she could be ready in ten minutes. As I hung up the phone, I thought to myself, *what the hell just happened?*

I never *did* go back to the office that day. At the park, we sat on the grass and studiously ignored both our sandwiches *and* our purported reason for being there. As she grew more comfortable in my presence, she became progressively more *playful* as well, climbing the trees and cavorting on the playground equipment. It was something I might have expected from an adolescent, but she was in her twenties. I found myself incredibly, irresistibly fascinated, amused, and yes... *smitten.*

We went back to her house, where we spent the rest of the day rolling around on the floor and bouncing off the furnishings the way cats tussle over a ball of yarn. The sex was an incredible mixture of passion and violence, a struggle to establish dominance, and an unrestrained expression of *raw hunger.* Despite a full day of biting, wrestling, scratching, hair pulling, spanking, blindfolds and bondage, we somehow managed to survive it and have a conversation later that evening.

I asked her how long she'd been in the BDSM lifestyle. *"BDSM?"* she responded with a bemused look on her face. "I don't know anything about that. I only know that I was *yours* from the moment we first met. I don't know *how* I knew it, I just *did.* I could *sense* it, somehow. I could *smell it.* I just trusted my instincts, and they told me to trust you. *I am yours."*

"In *that* case," I smiled, "Let's start by having you address me as *Master."*

"On the Internet, nobody knows you're a dog."

- - Peter Steiner cartoon
depicting an actual dog at the keyboard.
The New Yorker, July 5, 1993

CHAPTER 5: ONLINE BDSM RELATIONSHIPS

Many people get their very first taste of Domination/submission and the BDSM lifestyle via the internet. Web sites, chat rooms, fetish portals and virtual worlds have all combined to make the internet a veritable buffet of BDSM and kink in general. In fact, it is *so* plentiful and omnipresent, one often finds BDSM-related images and references in places it where they *shouldn't* be, such as on web sites and in chat rooms that are frequented by under-aged children.

If *you* happen to be one of those people whose only exposure to the BDSM lifestyle has been through the internet, you may very well find yourself wondering about the differences between the *online* BDSM lifestyle and the *real-world* one, and about the *validity* of your online experiences. Our goal in this chapter will be to try and answer some of those questions for you, and perhaps provide you with a road map that will help you to make the leap from *virtual* D/s relationships to the *real thing*, if that is what you seek.

The online BDSM culture is truly a double-edged sword in many respects. On one hand, it allows a person with absolutely no prior experience or knowledge of the lifestyle to dip his or her toe into the waters without fear of ridicule or harm. On the other hand, it allows a person with absolutely no prior experience or knowledge of the lifestyle to *misrepresent himself as an expert,* without worrying about any potential consequences. The horror stories one hears, again and again, are enough to make some people shun the online BDSM culture *entirely*. It is disturbingly common to hear tales of middle-aged submissive women who learn that their supposed Masters are actually *teenage girls*. Not only do men turn out to be women, but women are revealed to be men, and children routinely pose as adults. In short, the one thing that you *can* trust to be true when it comes to internet BDSM is: *Nothing is ever what it seems*.

My favorite story about online relationships concerns two overweight, middle-aged, heterosexual men who posed as twenty-something *lesbians* in order to engage in frequent cybersex with naïve bisexual or lesbian teenaged girls. What happened, *instead*, was they met and seduced *each other*, and *fell head over heels in love*. Imagine their mutual surprise, after *months* in a loving and ostensibly committed online relationship, when they discovered the awful truth. Apparently, karma is not only a *bitch*, but she has a wicked sense of humor.

Online BDSM culture and relationships can be illusory, deceptive, and abusive. They can also be entertaining, honest, and fulfilling *if* you approach them with open eyes, the right attitude, and take proper precautions. We'll discuss those precautions later in this chapter, after we've talked about some of the different venues where you may encounter the online BDSM culture.

Text-Based BDSM Chat

For most of the people who use the internet *today*, it's difficult to imagine that there was ever a time when the internet existed *without* the World Wide Web, robust graphics, or the high speed networks that made them all possible, *but there was*, and I was caught up in all of it from the very beginning.

My first exposure to the online BDSM culture was in the mid-1980s through an online service called *CompuServe*, which was the very *first* major internet service provider. In the beginning, CompuServe charged roughly *$5 per hour* to connect to their network and *overseas,* where I was stationed at the time, a person could easily spend $30 per hour in surcharges to connect through CompuServe's international nodes. Needless to say, at those prices, only the most obsessed and committed computer geeks bothered to do so. Yes, *people like me*.

The reason for my obsession was something CompuServe called *CB Chat*. It's humorous to think of it now, but at the time it was called *CB* chat because the marketing gurus at CompuServe believed that would be the best way to explain the concept of a *chat room* to people who had never heard of one before. The idea was to invoke the familiar notion of *CB, or citizens band, radio*. Yes, we're talking about the very same CB radio fad made famous by the popular 1975 song *"Convoy"* by one-hit wonder C.W. McCall, and the 1978 movie by the same name. By the way, if you're *not* familiar with the song, do yourself a huge favor and avoid the temptation to look it up on You Tube. It could be *days* before you get that earworm out of your head.

The chat rooms or *channels,* as they were sometimes called, were organized by topic or lifestyle, and I naturally gravitated to the BDSM lifestyle channels. There, I learned that the online BDSM culture – *even then,* in the internet's infancy - was *far different* from what I'd experienced in real-life and there were a *lot of new rules to learn*. A few years later, around 1988, other alternatives to CompuServe chat became available, including America Online (AOL) and a multitude of Internet Relay Chat (IRC) networks. Today, there are literally *thousands* of IRC chat networks in existence, with the four largest being EFnet, IRCnet, UnderNet, and DALnet. Many of the customs and online protocols that were developed by the CompuServe fetish community then were adopted by the users of these newer chat platforms, and most are still in practice, even now.

During the early days of the internet, certain protocols *had* to be followed in order to make sense of a BDSM culture *that could only be expressed in text.* There *were* no websites or social media portals like Facebook or Tumblr. The very notion of being able to have an internet-based *voice-chat, a la Skype*, was still *decades* away. Even the ability to attach a photograph to an email in order to send it to a friend was beyond the technical abilities of most people. In other words, if your message couldn't be expressed in letters, numbers, punctuation or symbols, you were quite simply *out of luck*.

So, we *adapted*. We learned to use *plain text* to provide all of the necessary vital clues to a person's status, relationship, sexual orientation, and standing in the online BDSM community to anyone who happened to be paying attention and knew what to look for. Dominants *capitalized* the first letter of their names; submissives used all *lower-case* letters. Submissives referred to any male Dominant who was not his or her own as *Sir*. Female Dominants were referred to as *Ma'am, Miss, or Mistress.* Personal pronouns such as *you, him, her, and they* were capitalized if you were talking *to* a Dominant. If we were talking *about* a Dominant, then we capitalized the *Him or Her*. If we were unsure, or we were addressing a mixed group, we sometimes used torturous grammatical monstrosities like *Y/you, T/them, or* even *E/everyone*. You could always identify the chronically clueless by their admirable but terribly misguided enthusiasm in misapplying this particular protocol, which would sometimes resulted in grammatical abominations like, *"H/hello E/everyone, H/how A/are Y/you A/all T/this E/evening?"* Nice try, but no cigar.

We couldn't always figure out a person's *sex* without asking, but we *could* immediately tell who was *collared* by the addition of bracketed initials at the end of a collared individual's name. For example, if a submissive named *slavekitten* was collared to a Dominant named *DarkKnight*, her username would often look something like this: slavekitten{DK}. If slavekitten were to log on one day without the {DK} attached to her name, you instantly knew what that meant. She had been released from her collar.

Despite the advent of the World Wide Web and the tremendous growth of more technically sophisticated chat platforms the appeal of text-based chat has remained as strong as ever, with over 3,200 IRC chat servers currently hosting *hundreds of thousands* of chat channels each day. The most popular IRC program is mIRC, which can be downloaded for free from practically any freeware or shareware download site. Some popular BDSM-related websites maintain their own custom web/IRC interfaces, which allow visitors to use their web browsers to access the site's IRC chat servers. To learn if your favorite BDSM web portal has an IRC chat server, just look for a search box on the site, and search for the term "IRC chat."

Virtual Worlds BDSM Chat

As computer technology and networking capabilities increased, so did our ability to explore a robust and growing BDSM culture online. The first networked *virtual worlds* were developed in the 1970s by the Department of Defense and deployed on ARPANET (Advanced Research Projects Agency Network), the precursor to what eventually became the modern internet. By 1978, the first non-commercial virtual world to be deployed on the internet was called MUD1, which ironically stood for *Multi User Dungeon*. The *dungeon* in this particular instance was more of a *Dungeons and Dragons* sort of dungeon, than a *BDSM* one.

By the late 1980s, commercial versions of virtual worlds had begun springing up, most notably *Habitat* by Lucas Films, and WorldsAway/Dreamscape by CompuServe. These experiments in virtual worlds led the way for the immensely popular Massively Multiplayer Online Role Playing Games (MMORPGs) that followed, like *Ultima Online* and *World of Warcraft*. Today, the most popular virtual world chat platforms are *IMVU for Windows, Second Life for Windows, Play Station Home,* and *The Sims Online.*

Virtual world chat programs added an exciting *visual* dimension to what had previously been limited to letters, numbers and symbols. Suddenly, you no longer had to guess or ask about a person's sex, you could figure it out simply by looking at that person's 3D *avatar.* Of course, nothing prevents a person from misrepresenting his or her sex by choosing an avatar of the opposite sex, but why let a little thing like *that* dampen our enthusiasm for the magic of 3D virtual worlds? The process of choosing an avatar to represent you in this virtual world also came with an *added bonus:* the ability to be the person you always wanted to be. In virtual worlds, we are unencumbered by age, obesity, bad teeth, bald spots, muffin tops, spare tires, small boobs or tiny penises. Everyone is *perfect*, or at least as perfect as they want and can afford to be, which for the most part, is *pretty darn perfect*.

For *some* people, this illusion of instant bodily perfection can be *pretty heady stuff.* Combine that with a large dose of internet anonymity, the allure of consequence-free 3D graphic cyber-sex, and a ready supply of naïve hormonal teenagers, and you end up with a recipe for a potentially problematic detachment from reality that *could* be downright catastrophic for *any* relationship, D/s *or* vanilla. Adding a BDSM relationship dynamic to the mix can be a little like throwing a bucket of gasoline onto an already out-of-control fire.

The sophistication of the 3D graphic cyber-sex available in these online virtual worlds is *astounding*, however, even at its best it is still only as good as one's *imagination*. In that sense, it is really not much different from phone-sex, sexting, or *cartoon porn* – perhaps better than nothing, but that isn't exactly *high praise.* Some virtual worlds impose bewildering rules on what is, and isn't, allowed sexually. One of the largest online virtual worlds, for example, forbids *erect penises* and/or *any hip to hip contact between avatars.* In fact, if you want your avatar to have a penis *at all,* expect to hand over some *real cash* for the privilege, since *starter* avatars come *penisless* in almost all virtual world chat programs.

Unfortunately, when it comes to *virtual sadomasochistic* sex, things get even *more* complicated and frustrating. For sadists who get off on inflicting pain on others, and masochists who enjoy the sensations of pain, a virtual world where no one feels pain *at all* can be just a little exasperating. *Imagined* pain and pleasure are poor substitutions for the real thing, unfortunately. *Bondage* loses much of its appeal when a person can free himself from his restraints with a simple click of his mouse, and simulated impact-play has all the emotional *impact* of swiveling Ken's little plastic arm to spank Barbie's perfect little plastic ass.

In short, BDSM play in these virtual worlds leaves a *lot* to be desired. The product designers typically have little or no experience or knowledge about the lifestyle or its practices and so what you end up with, more often than not, is a ridiculous caricature of what some nerdy developer in Taiwan *imagines* happens during BDSM sex. What is typically your first clue that the animator is *vanilla?* Apparently their view of BDSM sex involves *lots of crying, and no orgasms.* Go figure.

It also seems to consist almost exclusively of tying people to beds and/or giving spankings. Beyond those two activities, it's a virtual *fetish wasteland.* Suspensions? Nope. Edge play? Nope. Fire play? Nope. Violet wands, breath play, anal play, breast flogging, or pussy spankings? No, no, no, no, and *not even anything close*. Those poor Taiwanese animators *really* need to get out more.

One of the unique features of the online BDSM culture that you'll encounter in many virtual worlds is the *slave market*. Slave markets exist almost exclusively in BDSM chat rooms for the simple reason that they would be impractical or illegal *anywhere else*. They typically consist of chat rooms with kneeling-pillows, upon which hopeful, unowned slaves kneel and wait to be interviewed by Dominants who imperiously sit on nearby thrones. The rooms are called *markets*, even though no one buys – or even rents – anything, or anyone. Many of these so-called slave markets require visitors to announce their *"status"* to the existing occupants of the room and to request permission to enter. This status theoretically consists of whether you're a Dominant, submissive or switch, whether you are owned or unowned, and what – *if anything* - you happen to be seeking. An example might sound something like this: "I am an unowned submissive seeking a Mistress. May I enter?" Not all slave markets require such formality, but when in doubt, it is usually best to err on the side of high protocol.

Upon being granted permission to enter, Dominants should inquire as to which seats or thrones are appropriate to sit on. Submissives should assume that kneeling-pillows are their only seating option, though there may be certain pillows that are reserved for moderators or chat room regulars. If the seating arrangement consists of something *other* than thrones and pillows, it's probably a good idea to ask the current occupants of the room where you should sit.

You may be asked to tell the other people in the room a little about yourself; actually knowing how to respond to this question can go a long way towards establishing your credibility and making new friends. The absolute *worst* thing you can do is attempt to bluff your way through an initial conversation of this sort. There's no shame in admitting you don't know much about the lifestyle, as long as you are open and honest about it. Misrepresenting your experience and knowledge is considered not only *extremely bad form*, but can be emotionally devastating to your potential partners and potentially *dangerous* to everyone involved.

Spotting an Online BDSM Phony

One of the most useful skills that can be developed and honed by members of the online BDSM community is *the ability to spot a phony*. When the online environment allows virtually *anyone* to pretend to be *anything,* a person's credibility becomes his or her only currency. We should take a moment to clarify what we mean when we use the word *phony* in this particular context. If we assume that the *online* BDSM culture is *"real" in its own unique way* (at least to the people who are a *part* of it) then obviously *the people who are a part of it* should be considered real, as well. In other words, the mere fact that a person has no *real-life* BDSM experience does not mean he or she is a phony. Sometimes, real-life circumstances prevent people from acting on their wants and needs. Even so, it may be entirely possible that the person has *many years* of experience in online BDSM relationships and has much to offer someone who may be new and desirous of a mentor.

So, what constitutes an online BDSM *phony,* then? For *our* purposes, we'll define an online BDSM phony as a person who knows little or nothing at all about the BDSM lifestyle – *online or real-life* – yet attempts to present himself as experienced and knowledgeable. The most common example of this kind of behavior is what happens when a young, sexually frustrated person stumbles upon the existence of the online BDSM culture and naturally assumes that simply *calling* himself a *"Master"* (or *"Mistress"*) will result in a treasure trove of slaves offering sexual favors and unconditional adoration.

It never seems to occur to these individuals that there may be more to being a Dominant than *simply calling yourself one*. The clueless would-be Dominant immediately launches himself into slave markets and other BDSM-related chat rooms to proudly announce, *"I am a Master! Who wants to be my slave?"* To fully understand the sheer, unthinking vacuity of such behavior, try to imagine a person walking into a popular real-world nightclub, standing just inside the entrance, and calling out loudly to everyone within, *"I am a studmuffin! Who wants to be my love-bunny?"*

The first few words out of a person's mouth are usually all one needs to hear in order to know just how much credibility he or she deserves in the online BDSM culture. There are, however, some people who are quite skilled at the art of online *duplicity*. They can mimic the customs and protocols that are common in the online BDSM lifestyle, but they can't discuss knowledge of the lifestyle *that they don't have.* Their ignorance of the lifestyle very quickly becomes apparent to anyone who is *paying attention*. A skilled interviewer, whether Dominant or submissive, can usually expose the phonies by asking simple, polite questions in a *particular way.* The questions should be carefully worded to be *innocuously inoffensive* to authentic members of the online BDSM lifestyle, yet exceedingly difficult for anyone *pretending* to be something that he is not.

Here are just a few examples:

- Never ask, "Are you a Dom or a sub?" This allows a clueless imposter to simply *pick one of the above.* Instead, ask, "Are you a switch?" A knowledgeable person will typically respond with one of the following: *No, I am a Dominant. No, I am a submissive.* Or, *Yes, I am!* A phony will invariably be dumbfounded for a moment and ask, *"What's a switch?"*
- Always ask, "How long have you been in the lifestyle?" Don't refer to it as the *BDSM lifestyle.* Anyone who is actually in the lifestyle will *naturally assume* you mean the *BDSM* lifestyle. A phony, even as he or she sits in a *slave market,* will often inanely respond with, *"What lifestyle?"* While you're at it, check his answer against his supposed age. A twenty-year-old who claims to have been in the lifestyle for fifteen years is not only *a liar,* he's also a math-challenged *moron.*
- Try asking a *philosophical* question - perhaps something like, "Do you think D/s is a matter of *who you are, or what you do?*" A knowledgeable person will enjoy a chance to give his opinion on the subject, and you *may* even gain some insight from his response. A phony will ask, *"What's D/s?"*
- Ask questions of *preference*: "What's your favorite kind of scene?" It's a simple question for someone in the lifestyle – even for those who may be very new, or may be limited exclusively to the online lifestyle. A phony, however, will often be completely unfamiliar with the way the word is used in this culture, and will typically respond with, "What do you mean by *scene?*"
- Consider asking a *trivia* type of question: "We're having a disagreement about what the *D* in BDSM stands for. What do *you* think?" Feel free to consider *any* response that actually involves a word that starts with the letter *D* as acceptable.

Sometimes, it is the perplexing and often amusing questions that someone *asks* in these online chat rooms that expose him as a phony. The following is a list of *actual questions* that have been posed to me by allegedly *"highly experienced"* online Masters and Mistresses who claimed to have *years and years of BDSM experience*. Seriously, I couldn't *make this stuff up*:

- Do *your* slaves let you have sex with them? I was just wondering.
- How do you keep your slaves from running away? I'm having a bit of a *problem* with that.
- Would it be easier to get more slaves if I created second account as a sub and collared myself?
- How many slaves do *you* have? I have 23. *More*, if you count the ones whose names I don't remember.
- All my slaves turn out to be, like, *thirteen years old*. What am I doing wrong?
- I really want to be a *real-life* Master. Real-life Masters have lots and lots of sex, *right?* How much sex, *exactly*, are we talking about, here?
- How do you get your submissives to respect you? This is way harder than I *thought* it would be.
- Do you practice forced collaring?

Obviously, it's not particularly difficult to separate the wheat from the chaff in these kinds of conversations. The only *real* issue becomes, how do you *handle* a phony once he or she is exposed? Do you tell the person how you tripped him up? If you *do*, then the imposter simply chalks it up as a *lesson learned*, and tweaks his performance to better deceive the *next* person who comes along. If you *don't*, you are often left with the irksome feeling that you've allowed someone to think he has gotten away with deceiving you.

Sometimes, the best solution is to simply inform the individual that you weren't fooled. Then, if you have the power to do so, *boot and ban*.

Challenges

Despite all of the apparent pessimism you've thus far been bombarded with in this chapter, online BDSM relationships actually *do happen*, and sometimes, even *flourish*. The keys to having a successful online BDSM relationship generally come down to the following three factors: Determining *beforehand* where the line is that separates your *virtual BDSM life* from your *real-world* life, deciding for yourself the importance of the *reality behind the avatars*, and asking yourself, "Why am I doing this, and where is it going?" The answers to these three questions *aren't easy*, nor *should* they be. In fact, if one or more of the questions *seems* easy for *you,* then I would suggest that you've probably seriously underestimated the complexity and gravity of the issues involved.

The wildcard that is often overlooked when it comes to online relationships in general, and online BDSM relationships in particular, is the role that our *emotions* play in our perceptions and decision-making. We often go into these things with *one* set of expectations, only to discover - *after we have fallen in love* - that a completely *different* set of expectations has suddenly appeared out of nowhere and taken precedence. If either partner is unprepared for it when that happens, it can not only be potentially devastating to the online relationship, but it can lead to significant problems in their *real-lives*, as well.

The Virtual Line

There are many who will probably disagree with me on this, but I believe that there are *three kinds of people* who seek out the online BDSM culture.

The Reality Geek. This first category consists of those who live a BDSM lifestyle in real-life and simply want a convenient and entertaining way to connect online with like-minded friends, or make new ones. For those people, the line that separates their virtual lives from their real ones may be flexible, fuzzy or may not exist *at all*. There is little or no *cognitive dissonance* between the two environments. In fact, for many of the people in this category, the internet is not considered a virtual world or as a completely different environment *at all*. It is viewed simply as one more facet of their *real-world environment*; another mode of communication that is not unlike *talking on the telephone or texting*. Just as most people would never characterize a telephone conversation as an *alternate life*, the people in this group typically don't think of a graphic internet chat room as one, either.

The Toe-Dipper. This second group consists of people who wish to explore the lifestyle virtually before making the plunge into the real-life culture. For these people, it may be necessary due to their present circumstances, or simply preferable, to learn as much as they can *virtually* before considering a decision to adopt the lifestyle in reality. The individuals in this group must, out of necessity, consider the internet and their real-lives as *two separate realities* with no significant overlap. For them, the separating line is usually quite distinct, even though it may move or get fuzzier over time as they grow more confident and become more willing to cross the line. In short, the separating line is there, but it is often moving or *temporary.*

The Fantasizer. Third and finally, there are those who, for whatever reason, *cannot or have no desire to* live a BDSM lifestyle in reality, and so they do it *virtually*. There are many good and valid reasons why this may be so, and it isn't our place to judge another person's reasons for doing so. Long ago, I had a friend in the online BDSM lifestyle who, I learned *years later*, was a paraplegic, and had been confined to a wheelchair since his childhood. Another acquaintance was afflicted with agoraphobia, and hadn't left her apartment in almost a decade. There may also be family or career considerations which make the pursuit of BDSM in reality an impractical lifestyle choice for some. It should suffice to know that if these individuals believe there are good reasons to keep their two lives separate, then there is an equally good reason to establish a firm separating line between them. For these individuals, that line is usually non-negotiable and impermeable.

The online *environment* may be *virtual*, and the emotions experienced there are *real,* but what about everything *in-between?* What should be allowed to cross over from the virtual world to the real one, or vice-versa, and what shouldn't? Where do you draw that line? Should you give out your real name or telephone number to a stranger in a chat room, reserve them for the people you trust, or not give them out at all? Do you tell your online friends what you do for a living in real-life? Do you allow your online Master or Mistress to tell you what color you should dye your hair? Should that cross-over influence extend to controlling your real-life finances, or disciplining your children?

Cross-over influences happen all of the time - sometimes in dribs and drabs and others times in a flood - yet we very rarely consider the potential consequences. It is easy to believe, while basking in the aura of NRE *(New Relationship Energy)* that the person with whom you've just become involved is practically perfect in every conceivable way, and would *never* do anything to hurt you, but let's take a look at the *actual odds.*

The overwhelming majority of *all* relationships – *online or in real-life* - will fail for one reason or another, and many of those will *end badly.* There is very little hard data available on the success rates specifically for online BDSM relationships, but the phenomenon of online relationships in *general* have been studied extensively. A 2005 study of online relationships by Dr. Jeff Gavin, of the University of Bath in the U.K. revealed some fascinating data on relationships that began online and then made the transition to *real life:*

- When a couple met first online, and went on to meet in real-life, there was a 94% chance that they would meet *a second time* in real-life.
- Within that group (that met at least *twice* in real-life), 18% of the relationships lasted over one year, with the average relationship lasting seven months.
- Of the relationships that were no longer together at the end of the study, only 4%, or roughly *one in twenty-five*, had lasted two years or more.

- Surprisingly, men were significantly more likely to stay committed to an online relationship than women.
- *Not* surprisingly, the more a couple engaged in online chat or telephone calls, the better they were able to understand and depend upon one another emotionally.

A study by the Oxford Internet Institute surveyed a random sample of 24,000 men and women in 2011 and found that the odds for a successful relationship that begins online were *significantly higher* for middle-aged people *(aged 40 to 69)* than they are for younger adults. This was somewhat counter-intuitive to the prevailing notion that younger people would be more likely to start a relationship online and would be *better* at it. Of the 24,000 respondents to the survey:

- 30% of the respondents had tried online dating or online relationships.
- 15% had met their current partners online.
- Of the middle-aged group *(age 40-69)* 36% had met their current partner online.
- Of the younger adults *(age 18-39)* only 23% had met their current partners online.

Finally, a 2010 study entitled "Strategic Misrepresentation in Online Dating" by Jeffrey A. Hall and others examined and attempted to validate the online profiles of over 5,000 people who were registered on online dating sites. They found that among that group of people, people who were required to post *actual* photographs of themselves and allegedly had *every intention* of taking their new relationships real-life, the percentage of profiles containing *"strategic misrepresentations of the truth"* (otherwise known as *bald-faced lies*) was an *astonishing* 81%. The inevitable question that naturally comes to mind as a result of a study like this is a frightening one: If 81% of *those* people are *lying* on their online profiles, imagine what the percentage must be for individuals who *do not* have to post a photograph, and have *no intention whatsoever* of ever meeting you in real life. It's a scary thought, *indeed.*

If we assume that online BDSM relationships are, *by their very nature*, more difficult and significantly more likely to fail than a typical *vanilla* online relationship, then we're left with some pretty depressing prospects. Just in case you weren't taking notes, let's recap:

- The percentage of *vanilla* online dating profiles with a significant number of *lies* in them was 81%. This suggests that the number for *anonymous* BDSM *chat room* profiles is likely even *higher*.
- Just 4% of *vanilla* relationships that start online last two years or more, which suggests that for BDSM relationships, that number is probably closer to 2%.
- If you are age 40-69, you are 56% *more likely* to be in that *semi-successful* 2% .

Depressed yet? If you *aren't*, you haven't been paying attention. If these statistics and our estimates are accurate, then the odds of your online BDSM relationship lasting over two years are roughly *50 to 1*. On the *bright side*, your odds of being killed by lightning are encouraging, at 2.3 million to 1. This brings us back to the question we posed earlier, which is: What kinds of things should be allowed to leak from one world to the other, and where should we draw the line? If your online BDSM relationship has a very high probability of *failing* in the not-too-distant future (and it *does*) then it may not be wise to hand that person the potential ability to wreak havoc in your real-life circumstances, relationships or career.

You may *think* you're giving away meaningless snippets of personal information that can't be assembled into anything that can be used against you once the relationship sours, but *think again*. One online submissive thought she was being clever and careful by giving her online Master just her *first name* and the state she lived in. She didn't realize that a simple public records database search would reveal that there were just three people in the *entire state* with the same unique first name, and *two* of them were over *seventy years old*. After their angry break-up, her spiteful former online Master needed just five minutes to find her full name, home phone number, and her home address, where she lived with her unsuspecting vanilla husband and three elementary school-aged children. What followed was a month of harassing phone calls and even a clumsy *blackmail attempt*, which finally led the beleaguered couple to seek a restraining order.

There are *lots* of different ways that your expectations of anonymity can be *demolished* in a heartbeat. If you're one of those people who has nothing to lose, or you simply aren't worried about keeping your virtual life separate from your real one, then that may not be a problem. On the other hand, if you're the sort of person who likes to keep your former *virtual* lovers away from your *real-life* front door, the following tips can save you a *lot* of future headaches.

- If you give someone your phone number, a reverse telephone number search may reveal your real name, address, and even the names of the other people living at that address *with you*, including possibly your *children*. That information isn't always available for free, but you should never assume that a determined individual wouldn't be willing to spend the required $3 to purchase the information.
- If you send someone your photograph, a reverse photo search can be done on websites like Google or Tineye. These reverse photo searches could lead someone to your Facebook, Twitter, Myspace, Tumblr, or other social media websites that contain sensitive personal information about you. It can sometimes even send a snoop directly to your *employer's website* if your photo appears anywhere on the website.
- Practically every photograph contains embedded, hidden *meta* information called EXIF data. Using an EXIF data reader can reveal this information. EXIF data can include not only information about the camera used to take the photo, but sometimes, even the exact *latitude and longitude* where the photo was taken. In other words, if the photo was taken at your home, you may have just unknowingly handed someone your *home address*.
- Giving someone your *email* address may seem like a *perfectly safe thing to do*, until you realize that *Googling* an email address can reveal a wealth of information about you that you never even knew

existed. Think of all the times you've been asked to leave your name and email address in order to purchase something, leave a comment, post on social media, generate forum messages, ask questions online, or submit technical support trouble tickets. Eventually, a determined snoop will find *something* that has *both* your email address *and* your real full name on it, and the *rest is easy.*

- Every internet connection you make originates from a unique internet protocol (IP) address. Most of the websites and online applications that you use will automatically record your IP address when you connect to them. An IP address usually looks something like this: 12.345.678.910. The final few digits of your IP address may change each time you connect to the internet, but the *first* three groups of numbers *never do*. That's because they are *unique* to the servers used by your hometown Internet Service Provider (ISP), and can be readily identified by anyone who knows how. The internet has *scores* of free and easy-to-use IP tracing websites and utilities.

The bottom line is: *You are never as anonymous online as you think you are*. My intent in telling you this is *not* to frighten you to the extent that you are tempted to avoid *any involvement at all* in internet relationships or the online BDSM culture. No, *not at all.* My intent is to encourage you to go into it with *open eyes*. I want you to know how to take proper precautions when you *can*, and to understand the possible consequences when you can't, or *choose not to.*

The Reality Behind the Avatars

We've discussed the *virtual line* that many people use to keep their virtual world and their real lives from spilling over into each other's domain, and the many good reasons for establishing those limits. The existence of that line *shouldn't,* however, prevent anyone from acknowledging and appreciating the fact that there are *real people* behind those engaging little cartoon characters we call *avatars*. There's absolutely nothing wrong with expressing your wildest fantasies in an online virtual world, as long as you don't forget that *other people are doing precisely the same thing*.

Unfortunately, it is maddeningly common for some people to *completely reinvent themselves* online while simultaneously *expecting everyone* else to be *scrupulously honest* about their age, gender, body type, relationship status, location, finances, and other kinds of personal information. Not only is this sort of rampant deception generally the rule rather than the exception, but there are many who seem to be completely oblivious to the inherent improbability of establishing a meaningful relationship based on their *bogus online personas*. Ironically, there are people who spend months, *even years*, carefully crafting a phony online persona and searching online for that special someone who is *real,* only to discover after finding that person that he or she was looking for someone real, *too*. Whoops.

Let me reiterate the point I'm trying to make, here. I am *not* advocating that you should make your online avatar a virtual mirror image of your real-world self in every way. After all, *most* people are drawn to online virtual worlds primarily for entertainment and for the exploration of their fantasies. Making our virtual world and our virtual selves look and act exactly like our real selves would seem to be a sure way to suck all the fun out of what would otherwise be an amusing activity. What I *am* saying is this: If you're using a virtual world environment to search for a *real-life partner*, your probability of success will be *directly proportional* to the amount of reality that *you inject into your own profile and behavior.*

It won't do you any good if someone falls in love with an artificial construct that *isn't anything like you*.

Where Is It Going?

Major League Baseball manager Yogi Berra once said, "If you don't know where you're going... you might not get there." This is never truer than when it comes to online BDSM relationships. It's incredibly easy to find yourself entangled in an online relationship before you even realize what has transpired. If you find yourself waking up or going to sleep with thoughts of your online paramour, spending time online simply in the hope of seeing that person log on, or putting real life responsibilities off to spend time chatting with that person, it's time to face the awful truth: Surprise! *You're in an online relationship.*

The question you *should* ask yourself is: Is this a relationship that is destined to go anywhere I want to be? It helps, of course, to have some idea where you want to eventually end up; the operative word being *eventually*. You may not be able to make certain changes in your life *right now*, but choosing any path that leads in a direction that doesn't move you *closer* to your goals would be counter-productive, at best.

It's been said that men often marry expecting that their spouses will never change, but women marry expecting that their spouses *will.* Both strategies are completely unrealistic, but they handily demonstrate the prevalence of denial and self-delusion that is common at the start of many relationships. If you think online relationships are particularly susceptible, you're right. And online *BDSM relationships* are *doubly so.* As we mentioned earlier in this chapter, the odds of your online BDSM relationship lasting two years or more are roughly *1 in 50.* For the math-challenged, those are *not* great odds.

Improving the Odds

How can you improve those odds? The first step is to take a long hard look at yourself and to conduct a critical self-assessment. If you don't know yourself, and are not comfortable in your own skin, you can't possibly expect anyone else to be able to get to know you, either. If you don't know what you want, or what you need in a mate, chances are you're not going to find it. If you can't differentiate between what is good for you and what isn't, you'll probably end up with a lot of the latter, and less of the former. This self-assessment isn't always easy to do on your own. You may need to enlist the help of a trusted friend or associate, or perhaps even a trained counselor or therapist to help you to see yourself more objectively.

It's often easy to convince ourselves that we've simply been the victim of "bad luck" when it came to our past relationships, but more often than not, the seeds of those failures can be traced to misperceptions or misconceptions which, in turn, produced a series of *bad decisions*. If insanity can be defined as doing the same thing over and over while expecting different results, then when it comes to *failed relationships*, we all may be just a little insane.

Once you've done your critical self-assessment, you should take inventory of your needs and wants, being careful to differentiate between the two. Then go back down those lists, item by item, and rate your own willingness or ability to compromise on each. It might be useful to use a numeric scale ranging from one to five. A *one* means that you're a *complete pushover* when it comes to this issue; if your heels were any rounder, you'd probably just keep rolling. A *five* indicates that you have *no willingness compromise, whatsoever:* "Stubbornness is your *superpower* - you were bitten by a radioactive mule." *(Hat tip to author Shannon Hale. I just love this description.)*

The next step is where things get a little more complicated. Attempt to do the very same thing for your potential partner. While it would certainly be helpful at this point if you were a *mind-reader*, chances are pretty good that you aren't. Therefore, the next best strategy is to simply *ask* your potential love-interest. There are lots of different ways you can phrase these questions, but the easiest is typically something like, "Wow! So, you're into foot-worship! Have all your past lovers been into that, as well? Or is this something you are able to compromise on?" When you phrase it that *way*, it just sounds more like rapt fascination and less like a *job interview.*

Once you are able to compare these two lists, noting your abilities to compromise on key relationship issues, it becomes relatively easy to know if the two of you are traveling along *intersecting paths*, or moving in *opposite directions*. If it appears that the two of you are moving in opposite directions, it doesn't mean your potential mate is a *bad person.* It simply means that your time would be better spent talking to someone with whom you actually have a *sliver of a chance* of success at a lasting relationship. Focus your time and energy where it has the greatest potential for success.

Warning Signs

If you are *already* in an online relationship, and you're beginning to wonder if it's a good place to *stay,* then I would recommend learning to spot the early warning signs of an impending train wreck. It's always frustrating to look back *after the fact* and realize that the danger signs were always *right there in front of us,* frantically waving big yellow flags but, at the time, we were completely oblivious to them. Chances are actually pretty good that you'll ignore them the next time around, as well - *even after reading this* - but at least *now*, you can't say you weren't warned. As always, my use of the masculine pronoun *"he"* is *not* intended to suggest that any of these characteristics apply solely to the male gender. It's simply a grammatical convenience. If the shoe fits - *male or female* - drop the romance and *back away slowly.*

Here are some of the yellow flags you might want to be on the lookout for:

He continues to be overly secretive about his *real name*, even after you've been in a committed relationship for months. No one should be giving out their real full name to *strangers* over the internet, but once you're *officially a couple* and you're allegedly making plans for a lifetime together, it's a pretty safe bet that the need for name secrecy has passed. While there may actually be legitimate reasons for a certain level of caution, he should be able to articulate those reasons to you, and they should *make sense.* Don't let him get away with, *"I'm a secret agent. If I tell you, I'll have to kill you."* After all, intelligence agencies go to a great deal of time and trouble to create believable *cover identities* for their agents, just so they'll be able to give you a plausible name and occupation. Don't let your tax dollars go to waste!

His profile photo has a *copyright* mark on it. The same goes for a trademark, corporate logo, or website address. You'd think this would be a *huge* yellow flag that would be pretty hard to ignore, but you would be absolutely *amazed* at how many people find nothing unusual about it. Let me just spell it out for those who don't understand why this is weird. *Normal people usually don't copyright or trademark their personal photos.* The presence of that little symbol, or logo, or URL on the photo *usually* indicates that the photo was simply *right-click stolen* off of a random website.

His photo is posted to a photographs-only site like Flickr.com, but *not* anywhere else. Why should this be a yellow flag? Simple. Because, as a general rule, people discover the utility of certain internet sites in a *certain sequence*, starting with the simpler ones and graduating over time to the more complex. It's relatively *rare* for anyone to *start out* with complex photo sharing site without having *first* tried out more user-friendly social media sites, such as Facebook or Tumblr. In other words, someone with a Flickr photo-sharing account *almost certainly* has a Facebook or similar account. So, why might someone want to conceal his Facebook page from someone with whom he is in a committed relationship?

He doesn't have a phone. *Really?* We live in an age where *elementary schools* have to establish rules forbidding *8-year-olds* from taking their cell phones to school, but *he* doesn't have a phone. Your friendly neighborhood Wal~Mart sells pre-paid cellular phones for $10, but *he* doesn't have a phone. It's far, far more likely that he *does* have a phone; he simply doesn't want to give *you* his number. You probably won't even need to use up all three of your guesses to figure out *why not.*

He's only online very, very late at night, and into the wee hours. Translation: He has to wait until his wife is asleep. Award yourself extra points if he has to log off unexpectedly and without warning for no apparent reason, or because *"something came up"* at 3 AM. I don't know about *you*, but there's not a whole lot going on in *my* life at 3 AM.

Here's what that abrupt late-night log-off *really* means: *"Whoops. Accidentally woke up my wife."*

He isn't involved in any significant way with real-life local BDSM groups or activities. And *what a surprise,* he doesn't want *you* to get involved in any, either! Typically, he will justify this restriction by characterizing everyone in these groups as jerks and phonies, and claiming that he simply doesn't want them to teach you any bad habits or take advantage of you. Translation: "I have no idea what I'm doing, and if you start hanging out with people *who do*, you might figure that out. If *anyone* is going to take advantage of you, *it should be me."*

He has long spells - some lasting weeks or longer - where he simply seems to drop off the face of the earth. There's never any warning before it happens, and *nothing at all* during the dry-spell. No phone calls, text messages, nor even an email. When he returns, the explanation strains credulity. It's usually something like his laptop stopped working, or his grandmother died. The explanation makes very little sense, since *most* people these days have multiple ways to stay connected, including their telephones or friends with phones or computers. Even if he claims to be completely *phoneless and friendless,* there are *always* computers with free internet available for use at the public library. As for granny's untimely death, she's been dead for *three weeks now.* He couldn't find *thirty seconds* in his busy schedule to send you a message saying, "Grandma kicked the bucket?" *Please.*

It's *far* more likely that his absence was caused by one of two scenarios. The first is he is a cheater who got busted by his spouse and had to *lay low* for several weeks, until she let her guard down again. The second is he simply didn't want to be involved with you anymore, but didn't have the balls to *tell* you so. If this second scenario turns out to be the right one, you shouldn't be surprised if you learn that he's been *online the whole time*, but on a different account or under a different screen name.

His remarks about the time, local news events or the weather don't match up well with *reality.* There are lots of things people can be *expected* to be inconsistent about, but *the time* is rarely one of them. For most people, meals, work shifts, and sleep generally occur at fairly regular and predictable times and intervals. You can fool your body (and even your gullible online friends) for short periods of time, but eventually it all catches up with you. Anyone who claims to be in a time zone that differs from yours by six or more hours, and yet is *miraculously* able to keep exactly the same hours that you do, day after day, for weeks or months at a time without any ill effects, is most likely being deceptive about his actual location.

Local culture, customs and news is another easy way for deceptive people to get tripped up. It's one thing to *claim* to live in London, but it's another thing *entirely* to have any idea of what is actually *going on* in London. While chatting online, it's very common for people to talk about what is happening *where they actually live,* rather than what's happening in their *fictional community.* They tend to forget that you have access to the news too, and can actually check out their stories. They also sometimes assume that everyone is as ill-informed about the rest of the world as *they* are, which makes sniffing out their cultural blunders all the easier. A Londoner who isn't familiar with *"bangers and mash"* probably *isn't a Londoner at all.*

Don't forget to talk about the weather. Deceivers typically forget that *anyone* can pull up a national weather map in order to see what's happening in their supposed neighborhood. If someone tells you about a massive storm front pummeling his area, but the national weather maps show nothing but *sunny skies* where he *allegedly* lives, something's not right.

If a story doesn't seem to make a whole lot of sense, it's not just because the storyteller is odd or eccentric; it's usually because the storyteller hasn't sufficiently thought things through. An online friend once told me that she had been *shot in the arm during an attempted armed robbery* while working at a bar the previous night. Several hours later, she was talking about *going back to work that very evening.* I don't care *how* tough you are, or how superficial your gunshot wound might be - nobody goes right back to work the next day after being shot. *Nobody.*

Another online friend, who allegedly lived half a world away, mentioned in one of our conversations that she was downing a few shots of tequila as we chatted. A quick glance at my world-clock told me that it was 7:00 AM on a weekday where she was *supposed* to be. Considering the fact that she supposedly had a twelve-year-old daughter that she drove to school daily and a job where she allegedly worked *banker's hours*, it's not hard to see how the entire flimsy concoction immediately began to fall apart under its own weight.

There are no silver bullets that will work in every situation, every single time. The important thing is to *pay attention to the little things*. When something doesn't make sense, there's usually a *very good reason*. Take note of the inconsistencies. One or two may turn out to be nothing at all, *but dozens?*

A person who is telling the *truth* doesn't have to have a good memory, but a *liar* has to have an *exceptional* one, and most liars *don't*.

The Rewards

You might think, after wading through all of the *negatives* that we've discussed thus far, that online BDSM relationships are not worth the effort, but that isn't *at all* the conclusion you should take away from this chapter. Some of the most fulfilling and lasting D/s relationships I've ever been in began in one fashion or another in an online environment. There really *are* a lot of positive aspects to seeking or exploring a relationship online.

Ironically, one of those positive aspects is the paradox that allows people to *be themselves* behind a cloak of relative anonymity. It's been proven time and again in psychological studies that people will typically reveal *more* of their inner thoughts and feelings when they believe they are anonymous. Most of us are taught from an early age to stifle or conceal our sexual urges, kinks, and fetishes. Under the banner of *equality*, we are indoctrinated for most of our lives to reject the notion that some people *born leaders* and others *born followers*, or that there may actually be real and significant *differences* between men and women. In their quest to eliminate *real abuse*, many in our society *stigmatize* those who may find pleasure in pain, enjoy corporal discipline, or find fulfillment in giving themselves fully and *without reservation* to the person they love. Is it any wonder that many people have difficulty finding an outlet for exploring and expressing such things? The online environment allows them to do just that.

Anyone who has ever been involved in an online relationship can tell you that not only can it be a very *freeing* experience, but it can also be a very *deep* one. The medium forces you to focus on what is in your heads and hearts rather than on things like appearances, age, physical characteristics, sex appeal, or social and financial status. For many people, it will be the first time in their lives that someone is willing to overlook those *superficialities* to see through to their souls, and *that* can be quite *intoxicating.*

Another positive aspect of exploring an online BDSM relationship is its relative *safety.* Obviously, you're not going to get physically injured or contract a sexually transmitted disease from a *chat room.* That safety feature begins evaporate, however, the closer you get to actually meeting for the first time. In *Chapter 8: The First Meeting* we'll go over some of the steps you can take to preserve that safety advantage.

The safety advantage of online BDSM relationships goes far beyond the obvious fact that you can't get physically injured by online role-play. It also forces us to do something that most of us don't really do very often. It makes us *think through all of the little steps that are part of a process.* It's incredibly easy for most of us to *fantasize* about doing something without ever really considering the steps which must be taken to accomplish it. *Nothing* is ever as easy as we think it is! It may be *one* thing to *say,* "I'd love to tie you to a chair and make love to you!"

and another thing *entirely* to accomplish such a thing. Even if you're just *role-playing* out the scenario in an erotic online chat, you're forced to step through the process in your mind until you realize that making love to someone whose butt is firmly planted in a chair might actually be *harder than you thought.*

Time is another real advantage of an online BDSM relationship. *Time is your friend.* Time has a way of working *real magic* when it comes to separating the wheat from the chaff. The faster you move from the first online *hello* to a committed *real-life* relationship, the greater the probability that it will end in an epic *train wreck.* Sure, there are always *exceptions* to this rule (which I am sorely tempted to call *Makai's Law),* but the laws of probability are immutable and unyielding. You should view any online relationship as an opportunity to *really* get to know one another at the deepest levels *before* you start sharing the rent. If it is a relationship that is truly meant to be, then the time you spend doing so will be a *wise investment.*

Some of the most rewarding relationships I've ever been in began online and eventually transitioned successfully to real-life, committed relationships. Is it my preferred way to begin a relationship? No, it is not. But, then again, you don't always get to choose *how, when, and with whom* you fall in love. *Love chooses you*, and it has an annoying habit of doing so in agonizingly unpredictable ways.

The keys to succeeding in any online BDSM relationship are to go into it with open eyes, be aware of the many possible risks and rewards, to have a plan, and to keep your expectations realistic.

# # #

My Two Cents on Online BDSM Relationships

Roxy, a young submissive who was new to the online BDSM lifestyle and had no real experience whatsoever with the *real-world* one, seemed preoccupied and pensive as her avatar kneeled stoically on a pillow in a quiet corner of the BDSM chat room. She was usually a cheerful girl with a bubbly demeanor but *today*, she was anything *but*. Something was *obviously* very wrong.

"How's your trial with your new Master going?" I asked. She'd met Drago in this very room, just one week earlier, and had agreed to a trial with him after only a few minutes of conversation. At the time, I'd considered it a rather rash and unwise decision, but it really wasn't my place to say so. Roxy was silent for a moment, and then hesitatingly replied, *"Meh.* I told him to *go fuck himself."*

I nodded silently in response, *not* giving voice to the first thought that had popped into my head, which was: *Not entirely unexpected.* Instead, I diplomatically said, "I'm sorry to hear that. I'm guessing the trial is off, then?" She gave a little nod and replied, *"I guess so."* A moment passed, and she tentatively added, "Umm... He *threatened* me. Do you think I should be *worried?"*

"What do you mean, *threatened you?"* I asked. "What did he *say, exactly?"*

Roxy answered, "He said he would hunt me down in real-life, and kick my ass. He said he would make me sorry that I had spoken to him like that." Long pause. "He can't really *do* that, *can he?"*

"It's *depends,"* I replied. "Which part? Hunt you down, kick your ass, or make you sorry? I'm pretty sure he could accomplish *all three.* But then again, considering how hard headed you can be, that whole *making you sorry* part may be a little harder than he *thinks."*

Clearly, she *didn't* like what she was hearing. "Are you saying that he really *could* find out where I *live?* There is *no possible way!* I have never even told him *what state I live in*. At most, he knows my first name, and that isn't even my *real* first name, it's a *nickname."*

I sighed. I have always hated the painful process of trying to convince someone that she isn't really as clever or as anonymous as she *thinks* she is. Once they're shown just how vulnerable they *really* are, some people simply log off and *never come back*. It's that much of a *shock* to them. But the alternative is to stand by and do *nothing* while they risk being hurt or even killed by some crazed *whack-job*. It had to be done. "Don't go anywhere," I said. "I'll be back in five minutes."

When I returned a few minutes later, I showed her what I'd found: Her full legal name. Her home address and telephone numbers, both her landline *and* her cell phone. Her email address, Facebook, Pinterest *and* Tumblr accounts. Vacation pictures and names of her and all of her family members. And I found it all in less than five minutes. How? Simple, really. The trick is to find a single thread and pull on it until the entire illusion of anonymity unravels.

In her particular case, a simple reverse search of a photograph associated with her account led me to her social media accounts like Facebook and Tumblr. *Those* sites gave me her email address and the name of her home town. From there, it was easy to get her real name, home address, and telephone numbers.

Predictably, Roxy was *not at all amused.*

"The difference between involvement and commitment is like ham and eggs. The chicken is involved; the pig is committed."

- - Martina Navratilova

CHAPTER 6: THE COLLAR

What is a collar?

Ask the average person on the street, and he'll tell you that a collar is something that the owners of cats and dogs put around their necks of their pets; they're usually made of leather and have D-rings which make it easier to attach a leash and any dog-tags which might help to identify the pet in the event it becomes lost. Ask someone in the D/s or BDSM lifestyle for *their* definition of a collar, and you're likely to get a completely different answer. In fact you'll probably get *a lot* of completely different answers, because even *within* the lifestyle, there are divergent opinions on the significance and meaning of collars.

It might be overly simplistic to put forth the idea that the common denominator that binds all of those differing opinions on collars is the notion that a collar represents a commitment of some sort on the part of the wearer and the one who bestows the collar, but even *that* becomes problematic when one considers the fact that collars have become a vanilla counter-culture *fashion accessory* for many. You'll also find, even *within* the BDSM culture, that there are some who wear a collar as a fashion statement, socio-political statement, or purely for utilitarian *play purposes*. Obviously, there isn't a *one-size-fits-all* definition that could put any raging collar controversies to rest, but we *can* focus on some of the most common characteristics, types, and assumptions about collars in the BDSM culture.

Symbolism of the Collar

To *most* of the people in the BDSM lifestyle who assign meaning to a collar, it is symbolic of *ownership* and represents a *mutual commitment*. It is usually the *degree* of ownership and/or commitment that typically becomes a point of contention in BDSM relationships. For some, particularly in the *online* BDSM community, a collar may be nothing more than a *role-play accessory* which has no more significance than an imaginary sword used in *World of Warcraft.* For others who may be living the lifestyle full-time in a *real world* setting, a collar could represent something that – in terms of importance and level of commitment - surpasses even *marriage*.

Since collars are entirely *symbolic* in nature to the people in this lifestyle, it is *extremely important* that anyone considering entering into a relationship that involves a collar, or even the *possibility* of a collar in the future, have a frank discussion with his or her partner about *exactly* what that collar symbolizes for everyone concerned. Imagine the potential problems which are bound to occur in any relationship where a Dominant believes the collar symbolizes *absolute ownership* requiring unquestioning obedience from the wearer, while the submissive simply thinks of it as a coveted status symbol or fashion accessory. Unfortunately, this sort of thing happens *all the time*.

The actual, physical collars that are used by those in BDSM relationships, if they are used *at all*, may consist of literally *anything* that is worn around the submissive's neck. For most people, the *stereotypical* collar generally conjures images of a black leather pet-style collar with a buckle and D-rings; perhaps even decorated with adornments such as rhinestones or metal studs. But in *reality*, a collar is just as likely to be a fashionable choker or ribbon, or even a conventional looking gold or silver chain with a pendant. The bottom line is a collar may be anything that the individuals in a relationship mutually agree upon. This applies equally to the rules governing the wear of the collar. For some, a collar is something that should never be removed, under any circumstances. For others, the collar is worn only in the bedroom or at BDSM group functions. It is generally a good idea to ensure that any rules specifying what is or isn't appropriate, when it comes to when, where and how the collar is worn in your relationship, be established *before* the collar is padlocked around your neck.

As long as we're discussing *physical* collars here, we should take the opportunity to discuss something that is, for many, the bewildering and often frustrating phenomenon of *online collars.* An online collar, for our purposes, is defined as a collar that represents the relationship between two people who have *never actually met in real life.* This would also include solid, three-dimensional collars that are sent by Dominants to submissives whom they have never actually met, in reality. At the risk of engaging in a generalization that will probably anger and offend some readers, here's what I think of online collars: They are just like *real-life* collars, except *less so*. By that, I mean that they are less *real* and less *significant* in practically *every possible aspect*, save one – the *emotions* associated with it. The emotions associated with an online collar can be very real and very strong, however, almost by definition, the *commitment* is not yet strong enough to merit *meeting in real life*. Do online collared relationships *ever* successfully make the difficult transition to real life? Of *course* they do. Unfortunately, the odds of it happening are *extremely* low.

Types of Collars

A collar represents, for the individuals involved, *whatever they agree that it represents.* In other words, no one should attempt to define the symbolism, meaning or significance of another person's collar. It would be very much like trying to tell a *married person* what her wedding ring is supposed to symbolize. Each collar means something different to the person wearing it. Even so, there are several *generic classifications* of collars which you may encounter that typically have the same meaning to just about everyone in the BDSM lifestyle. In other words, if you want your collar to mean *something else entirely*, it's probably not a good idea to use one of the following names for it:

Velcro Collar

Velcro collars *don't really exist*, at least not in the sense that the term is generally used in the BDSM community. It's a derogatory term used by people in the lifestyle who take their collars very seriously to describe the practice of collaring *indiscriminately and often*, without regard to whether or not there is any real relationship at its core. The rapid growth of BDSM related internet chat rooms, games, and instant messaging programs have contributed to an online environment where casual and often anonymous experimentation occurs with few significant or lingering consequences. As a result, it is not at all unusual to see brand new, curious or naïve self-proclaimed Dominants collaring several new submissives *each day*. The commitment associated with accepting such a collar is typically limited to a one-night-stand of *cybersex*, after which the status of the *pseudo-relationship* is dubious, at best.

One of the things that make so-called Velcro collars a common phenomenon, at least in the *online* BDSM community, is the unfortunate tendency on the part of new submissives to believe that they must find a Master *immediately*, and *at all costs.* This is not only *foolish*, but can be extremely *dangerous*, especially for brand new, naïve submissives who haven't yet learned how to protect themselves from the predators and abusers who are sometimes drawn to the lifestyle like moths to a flame. It's reminiscent of the old Steve Martin joke about how to be a millionaire. *("First, get a million dollars.")* Similarly, there are many curious people exploring the lifestyle right now who believe that the key to becoming a submissive is, *"First, get a Master."* The truly unfortunate thing about it is, it's *not a joke.*

Play Collar

A play collar is any collar that is worn primarily for *utilitarian purposes* during a BDSM *play* session. Typically, play collars are constructed of leather or metal, but they can literally be made of any material that is appropriate for the type of play that is going to take place. The most common type of play collar used in *bondage* scenes are constructed of durable leather and heavy-duty steel D-rings which facilitate the attachment of chains, straps, rope, or other restraints to the collar. Other types of play collars may include *posture collars, neck corsets, steel lockable collars, rubber or PVC collars, medical (cervical) collars, ball gag collars, bit gag collars, or hooded collars*. For obvious reasons, play collars are *not* common in the *online* BDSM culture.

Collar of Consideration

A collar of consideration is a *provisional* collar that is offered by a Dominant to a submissive that he is considering as a potential submissive who will presumably become eligible for a collar of greater significance and commitment at the end of the probationary period. It is typically used to give some recognition to the process of getting to know each other by formalizing a *tentative* commitment by a submissive to discontinue shopping for a Dominant while being considered by this one, and by the Dominant to treat her *as his own* for the duration of the agreement. The terms of this tentative agreement should be negotiated *prior* to the collaring, and are typically set to expire after a relatively short period of time. This is designed to prevent a submissive from being strung-along by an indecisive Dominant for an indefinite period of time. If, at any time during the agreed-upon consideration period, either party decides that a more serious relationship is not worth pursuing further, that party is permitted to unilaterally withdraw from the agreement without fault or blame. Collars of consideration are far more common in the *online* BDSM culture than they are in *real-life.* There are many reasons for this, including the inherent difficulty of getting to know someone in a purely online environment, the added complications related to *role-playing,* and an overabundance of the merely curious and clueless.

Collar of Protection

A collar of protection is similar in many ways to a collar of consideration, and in fact, there are usually a lot of areas of overlapping functionality. Most collars of consideration are *also* collars of protection; however, *not all* collars of protection are collars of consideration. The reason for this is simple. Sometimes, a Dominant will extend his *protection* to a submissive out of friendship or charity, even though *neither person* has any intention whatsoever of establishing a more serious relationship with the other as a consequence. The actual nature of the so-called *protection* offered to the submissive in these circumstances can vary widely from person to person. As a general rule, it includes offering advice and guidance, approving play partners and events, and interviewing and/or approving prospective Dominants who may wish to consider the submissive. A typical recipient of a collar of protection is a submissive who is brand new to the lifestyle, or perhaps one who has recently been *released* by her Dominant. One of the most useful aspects of a collar of protection is simply the way it serves notice to other Dominants that *this* submissive is *being looked after* by someone who is experienced in the lifestyle and has her best interests at heart.

Training Collar

A training collar is, for *many* submissives, the logical second step that follows a short period of consideration and decision to move forward into a more serious and committed relationship. It serves as recognition that, while a more intense and formal relationship is *desired* by both parties, there is still much to be learned by the submissive before a formal collar can be offered. Previously, if the submissive wore a collar of consideration or a collar of protection, her actions would not reflect upon the Dominant in any significant way. Now, however, every action by a submissive in a training collar reflects *directly* upon the Dominant, telegraphing to everyone his competence - *or lack thereof* – as a trainer of submissives. This can also be a period of great stress and contention as the Dominant and submissive adjust to their new roles in the relationship, and learn to reconcile their expectations and preconceptions with reality. Even those who have a great deal of experience in D/s and BDSM relationships will have a lot of adjusting to do, since no two D/s relationship dynamics are the same, and each individual has his or her own quirks, limitations, and unique character traits.

The training phase is also where a Dominant and his submissive should work out the details of how they will handle *conflict*, what the *rules and protocols* that are unique to this relationship will be, how *discipline* will be applied when and if it becomes necessary, and what levels of *trust* must be achieved before the relationship can proceed on to the next level. Some of the other challenges which usually must be overcome by a submissive in training include learning how to properly process *fear, doubt and distrust, rendering proper respect, avoiding excessive argumentation, and utilizing tact.*

Training collars are rarely assigned specific *term limits*, since the idea is to accomplish specific *training goals* during this phase. If those goals haven't been met, the training theoretically continues *until they are*. It is therefore important to negotiate, from the very start, *exactly* what those goals should be, and what happens if they aren't achieved.

Formal Collar

A formal collar may be known by a host of other names, including slave collar, full collar, or true collar. If one were to consider a collar of consideration to be analogous to a vanilla *friendship ring*, and a training collar comparable to an *engagement ring*, then the formal collar is the BDSM version of a *wedding ring.* It is symbolic of what is usually *intended* to be a lifelong committed and loving relationship between a Dominant and his submissive. Formal collaring ceremonies, similar to weddings, are often performed to commemorate and consecrate the beginning of the relationship. Collaring ceremonies typically include an exchange of vows, spiritual messages, and/or uplifting music, just as one might expect to see at a vanilla wedding ceremony. Some couples go so far as to have both a collaring *and* a wedding simultaneously, combining the two events into one. The symbolism of a formal collar obviously means different things to different couples, but it is often referred to as the ultimate gift of one's submission and self to another; a manifestation of complete and total *power exchange.* Whatever form the relationship dynamic takes, it represents the highest level of commitment, love, respect, trust and devotion possible between two people.

House Collar

A house collar is essentially a *temporary collar of protection* that is offered to a submissive by a house, clan, family, organization, dungeon, or club for the express purpose of identifying the sub as someone who is being looked after by the *group or establishment*, and should not be aggressively courted without the establishment's approval. House collars are often used as an effective way to offer a measure of security to unattached women, who are sometimes seen as *vulnerable* in BDSM environments that typically favor *couples* and/or aggressive Dominants.

Everyday Collar

An *everyday collar* is anything that can be worn in a vanilla environment to symbolize your D/s relationship. For many D/s couples, their everyday collar consists of a simple choker or traditional-looking necklace, with or without a pendant. An everyday collar need not necessarily even be worn around the neck; some people substitute a ring, bracelet, ankle bracelet, or tattoo. The important thing is that, at least in the minds of the D/s couple in question, the item designated as the *everyday collar* is firmly associated with and symbolic of their relationship.

I'm often asked whether a collared submissive must wear a physical collar of some type to symbolize her commitment to her Dominant. The answer, of course, is *"it depends."* It depends on her Dominant, and her own personal preferences. It's very much like asking, "Does a married woman have to wear a wedding ring?" There are a lot of people who would reply, *"Absolutely!"* And yet, there are also those who'll say just the opposite. A recent survey conducted by a wedding industry media group found that 28% of women said they would *turn down a wedding proposal* if they didn't like the ring! That says a lot about the importance - *to some* – of the actual ring that symbolizes their union. There are no statistics available on how many submissives would turn down a *collaring proposal* if they didn't like the *collar.*

Let's reiterate what we said about the symbolism of a collar at the beginning of this section. Each *individual collar* will have its own symbolic meaning that is *unique* to the individuals in the relationship it represents. There are, however, *general categories* of collars which generally conform to the expectations and assumptions of the larger D/s and BDSM communities. If you happen to refer to *your* particular collar as a *"training collar,"* you should do so with the full awareness that the terminology you're using will imply some *very specific things* to *others* in the lifestyle. There's absolutely nothing wrong with blazing your own path as you explore and grow in the D/s lifestyle, but it can be *considerably easier* if we're all at least speaking the *same language.*

Slave Contracts

In this and previous chapters, we've repeatedly emphasized the need for frank discussion and negotiations between any potential partners *before* entering into a D/s relationship. When these negotiations result in any sort of *agreement,* the terms of the agreement often end up in written form, and that document is sometimes referred to in the lifestyle as a *slave contract, D/s contract, or TPE (Total Power Exchange) contract.* For the sake of simplicity, we will be using the term *slave contract* for the remainder of this chapter, but *do* keep in mind the fact that, *when we do,* we are referring to a *wide variety* of D/s lifestyle contracts. You should also be aware that the topic of slave contracts is one of the most controversial subjects you're likely to encounter in the D/s lifestyle. We'll discuss the reasons for the controversy shortly. The predictable result of the controversy is a confusing hodge-podge of opinions – some authoritative, *others not so much* - on the utility and value of slave contracts.

Before we wade too deeply into the various types of slave contracts that you are likely to encounter in the lifestyle, we should first clarify a few things about *contracts in general.* There are a lot of misconceptions about contracts and *contract law* will certainly complicate any attempt to apply those concepts to the arcane realm of *slave contracts.* Let's begin by discussing some of the legal requirements that must be met for *any* contract to be valid and enforceable. They are:

- Competency. Both parties must be *legally competent* to enter into a contract. That means they must be over the age of 18, may not be mentally incompetent, and they cannot be intoxicated or impaired.
- Mutual Agreement. Both parties must agree to *all* terms of the contract. If either party disagrees with *any* portion of the agreement without the mutual disagreement of the other party, the *entire contract* is void.
- A Legal Objective. A contract may not require the performance of an illegal act, nor have as its objective, an illegal act. Additionally, a person cannot enter into any contract concerning a right that they do not have.

- Consideration. Consideration is a legal term which refers to *something of value* that is exchanged as a condition of the contract. In most cases, the consideration involves *money* or merchandise. Love, affection, loyalty, and gifts do not legally qualify as consideration.
- Mutuality of Obligation. A valid contract mutually obligates both parties to *something.* If there is an absolute right to cancel by any of the parties, the contract is unenforceable and not legally binding.
- In Writing. *Verbal* contracts are legal and binding, but they are *virtually unenforceable.*

You don't have to be a practicing attorney to notice a few things that immediately leap off the page at you, particularly if you're reading it in the context of *slave contracts*. First, anyone under the age of 18 is not legally competent to enter into a contract of any kind, and yes, this includes people who *pretend to be older* in internet chat rooms. Second, all contracts must have a legal objective. In 1865, the 13th Amendment to the U.S. Constitution made slavery illegal in the United States. That makes any *slavery contract*, by definition, a contract that is not legally binding. Many slavery contracts also have provisions requiring the slave to be available to the Dominant for sex. Since the Dominant has exchanged something of value (the collar) as *consideration*, the contract *could* actually be considered a contract for *prostitution* by many states. Finally, many slave contracts contain clauses that essentially grant the right to either party to walk away from the agreement unilaterally, without penalties of any kind, which makes it a contract that is not legally enforceable.

The bottom line? Slave contracts are neither legal nor enforceable in any court of law in the United States. Now, you may well ask, isn't *marriage* a contract that often defies many, if not all, of those legal requirements? After all, people under the age of 18 marry *all the time* and, in most states, sex is a *requirement* for the consummation of the marriage. Additionally, most marriages don't have a *written contract* spelling out all of the rights and obligations of the partners, and if you ask around, you'll probably find no shortage of people who are willing to equate marriage with slavery. So, why are *slave contracts* illegal, while marriage contracts are not? Here's why: A *slave contract* is a contract solely between *two people*; a *marriage contract* is a contract between a couple *and the government.*

This subtle difference is, frankly, the same issue that is at the heart of the gay marriage debate currently raging in the American political arena. Nothing stops same-sex couples from entering into contracts that grant each partner the same legal rights and privileges that heterosexual partners are legally able to *grant one another.* In fact, a contract such as a *general power of attorney* grants more rights and privileges than any marriage does, such as the right to sign your partner's name to a contract, or to access his or her private bank accounts! The issue at the heart of same-sex marriage is *government recognition and participation* in same-sex marriages, and the couple's entitlement to the legal rights and privileges *that governments grant* as a condition of that contract. Some activists ask, *why does the government recognize and reward some types of marriages, and not others?* What are the legal or ethical arguments against *slave marriages, plural marriages, arranged marriages, corporate marriages, child marriages*, or even *inter-species marriages?* And no, simply posing the *question* should *not* be interpreted as advocacy for any of those notions, some of which are admittedly somewhat extreme. But perhaps it *would be* appropriate to ask, *why is the government involved in the business of marriage at all?*

Slave contracts are fairly common in the D/s lifestyle, though you are far more likely to encounter them in the *online* BDSM culture than you will in real-life. The reality that slave contracts are neither legal nor enforceable makes little difference in an online environment where Masters often don't even know their slave's real *name, age, or gender.* The *real* problem with most slave contracts *isn't* the fact that they're not legal; it's mostly related to the fact that even if they *were* legal, they'd *still be unenforceable.*

Take, for example, the following verbiage which has been taken directly from a slave contract that is commonly used:

> *"The parties shall conduct themselves in light of their goals at all times. The goals of the parties are detailed in Section 2(b) of this contract."*

There's a glaring problem with this sort of fuzzy language; it has no real legal definition. What, exactly, does it mean to conduct one's self *"in light"* of something? How do you measure it? At what point does one's behavior pass from being in light of a goal to *not* being in light of a goal?

> *"The parties shall treat each other with mutual respect and honesty at all times."*

That seems pretty straightforward. You're probably thinking, what could possibly be wrong with *that?* Well, for one thing, contracts are designed to spell out the *individual responsibilities* of each party. That way, when *one* person fails to meet his or her obligation, that person is in breach of the contract. If a contract specifies *mutual* obligations, as this one does, there is no way *one* person can be held responsible for a mutual obligation. The other major flaw in a line like this one is there is no definition of what constitutes *respect.* A Dominant may believe that *respect* demands that his submissive drop to her knees and genuflect whenever he enters a room; *her* idea of respect may differ somewhat from that.

> *"The parties shall never abuse each other, violate the trust of the other, play mind games or engage in emotional manipulation with one another, other than as part of play between the parties."*

Aside from the fact that there are no definitions for the terms *abuse, trust, mind games*, or *emotional manipulation*, the most conspicuous flaw in this contract verbiage is the *"other than as part of play"* clause. What this means, essentially, is that you're allowed to do anything listed previously, as long as you later claim *you were only playing.*

> *"Since the body of the slave now belongs to the Master, it is the Master's responsibility to protect that body from permanent bodily harm. Should the slave ever come to permanent bodily harm during the course of punishment or in any other slavery related activity, whether by intention or accident, it will be grounds for immediate termination of this contract, should the slave so desire. Permanent bodily harm shall be determined as: death, any damage that involves loss of mobility or function (such as broken bones), any permanent marks on the skin (such as scars, burns, or tattoos, unless accepted by the slave), any loss of hair, (unless accepted by the slave), any piercing of the flesh which leaves a permanent hole (unless accepted by the slave), any diseases (including sexually transmitted diseases).*

At least, in *this* instance, the contract writer made a half-hearted – *though highly incompetent* - attempt to define the terms being used. One of his definitions of *"permanent bodily harm"* is "*death*." Would *you* be comforted to know that in the event that your Master *intentionally or accidentally causes your death,* that you have grounds for the "immediate termination of the contract?" Somehow, *I doubt it.*

> *"The slave may not seek any other Master or lover, nor relate to others in a sexual or submissive way without the Master's permission. To do so will be considered a breach of contract, and will result in extreme punishment. The Master may accept other slaves or lovers, but must consider the slave's emotional response to such actions and act accordingly. Under no circumstance will the Master allow such actions to unbalance the slave emotionally, nor allow such actions to result in ignoring the slave."*

Not only are we left to hypothesize on the true meaning of *"relate to others in a sexual or submissive way,"* but we're also left scratching our heads over what it means to *"consider the slave's emotional response."*

The Dominant would obviously be free to say, "I *have* considered it, and am *dismissing* it as unimportant." Just to make thing fair, however, the *submissive* has a nifty little legal loophole of her *own.* No matter *what* the Master does, the submissive can always claim that his actions have *emotionally unbalanced* her, since there is no definition of *what that means.* Aren't slave contracts *fun?*

So, let's recap. Slave contracts *aren't legal*, and even if they *were*, they would be largely *unenforceable* due to fuzzy language and the general impossibility of defining such things as *love, respect, abuse, manipulation, mind games, or emotions.* Even so, slave contracts have always been around, and *always will be*. Get used to seeing them, and discussing them, and try not to laugh out loud *when you do*.

The following are a few of the different kinds of slave contracts you may find being used:

Master/slave Contract

The Master and his slave enter into an agreement which requires the slave to relinquish all personal rights, property, finances and decision making powers to the Master. Typically, the slave is required to consider her "mind, body, and soul" to be the Master's property, practice full disclosure of her thoughts and actions at all times, and give up the right to say "no" to any of the Master's directives.

Dominant/submissive Contract

The terms of a Dominant/submissive contract are typically less stringent than those of the Master/slave contract. A Dominant/submissive contract gives the submissive the ability to choose which particular aspects of their lives she'll turn over to her Dominant to control. It also often defines which parts of the relationship are real versus the parts that are role-played, and may set limits on what is, or is not, acceptable behavior for either partner. Though many submissives consider themselves *"owned"* by their Dominants, the reality is, they are submissive *partners*, not *property*.

Online Relationship Slave Contract

As we stated earlier in this chapter, slave contracts are far more common in the online BDSM culture than anywhere else, for fairly obvious reasons. An *online relationship slave contract* serves several purposes that are practically tailor-made for the internet culture. For example, when contact with your partner may be limited to just a few minutes or hours each day *or less*, it may be difficult to communicate one's expectations and assumptions to your partner in the limited time that you have. It therefore becomes useful to have a document that can be referred to and studied when your partner is not online. It serves an *educational* function. The online slave contract also gives the partners in an online relationship something that is seemingly tangible and authoritative, in an environment where practically *nothing else is.* It makes the whole thing *seem more real.* Finally, online slave contracts help to instill a sense of obligation and responsibility towards the relationship, even though the internet culture in general seems to encourage just the opposite. The lyrics of a song called *"Do You Want to Date my Avatar,"* by Felicia Day and the Guild, illustrate this tendency perfectly: *"And if you think I'm not the one, log-off! Log-off, and we'll be done!"*

The major differences between online slave contracts and real-world contracts are the provisions which make certain allowances for the fleeting nature of online relationships, the time constraints, the anonymity of participants, and the disclosure of personal information. Since many online relationships exist in *secrecy* and in *addition* to the participants' real-world relationships, the potential for wreaking havoc in each other's personal lives is almost always high. Hence, there are almost always clauses in these kinds of slave contracts which emphasize the importance of discretion and privacy.

Owner/pet Contract

An Owner/pet contract is similar in some ways to a Master/slave contract, particularly in the sense that a pet is usually considered the *property* of his owner. But it is also similar to the Dominant/submissive contract in the way it specifies which parts of a pet's life are to be considered under the jurisdiction of the Owner, and sets limits.

There is one major factor which makes all Owner/pet contracts unique, and that is the amount of attention which must be devoted to the *role-play aspects* of the Owner/pet relationship. After all, slaves like to consider themselves *real slaves*, and submissives can actually be *real submissives*, but a *ponygirl* is not a *real pony*, and no *contract* can make her one. Therefore, a great deal of verbiage must typically be devoted to accommodating those differences.

Scene Contract

A scene contract typically applies to a single event or BDSM scene, but it can also be applied to specific individuals with whom you play on a frequent basis, even though there may be no significant relationship between them. Scene contracts are usually negotiated prior to an event, and should spell out what is supposed to happen during the scene, identify hard and soft limits, list safety precautions such as safe-words, and specify whether or not sexual or body-fluid contact is permitted.

It's Your Collar, Your Commitment

In this chapter, we've discussed the various types of *commitments* that can be made by anyone who might be considering entering into a D/s relationship. We cannot stress enough the fact that *no two relationships are alike*, and any attempt to force *your* existing or potential relationship into a cookie-cutter D/s relationship mold will likely result in a great deal of heartache for everyone concerned. The *one-size-fits-all slave contracts* that litter the internet as downloadable forms generally aren't worth a damn.

This lifestyle is full of people who will try to define *your* relationship dynamic according to *their* world-view or try to make *your* collar conform to their *own* notions concerning such things. Don't buy into their delusions, and don't allow them to project either their naïve optimism *or* their gloomy cynicism onto *your* symbol, *your* collar, or *your* relationship dynamic.

Beware of those who would preach of a *"One True Way,"* as no such thing exists, *nor should it.*

# # #

My Two Cents on Collars

Ever since she was a little girl, Jade had always been fascinated with dragons. In college, she studied ancient mythology and as an adult she decorated the shelves at home with dragon figurines. A painting of a dragon hung on the wall above her bed, and a pewter dragon wrapped itself around the hilt of a large steel sword propped in a corner behind the bedroom door. Jade didn't particularly care for *tattoos*, but if she was ever going to get one, it would most assuredly depict a *dragon*.

Jade not only *loved* dragons, but she had always *identified* with them. That became less certain, however, after she experienced an odd dream. Jade always took her dreams seriously, particularly in light of the fact that the women in her family have always had a long history of prescient gifts bordering on clairvoyance, manifested mostly in visions and dreams. But this dream confused her. It had come at a turning point in her life. She and I had met and grown close while playing an online game, and we progressed over the following months to phone calls, video chats and planning a future together. As we were planning our first real-life meeting, she had this dream. Her dream was of a *phoenix*, the mythical bird of ancient Greek legend that was consumed by flame and reborn from the ashes to start life anew. She had always loved and identified with *dragons,* yet this dream seemed to imply that she was *the phoenix*, reborn out of the ashes of a former life, which had disappointed in so many ways. If that were the case, then perhaps her dream was trying to tell her that the dragon represented *her new Master*.

Interestingly enough, the symbolism of the dragon and phoenix had some significance to *me*, as well. When Jade told me of her dream, I was immediately reminded of the *Asian* depictions of these mythical creatures that I'd grown up with in Japan and Hawaii, where Asian traditions are commonplace. Asian folklore involving dragons comes primarily from China, where the dragon represents the highest-ranking animal in the Chinese hierarchy of animals. Historically, the dragon was revered the symbol of the *Chinese emperor*, while the *empress* was represented by the mythical *fenghuang*, more commonly known to westerners as the *Chinese phoenix*.

I researched the symbolism of the dragon and phoenix together. I learned that in both ancient and modern Chinese culture, the dragon and phoenix together are considered a *yin and yang* metaphor, and because they are symbolic of the blissful relations between a man and wife, they are often used as symbolic of *weddings* and *new beginnings*.

Each part of the Chinese phoenix's body was associated with a particular virtue. The head represented *virtue*, the wings represented *duty*, the back represented *propriety*, the abdomen represented *belief*, and the chest *mercy*. In both China and Japan, the phoenix exemplified the *sun, fire, justice, obedience and fidelity*. The more I learned about the symbolism of the dragon and phoenix together, the more I believed in and appreciated the power of Jade's dream. I set out to find the perfect collar for Jade, one that would not only honor her dream and her new beginnings, but would represent all of the things that we hoped for in our relationship as Master and submissive.

A few weeks later, at our first real-life meeting, I presented Jade with her new collar – a simple gold chain with a pendant comprised of a disk-shaped ring of jade with a center inlaid with an 18K gold depiction of a dragon and phoenix together. From that day forward, for the next six years, that collar was never dishonored and never left her neck until the day we were compelled to go our separate ways.

Even then, her collar did not lose its meaning or significance, and it never will.

"It is strange," he said,
"I have faced sleen and the steel of fierce enemies.
I am a warrior, and am high among warriors. Yet you,
a mere girl, would conquer me with a smile and a tear."

~ *John Norman, Slave Girl of Gor*

CHAPTER 7: THE GOREAN WAY

There are many in the D/s and BDSM lifestyles who believe that any discussion of Gor and Gorean tradition would be more appropriate to a forum related to fantasy and science-fiction than in any conversation about *relationships and sexuality*. In fact, there is no shortage of people who typically react to the merest *mention* of Gor almost *viscerally,* with much hostility and resentment. What causes them to respond so *negatively* to *anyone or anything* seemingly connected to the Gorean way? The answer lies in two little words: *the internet.*

For close to twenty years, internet chat rooms and online virtual worlds have been overrun by *millions* of *Gorean role players,* many of them *teens and young adults* seeking a fantasy role play world that would push their *sexual* limits in ways that *Dungeons & Dragons* never could. Even though the Gorean novels upon which this fandom is based had already been widely read for over twenty years, the sudden and geometric growth of *internet chat* in the 80s and 90s allowed virtually *anyone* to assume the role of a Gorean slave master *anonymously and, for the most part, unchallenged.* To muddy the waters even further, many of these role players, drunk with their very first taste of power over another human being, deliberately set out to blur the lines between their *role play* activities and *real life* by concealing their ages, experience levels, and the fact that most of them *were still in high school.* As a result, an *astonishingly* large number of curious and bored middle-aged housewives were sucked into the charade, and suddenly found themselves *slaves* to deceptive and sadistic *teenagers* who, more often than not, *had never read a single page* of any of John Norman's 32 Gor novels.

It would not be unreasonable to assume that *many* of the teenaged Gorean "Masters" *had never even had a real girlfriend* prior to becoming the proud owners of *actual women* who fancied themselves Gorean slave girls. Unfortunately, this *catastrophic combination* of rampant deceit, adolescent immaturity, inexperience in adult relationships, and even their *rank incompetence at role playing* over the past twenty years has left literally *millions of women* and the people who cared for them with an intense hatred for anything Gorean. As if that wasn't bad enough, the online Gor phenomenon demonstrated exquisitely poor timing by gaining popularity at the *peak* of the American feminist movement. Gorean notions of male dominance and the treatment of women as sex objects and property didn't earn them many friends among rank and file feminists.

The poor reputations rightfully earned by these *chat room Goreans* make it extremely difficult to present an unbiased portrait of the *actual Gorean way*, versus the *caricatures* and distortions that have shaped public opinion for so many years. It would be a little like trying to write a serious book about ghosts and spirits, using only *Halloween costumes* as your source material. Luckily, we have a way to bypass the role players and the bad publicity in order to go directly to the literary source of the Gor phenomenon, the thirty-two *"Counter-Earth"* novels by John Lange Jr., writing as *John Norman.*

John Frederick Lange Jr. was an aspiring science fiction novelist who greatly admired the works of Edgar Rice Burroughs *(b. September 1, 1875 – d. March 19, 1950).* There was, after all, a lot to admire about Burroughs, who was the celebrated author of twenty-six successful *Tarzan* novels and close to a dozen books about an earth man who becomes an unlikely hero called *John Carter of Mars.* Lange, who earned his Ph.D. in 1963 from Princeton University and currently teaches at Queens College, University of New York, is perhaps better known to millions of science fiction and fetish lifestyle fans as *John Norman*, the author of a series of pulp sci-fi novels about the planet *Gor.* Under that name, he published twenty-five *Gor* novels from 1967 through the mid-1980s, and an additional seven Gor novels in the following decades. The popularity of the *Gor* novels over the past four decades has spawned a cult-like following reminiscent of the millions of enthusiastic *"trekkies"* who are devoted to memorializing and making real, to the greatest extent possible, Gene Roddenberry's fictional *Star Trek* universe. The difference, of course, is that trekkies typically keep their *warp drives* and *sex drives* completely *separate.*

There are some of you reading this right now who would have preferred that I give anything having to do with Gor a far more cursory treatment in this book than I have. Much of that disinterest and animosity is a natural result of the events and resulting bad feelings which I have just described. Some of it is also the result of a general lack of awareness of the critical role that the Gor novels have played in the growth of the D/s movement in the past fifty years. A lot of what we take for granted in the lifestyle today got its start in John Norman's pulp fiction. Much of our lifestyle's customs, protocols, language and traditions *(such as collaring)* can trace its heritage *directly* to the Gor novels. Even so, it can be difficult to discuss this lineage and the impact it has had without encountering the lingering animosity and misinformation that plagues this particular D/s subculture.

Separating the common misperceptions and negative biases from what might be considered the *"real"* Gorean way has been an almost-insurmountable challenge in the writing of this chapter. My solution has been to rely less upon what people *think* Gor is about, and more upon what John Norman *says* it is about. For that reason, I'll be borrowing heavily from the Gor books *themselves* to illustrate the tenets, traditions, and values that are the *Gorean way.*

What is a Gorean?

Devotees of the *"Gorean"* subculture of the D/s lifestyle pattern their relationship and social dynamics, language, customs, protocols, and even their sexual activities after the manner of the people of the fictional planet *Gor*, which is sometimes referred to by the series publishers as *"Counter-Earth."* The planet, as envisioned by John Norman, is ruled by a technologically advanced insect-like race of Priest-Kings who have, over the course of eons, transported large numbers of humans from earth to populate the planet. One of those humans, a British professor named *Tarl Cabot*, is the main protagonist throughout most of the series of novels.

In the late 1960s, my father became a devoted fan of the Gor novels and as a result, he set aside for them an entire shelf of his massive library, which included books on practically every topic from Aristotle to Zombie erotica. As you might imagine, my reaction as a hormonally-charged teenager to the serendipitous discovery there of *"The Tarnsman of Gor"* and its sequels was a little like winning the *porn lottery.* While most of the other kids in my neighborhood were reading *Batman* and *Spiderman* comic books, I was perusing *"Outlaw of Gor"* and *"Slave Girl of Gor."* At about the same time, I had an incredible crush on the beautiful and talented *Barbara Eden*, star of the television series, *"I Dream of Jeanie."* I tuned in religiously each week in eager anticipation of hearing her giggle as she intoned those magical words, *"Yes, Master."* Is it any wonder that I turned out the way that I did? But, I digress.

A *Gorean* is someone who emulates the customs, culture and morality of the fictional planet Gor as it is portrayed in John Norman's novels.

Individually and collectively as a subculture, Goreans are far more prevalent *online* than in real-life. Even so, the influence and impact that they have exercised upon the D/s culture in general *cannot be understated.* It should be noted, however, that many of the overtly sexual beliefs and practices of the Gorean subculture come *not from the Gor novels at all*, but from a work of non-fiction by Lange, written in 1974 under the pseudonym *John Norman*, called *"Imaginative Sex."* We should also take a moment to acknowledge here that Lange has *never endorsed* the notion of adopting, *in any way,* the customs or ethics of the fictional planet Gor. Lange has studiously refused to sanction, recognize, participate or cooperate in any way with the popular subculture that his novels have inspired. The closest that he has come to doing so has been as a strong advocate for strengthening marriages through the use of fantasies and sexual role-play to bring about a couple's *"sexual liberation."*

As long as we're discussing some of the minor details which don't quite seem to fit the preconceived notions held by many about Gor, this is probably a good time to mention that Goreans generally consider themselves a part of the *D/s* culture, but *not* the *BDSM culture*. Their reasoning is typically based on the belief that Gor is a *philosophy* and a *way of life* that fits neatly within the D/s worldview, rather than an assemblage of activities, techniques or scenes. Most Goreans *(quite rightly, in my view)* see BDSM as *something you do*, versus D/s as being *something you are*. Even so, just as there will always be a great deal of *overlap* when it comes to BDSM and D/s, one should *also* expect to find aspects of Gor just about anywhere you look in *either* lifestyle.

What Do Goreans *Really* Believe?

If we're going to discuss what Goreans really *believe*, we must be willing to make a distinction between what is described in the Gor novels, what is actually *preached and practiced* by those in the real-world Gorean subculture, and how it is misinterpreted and caricatured by chat room role players who, more often than not, have never actually read any of the novels. As if all of that isn't *already* enough to make your head spin, we'll finish up with some real-life true stories involving the Gorean lifestyle. Good times ahead; *get in, buckle up, and hang on.*

Over the course of writing thirty-two novels about the planet Gor, Norman meticulously developed and refined his vision of Gorean culture and traditions. Considering the contemporary standards for the pulp fiction genre within which he worked, many found Norman's vision to be surprisingly consistent and cogent. This is significant when one considers the fact that contemporary Goreans attempt to emulate, as much as possible, the cultural beliefs and practices of Gorean society. According to Norman's novels, the "Three Pillars" of Gorean society are *Home Stone, Caste,* and *Natural Order.*

Home Stone. The *home stone* is representative of Gorean *sovereignty,* which can be applicable to a home, village, or city. It is typically a small stone marked with a letter or symbol, and displayed in the center of the sovereign territory it represents. It is, in some ways, analogous to the way we use *flags* as symbols of our sovereign nation-states. A practicing real-life Gorean would mostly likely adopt and apply this concept to reinforce the notion that he is the sovereign ruler of his home.

Caste. Goreans are defined primarily by their caste, which is based primarily on profession and city. There are some castes designated as *high castes* (comprised of those in governance and other elites) or *low castes* (comprised primarily of tradesmen and craftsmen). The application of this concept by real-world Goreans is generally manifested in the high esteem they typically place on a person's practical skills and warrior ethos.

Natural Order. In the Gorean culture, it is considered part of the *natural order* that males are considered to be naturally dominant, while females are considered to be inherently submissive. Even so, there are many significant *exceptions* to the rule, even on the fictional world of

Gor. The practical end result, however, is that most modern-day real-world Goreans tend to be rather dismissive of any notion of female domination, in any form.

Interestingly, despite the fact that the Gor novels are probably best known for their erotic depictions of *women in slavery*, there is a widespread misconception - *occasionally even among Goreans, themselves* - that *all* of the women of Gor are slaves. In actuality, even though the great majority of Gorean slaves *are* women, only about one woman in forty is a slave. Female slaves are individually called *kajira*, and *kajirae* in the plural. There are *male* slaves on Gor, as well, however they are far fewer in number and, unlike the women who are either bred for slavery or kidnapped from Earth, the male slaves of Gor typically become slaves as the result of war, criminality, or indebtedness. Male slaves are individually called *kajirus*, and *kajiri* in the plural. Slaves may be owned by free persons (men *or* women), entire households, or even municipalities.

The Gorean Slave

Gorean slaves are categorized in a variety of ways, such as pedigree, virginity, training and utility. In general, *barbarian* slave girls are women who have been abducted from Earth by the insect race of Priest-Kings on their voyages of acquisition. True *Gorean* slave girls are those who are native-born to Gor, whether they were born free or slave. Pedigree also is a factor when it comes to passion slaves and exotics, which are slave specifically bred by a slaver from slave stock to perpetuate desired traits and attributes.

Virginity, to absolutely no one's surprise, is a *big deal* on the planet Gor. A female slave who is a virgin is referred to as a *"white silk girl."* A female slave who is *not* a virgin is referred to as a *"red silk girl."* The distinction is largely semantic and ceremonial, as it is neither required, nor even customary, for white silk girls to wear only white, or red silk girls to wear only red. It is, however, common for the appropriate colors to be worn for special occasions, ceremonial purposes, and sometimes for a number of days following those events.

Slaves are also categorized by the types of training they have received. For example, most slave girls are expected to know how to *dance* in order to entertain their Masters, however a slave girl of Gor who has been formally trained and certified by a recognized school of dance has earned the right to be specifically referred to as a *Dancer.* A lady's serving slave, which is a slave who has been specifically trained in the skills required for attending to the needs of high-bred Gorean women, would be expected to know far more about the subjects of clothing, bathing, hygiene, serving, table service, and social protocols than any typical slave girl.

A Gorean slave's training, like her virginity, is *also* a really big deal. When we think of the word *training*, we *usually* think in terms of skills that require specialized abilities or an abundance of technical knowledge. This is typically *not* the case when it comes to the training of Gorean slaves. They must be taught *everything* they know *again* from scratch, and the most difficult part of that process is the *unlearning* of the old habits. A Gorean slave must be taught how to stand, sit, kneel, walk, speak, be silent, serve, entertain, assume various poses and positions as required, and perform a wide assortment of other mundane tasks in a *very specific fashion*. Even a task as seemingly simple as *entering a room* becomes infinitely more complicated, if you happened to be a slave girl of Gor:

> "Observe," once had said Elizabeth to me, to my amusement, in the secrecy of our compartment, "the twelfth way to enter a room."
> I had observed. It was not bad. But I think I preferred the tenth, that with the girl's back against the side of the door, the palms of her hands on the jamb, her head up, lips slightly parted, eyes to the right, smoldering at just the right temperature.
> "How many ways are there," I asked, sitting cross-legged in

> the center of the compartment, on the stone couch, "to enter a room?"
> "It depends on the city," said Elizabeth. "In Ar we are the best; we have the most ways to enter a room. One hundred and four."
> I whistled. "What about," I asked, "just walking straight through?"
> She looked at me. "Ah," said she, "one hundred and five!"
> (John Norman, Assassin of Gor, 1970)

Gorean slaves may be used for any purpose their Masters desire, whether it is for utilitarian purposes or for pleasure, she would be classified primarily by her assigned duties. This is the fourth way by which Gorean slaves at categorized: by how they are *utilized.* A slave who has been formerly trained as a *Dancer,* yet is employed by her Master as a *Bath Girl,* is for all intents and purposes, a *Bath Girl.*

The following is just a *partial* list of the various types of Gorean slaves, as described by John Norman:

Bath Girl. Bath girls are slaves who are kept either by the owner of a bath house or, in the case of public bath houses run by the village or city, city slaves. Sexual use of the bath girl by patrons is typically included in the bath house entry fee.

Below Deck Girl. When Gorean slaves are transported by ship, some are kept top-side, or *"on deck,"* while others are kept in the hold of the ship, or *"below deck."* The slaves *on deck* are given a certain degree of freedom in exchange for their labor, whereas the *below deck girls* are kept in cages and shorn of their body hair in an effort to discourage nits and lice.

Bond-maid. Bond-maids are slave girls who have been won in battle or captured by raiding parties. They refer to their Masters as "Jarl", and are typically more bold, boisterous and playful than the typical kajira, whom they view with some distaste. Their collars are made of iron, and riveted by hammer around their necks. The role of a bondmaid tends to be a favorite among those who are new to role-playing the Gorean lifestyle, as it provides a simple and convenient back-story *("I was taken in a raid, and forced to become a slave")* and it provides a semi-plausible explanation for behavior that would, in reality, be better suited to a BDSM *brat-sub* than a kajirae trained Gorean. The following passage from *Marauders of Gor* beautifully illustrates the typical behavior of bondmaids:

> A bond-maid thrust through the crowd. "Does my Jarl not remember Gunnhild?" she asked. She whimpered, and slipped to his side, holding him, lifting her lips to kiss him on the throat, beneath the beard. About her neck, riveted, was a collar of black iron, with a welded ring, to which a chain might be attached.
> "What of Pouting Lips?" said another girl, kneeling before him, lifting her eyes to his. Sometimes bondmaids are given descriptive names. The girl had full, sensuous lips, she was blond; she also smelled of verr; it had doubtless been she whom I had seen on the slope herding verr. "Pouting Lips has been in agony awaiting the return of her Jarl," she whimpered.
> The Forkbeard shook her head with his great hand.
> "What of Olga?" whined another wench, sweet and strapping, black-haired.
> "Do not forget Pretty Ankles, my Jarl," said another wench, a delicious little thing, perhaps not more than sixteen. She thrust her lips greedily to the back of his left hand, biting at the hair there.
> "Away you wenches!" laughed Ottar. "The Forkbeard has new prizes, fresher meat to chew!"
> (John Norman, *Marauders of Gor*, 1975)

Admittedly, it is extremely difficult for anyone familiar with the Gorean lifestyle to imagine *any kajira*, under *any circumstances*, trained or untrained, conducting herself in such a fashion. On the other hand, the role of a bond-maid is a tempting role indeed for anyone wishing to adopt Gorean ways and become a slave, *without becoming a kajira.*

Camp Slave. *Camp slaves* are slave girls who are kept in a military camp and who travel with the military unit in accordance with the terms of a contract between a slave merchant and the military leaders.

Chamber Slave. *Chamber slaves* are human slaves kept by the insect race of Priest-Kings for the sole purpose of servicing other humans who find their way to the Nest and become enslaved themselves.

City Slave. Refers to any slave that is owned by the governing body of a village or city.

Coin Girl. A coin girl is a slave who is prostituted for sexual favors as a means of generating income for her Master. She wanders the streets naked, wearing only a necklace with coin box attached, into which her customers are expected to deposit coins in exchange for sex.

> "Coin girls were a form of street slave, usually sent into the streets around dusk by their masters, who commonly own several of them, with a chain on their neck, to which would be attached, normally, a bell, to call attention to their whereabouts, and a small, locked coin box. And woe to the girl who returns with coins jangling in the box! To be sure, in some places, one might even have a paga slave, or a brothel slave, for as little as a tarsk bit."
> (John Norman, *Renegades of Gor*, 1986)

Draft Slave. A draft slave is one who is used primarily to pull carts.

Feast Slave. A slave who is specially trained to serve at large banquets or special events is commonly referred to as a *feast slave.*

Fighting Slave. Specially trained in the martial arts, fighting slaves typically serve as body guards and site security. They sometimes are pitted against one another, like gladiators, in various kinds of mortal combat for the entertainment of the free.

House Slave. A Gorean *house slave*, sometimes also referred to as a *tower slave*, is considered to be a slave of relatively low status, if there can be such a thing as status among slaves, *at all.* Their duties typically involve housekeeping, cooking, serving, sewing, washing and other domestic chores. The label is almost always preceded by the descriptive word *"mere,"* as it is in this passage:

> "Even though she had then been turned in effect into a pleasure slave, much as might be purchased in any market, he had, it seems, considered having her serve in his city as a mere house slave, or even, in spite of what she had now become, if it pleased him, denying her the collar, as a mere cleaning prisoner, a confined servant, a mere housekeeper in captivity." (John Norman, Vagabonds of Gor, 1987)

Kettle Slave. A *kettle slave* is a sub-category of *house slave* that is utilized primarily in the kitchen to perform food preparation, cooking, and cleaning. Kettle slaves are sometimes referred to as *pot girls*.

Love Slave. A love slave is a slave who has f*allen in love* with her Master, although there is some debate among Goreans about whether she must be loved by her Master, in return. In Gorean tradition, it is believed that the life of a love slave is necessarily harsher than for any other kind of slave. That is because her Master must always be vigilant against accusations of favoritism, and will often over-compensate for his secret desire to go easy on her. Love between Master and slave isn't always spoken of openly, but when it is, it is done so *powerfully*:

> He took me by the hair and thrust my head down to the furs. "A man can truly love only that woman," he said, "who is truly his, who belongs to him. Otherwise he is only a party to a contract."

"A woman," I said, "can love only that man to whom she truly belongs."
"To whom do you truly belong, Slave?" he asked.
"To you, Master," I said.
"You please me, Slave Girl," he said.
(John Norman, Slave Girl of Gor, 1977)

Luck Slave. A *luck slave* is a shipboard slave who - for whatever reason - is kept because it is believed she will bring good luck, and serves as a sort of mascot and pleasure slave for the crew.

Lure Girl. A lure girl is a slave whose primary purpose is to draw men from an enemy's camp into a trap. Once the trap has been sprung, the prisoners are often put to work as slaves, themselves.

Mat and Kettle Slave. Actually, a fusion of two different types of slaves - a mat slave is used primarily for sexual purposes, while a kettle slave is a kitchen domestic. In many households, a single slave may be forced to perform domestic kitchen duties as well as please her Master sexually, and so she is known as a *mat and kettle slave.*

Message Girl. A message girl refers to a slave who is utilized as a courier to transmit secret messages. The message girl's head is shaved and the message, which is sometimes encoded, is tattooed on her head. The girl chosen for this sort of duty is usually illiterate, even though it would be almost impossible for her to see the message on the back or top of her head, *even if she weren't*. Her hair is then allowed to grow back before she is sent to deliver her message. The recipient shaves her head to read the message, and then typically *keeps her* as part of the bargain.

Mul. Mul is the Priest-King word for the human slaves that serve them. Muls are bred in their nest by the insect-like race of Priest-Kings, and fed an extremely bland, pale, whitish, fibrous vegetable-like paste called mul-fungus. Obviously, you probably won't be meeting many *muls* here on Earth.

Paga Slave. Sometimes known as a *tavern slave*, the *paga slave* is owned by a tavern keeper and offered to patrons for the price of a cup of paga, which is a fermented brew made from yellow grain and consumed at room temperature. Think: *Tavern wench.*

Passion Slave. A passion slave is one who has been specifically bred and trained in the arts of lovemaking. As Gorean slave roles *go*, this one is immensely popular for fairly obvious reasons.

Personal Serving Slave. A personal serving slave is typically assigned to care exclusively for a specific individual who may or may not necessarily be her owner.

Pierced-Ear Slave. On Gor, ear piercing is a symbol of low status or degradation. A slave that is marked by the piercing of her ears is considered the lowest of the low, and will likely never win her freedom. In Norman's novels, this was often portrayed as a unique and ironic problem for slave girls formerly from Earth:

> "Many Gorean slave girls live in terror of having their ears pierced... Woe to the Earth girl brought to Gor whose ears are pierced. She will be sold publicly, as a pierced-ear girl." (John Norman, Prize of Gor, 2008)

Rent Slave. A rent slave is a slave who is regularly rented out to others as a way of generating income for her Master.

Seduction Slave. A seduction slave is typically a male slave who seduces a female free woman with the intent of placing her in a compromising situation that can be used to put her into slavery.

Self Contract Slave. A self contract slave is a free woman who enters into a temporary contract of slavery in order to satisfy a debt or to learn what it is like to be a slave. Needless to say, this is an *uncommon* practice among Gorean free women in John Norman's novels. It can, however, provide a credible backstory for a uniquely *temporary slave role* for a novice Gorean role player.

Silk Girl. *Silk girl* is a somewhat pejorative term used by the *bondmaidens* of the northern climes (who typically wear *wool*) for *kajirae*, who usually wear *silks*.

Silk Slave. *Silk slaves* are male pleasure slaves owned by free women. They are often chosen for their virility and rugged good looks, though some slave owners prefer silk slaves of a more *effeminate* variety.

State Slave. Refers to any slave that is owned by the governing body of a province, territory or state.

Whip Slave. A *whip slave* is one who has been delegated by her Master the authority to punish his other slaves with a whip or similar implement.

Work Slave. A *work slave* (sometimes referred to as a *field slave* or *stable slave*) is a somewhat generic label for any slave whose duties include laboring in the fields, cleaning stables, caring for livestock, or performing other manual labor.

The Gorean Collar

A pretty compelling case could be made that we all owe a great debt to John Norman for being the originator of the notion of *collaring* as the Master/slave alternative to traditional committed relationships. He was *certainly* largely responsible for the *popularization*, if not the origination, of the concept. Our Earthly BDSM culture may recognize only a handful of different collar types, but on the planet Gor, a collar has *dozens* of practical and symbolic purposes, not the least of which are their *aesthetic* qualities. In *Slave Girls of Gor (1977)*, John Norman wrote, "In the matter of collars, as in all things, Goreans commonly exhibit good taste and aesthetic sense." Elsewhere in the same work, Norman commented on the *emotional* utility that a collar may have for *both the Master and the slave:*

> "It is said, in a Gorean proverb, that a man, in his heart, desires freedom, and that a woman, in her belly, yearns for love. The collar, in its way, answers both needs. The man is most free, owning the slave. He may do what he wishes with her. The woman, on the other hand, being owned, is institutionally and helplessly subject, in her status as slave, to the submissions of love." (John Norman, Slave Girl of Gor, 1977)

New slaves - *particularly slaves brought to Gor from Earth* - are made to memorize the customs and cultural lore surrounding the history and purpose of Gorean collars, and are expected to be able to recite them upon her master's command:

> "What is the common purpose of a collar?"
> "The collar has four common purposes, Master," she said, "First, it visibly designates me as a slave, as a brand might not, should it be covered by clothing.
> Second, it impresses my slavery upon me. Thirdly, it identifies me to my Master.
> Fourthly," she said, "it makes it easier to leash me."
> (John Norman, Explorers of Gor, 1979)

Categories of Collars

Gorean merchant law defines a collar as anything that is worn about the neck of an individual for the primary purpose of marking the person as a slave, though as we are about to see, they can serve many other purposes, as well. Slave collars are not required by Gorean law, but they are strongly recommended. If a collar bears markings at all, it will typically identify the slave's owner, and bear the slaves given name.

Gorean collars can be made of just about any material. The most commonly used are steel, leather, rope, cord, and fabric. Gorean collars, like the slaves who wear them, are typically categorized by their utility and purpose. At times, those purposes can be so specialized, that some of the collars described in the novels would have no conceivable counterparts or utility on *Earth* except, perhaps, as collars which are used solely for role play purposes. On the other hand, many of the most strikingly beautiful and exclusive collar designs on Earth have been inspired by Norman's colorful descriptions. As you peruse the following list of Gorean collar types, see if you can tell which might be better suited for practical use in the *real-world.*

Beaded Collar

The beaded collar was typically worn by slaves of the "Red Savages of the Barrens." Many of these so-called *red savages, or Red Hunters,* were the direct descendants of *American Indians and Inuit* who had been brought to Gor hundreds of years ago by the insect-like race of Priest Kings in order to populate the barren planet. The collar itself is described in the following fashion:

> "She was barefoot. About her left ankle there was, about two inches high, a beaded cuff, or anklet. Her garb was doubtless intended to suggest the distinctive, humiliating and scandalously brief garment in which red savages are sometimes pleased to place their white slaves. One difference, however, must surely be noted. The red savages do not use steel collars. They usually use high, beaded collars, tied together in the front by a rawhide string. Subtle differences in the styles of collars, and in the knots with which they are fastened on the girls' necks, differentiate the tribes. Within a given tribe the beading, in its arrangements and colors, identifies the particular master. This is a common way, incidentally, for warriors to identify various articles... they own." (John Norman, Savages of Gor, 1982)

Among the Red Hunters who are specifically descended from *Inuit, their slaves and animals* are identified by an intricately knotted set of four leather strings, similar to a collar. These are called *bondage strings* and, like the beaded collar, the different types of knots used identify the specific owner.

Capture Collar

The capture collar consists of a loop of *chain* attached to two wooden handles in such a way that it is easy to block off a slave's air supply as a measure of physical control while maintaining a safe distance. It was described by the author thusly:

> "About my throat, closely looped, was a narrow golden chain. It was controlled by two narrow wooden handles, in his hands... It was a girl-capture chain... It is to be distinguished from the standard garrote, which is armed with wire and can cut a throat easily. The standard garrote, of course, is impractical for captures, for the victim, in even a reflexive movement, might cut her own throat."
> (John Norman, Savages of Gor, 1982)

Coffle Collar

A coffle is a line of prisoners, chained together. Therefore, a coffle collar is a slave collar with a sturdy ring attached to it which allows a chain to be threaded through the ring in order to control multiple slaves on the same chain. The chain may be permanently attached or removable, depending on the number of slaves in the coffle, and what they will be doing while chained in this fashion.

> "The collars had front and back rings, were hinged on the right and locked on the left. This is a familiar form of coffle collar. The lengths of chain between the collars were about 3 to 4 feet long. Some were attached to the collar rings by

> the links themselves, opened and then re-closed about the rings, and some of them were fastened to the collar rings by snap rings. Another common form of coffle collar has its hinge in the front and closes behind the back of the neck, like the common slave collar. It has a single collar ring, usually on the right, through which, usually, a single chain is strung. Girls are spaced on such a chain, usually, by snap rings." (John Norman, Savages of Gor, 1982)

Coil Collar

A coil collar is constructed from a *coil of marsh vine*. The material is flexible and not as sturdy as a collar made of metal, but is useful in establishing the ownership of a slave:

> "It was hot, and the coils of the marsh vine about my throat were hot. Beneath the coils my neck was red, and slippery with sweat and dirt. I put my finger in the collar to pull it a bit from my throat." (John Norman, Raiders of Gor, 1971)

Cord Collar

The cord collar consists of a light cord, which is tied about the slave's throat and has, dangling from it, a small disk which identifies the name of the slave's master. This type of collar is used in areas of Gor where metal is scarce or too expensive to be used for slave collars:

> "On some rence islands I have heard, incidentally, that the men have revolted, and enslaved their women. These are usually kept in cord collars, with small disks attached to them, indicating the names of their masters." (John Norman, Vagabonds of Gor, 1987)

Dance Collar

The dance collar is a collar designed primarily for its aesthetic value as adornment for Gorean dancers. It consists primarily of a collar with a largely ornamental light-weight chain attached, which sometimes is also attached to wrist cuffs. The design varies from region to region and from dancer to dancer:

> “A wrist ring was fastened on her right wrist. The long, slender, gleaming chain was fastened to this and, looping down and up, ascended gracefully to a wide chain ring on her collar, through which it freely passed, thence descending, looping down, and ascending, looping up, gracefully, to the left wrist ring. If she were to stand quietly, the palms of her hands on her thighs, the lower portions of the chain, those two dangling loops, would have been about at the level of her kneels, just a little higher. The higher portion of the chain, of course, would be at the collar loop.” (John Norman, Kajira of Gor, 1983)

Kur Collar

The Kurii are an egg-laying, bearlike alien race at war with the insect-like Priest-Kings of Gor. They are described by Norman as weighing 900 pounds, incredibly strong, and having seven clawed fingers on each hand. They occasionally enslave human women, but more often than not, it is for the sole purpose of keeping them as a *food source.* In fact, the Kurri maintain *slaughterhouses* just for humans. Some Kurri even like to *play with their human food.* In *Blood Brothers of Gor* (1982), a Kurrii is described as *swinging a kajira around in circles above his head* before finally devouring her. On the bright side, Kur slave collars are considered to be a great way to improve one’s *posture:*

> She approached me. From my pouch I drew forth a leather Kur collar, with its lock, and sewn in leather, its large, rounded ring. "What is it?" she asked apprehensively, I took it behind her neck, and then, closing it about her throat, thrust the large, flattish bolt, snapping it, into the locking breech. The two edges of metal, bordered by the leather,

> fitted closely together. The collar is some three inches in height. The girl must keep her chin up. "It is the collar of a Kur cow," I told her. (John Norman, Marauders of Gor, 1975)

Lock Collar

A lock collar is a typical Gorean slave collar which locks at the back of the neck. The lock usually has six pins or six disks within, which have symbolic significance:

> "A small, heavy lock on a girl's slave collar, incidentally, may be of several varieties, but almost all are cylinder locks, either of the pin or disk variety. In a girl's collar lock there would be either six pins or six disks, on each, it is said, for each letter in the Gorean word for slave, Kajira." (John Norman, Assassin of Gor, 1970)

Message Collar

A message collar is a sewn leather collar with a peculiar purpose. The slave that wears it is often presented by her owner as a gift to the recipient of the message:

> "Did you note the collar she wore?" He had not seemed to show much interest in the high thick leather collar that the girl had had sewn about her neck. "Of course," he said. "I myself," I said," have never seen such a collar." "It is a message collar," said Kamback. "Inside the leather sewn within, will be a message." (John Norman, Nomads of Gor, 1969)

Northern Collar

The northern collar is comprised of an unmarked flat black metal which is riveted with a hammer about the neck of a slave:

> "Look up at me," said the smith. The slender, blond girl, tears in her eyes, looked up at him. He opened the hinged collar of black iron, about a half inch in height. He put it about her throat. It also contained a welded ring, suitable for the attachment of a chain. "Put your head beside the anvil," he said. He took her hair, and threw it forward, and thrust her neck against the left side of the anvil. Over the anvil lay the joining ends of the two pieces of the collar. The inside of the collar was separated by a quarter of an inch from her neck. I saw the fine hairs on the back of her neck. On one part of the collar are two, small, flat, thick rings. On the other is a single such ring. These rings, when the wings of the collar are joined, are aligned, those on one wing on top and bottom, that on the other in the center. They fit closely together, one on top of the other. The holes in each, about three-eighths of an inch in diameter, too, of course, are perfectly aligned. The smith, with his thumbs, forcibly, pushed a metal rivet through the three holes."
>
> (John Norman, Marauders of Gor, 1975)

Plank Collar

A plank collar consists of a heavy wooden plank which is split lengthwise, with each half containing five semicircular openings. When the two halves are joined, they form wooden stocks for holding five slaves. The assembled plank is then chained down wherever needed:

> "The primary holding arrangement for women on the benches, however, [is] not chains. Each place on the bench is fitted with ankle and wrist stocks, and for each bench there is a plank collar, a plank which opens horizontally, each half of which contains five matching, semicircular openings, which, when it is set on pinions, closed, and chained in place, provides thusly five sturdy, wooden enclosures for the small, lovely throats of women. The plank

> is thick and thus the girl's chins are held high. The plank is further reinforced between each girl with a narrowly curved iron band, the open ends of which are pierced; this is slid tight in its slots, in its metal retainers, about the boards, and secured in place with a four-inch metal pin, which may or may not be locked in place." (John Norman, Savages of Gor, 1982)

Plate Collar

A plate collar is a heavy metal collar that is typically used on males or untrained female slaves as a way of discouraging escape. It is hammered onto the throat and only a blacksmith or skilled metal worker can remove it:

> "I could see the heavy metal collar hammered about the man's neck, not uncommon in a male slave. His head would have been placed across the anvil, and the metal curved about his neck with great blows." (John Norman, Hunters of Gor, 1974)

Turian Collar

The *Turian* collar, unlike most collars which fit closely to a slave's skin, is a round metallic ring that fits so loosely that the slave can turn within it. The Turian collar style is a popular design which is emulated by many real-world practitioners of the Gorean way.

> "She wore the Turian collar, rather than the common slave collar. The Turian collar lies loosely on the girl, a round ring; it fits so loosely that, when grasped in a man's fist, the girl can turn within it... Both collars lock in the back, behind the girl's neck. The Turian collar is more difficult to engrave, but... like the flat collar, will bear some legend assuring that the girl, if found, will be promptly returned to her master." (John Norman, Nomads of Gor, 1969)

Shipping Collar
A shipping collar is a usually a *temporary* collar used to identify a slave while he or she is in transit as cargo aboard a slave transport ship.

> "What sort of collar do you wear?"
> "A shipping collar, Master. It shows that I am a portion of the cargo of the Palms of Schendi."
> (John Norman, Explorers of Gor, 1979)

Sleeve Collar
A sleeve collar is one that is constructed from cloth, and is typically used as a covering or liner for the less attractive metallic collar worn by the slave. On rare occasions, the sleeve collar may be worn by itself, without the uncomfortable collar within.

> "I reached out, timidly, towards her throat. I touched the object there. "What is this?" I asked. "The silk?" she asked. "That is a collar stocking, or a collar sleeve. They may be made of many different materials. In a cooler climate they are sometimes of velvet. In most cities they are not used."
> (John Norman, Kajira of Gor, 1983)

Collaring, the Gorean Way
The traditions and lore associated with the Gorean custom of collaring slaves were described and expounded upon by John Norman as a recurring theme over the course of all thirty-two Gor novels. The widespread contemporary practice of *collaring* as a symbol of commitment within the BDSM culture owes a great deal to Norman's imagination and vision, even though he never advocated that the Gorean culture should be emulated in real-life.

A Gorean collar is symbolic of far more than simply the

unbreakable bond between a master and his slave. Gorean tradition celebrates what they consider to be the natural order of things, which includes a man's inherent dominance over women. According to folklore passed down through countless generations, this natural order was the result of an ancient war of the sexes:

> "In Gorean mythology it is said that there was once a war between men and women and that the women lost, and that the Priest-Kings, not wishing the women to be killed, made them beautiful, but as the price of this gift decreed that they, and their daughters, to the end of time, would be the slaves of men." (John Norman, Dancer of Gor, 1985)

The actual procedures involved in the collaring of a slave vary widely, depending on the culture, region, type of slave being collared, and the collar itself. At one end of the spectrum, the process is no more sacrosanct than the shoeing of a horse or the branding of a steer might be on Earth, as this passage from *"Marauders of Gor"* illustrates:

> "Do not move your head, bondmaid," said the smith.
> Then, with great blows of the iron hammer, he riveted the iron collar about her throat.
> A man then pulled her by the hair from the anvil and threw her to one side. She lay there weeping, a naked bondmaid, marked and collared.
> "Next," called out the Forkbeard.
> Weeping, another girl was flung over the branding log.
> (John Norman, Marauders of Gor, 1975)

At the other end of the spectrum, slave collarings are far more ceremonial in nature and demonstrative of an emotional bond and commitment between master and slave. The following passage is not only typical of many of the collaring ceremonies described by Norman in his novels but the wording is, in some ways, almost identical to many of the contemporary real-life collaring ceremonies conducted right here on good ol' *planet Earth:*

> "Assume the posture of female submission, I told her. She did so, kneeling back on her heels, her arms extended, wrists crossed, her head between them, down. She was weeping.
> "Repeat after me," I told her. "'I, once Miss Elizabeth Cardwell, of the planet Earth--'"
> "I, once Miss Elizabeth Cardwell, of the planet Earth--" she said.
> "--herewith submit myself, completely and totally, in all things--"
> "--herewith submit myself, completely and totally, in all things--" she said.
> "'--to him who is now known here as Hakim of Tor--"
> "--to him who is now known here as Hakim of Tor--" she said.
> "--his girl, his slave, an article of his property, his to do with as he pleases--"
> "--his girl, his slave, an article of his property, his to do with as he pleases," she said.
> Hassan handed me the collar. It was inscribed, "I am the property of Hakim of Tor." I showed it to the girl. She could not read Taharic script. I read it to her. I put it about her neck. I snapped it shut.
> "I am yours, Master," I said to the girl.
> She looked at me, tears in her eyes, her neck in my locked collar.
> "I am yours, Master," she said.
> "Congratulations on your slave!" said Hassan. "She is lovely meat. Now I must attend to my own slave." He laughed, and left.

> The girl sank to the straw, and looked up at me. Her eyes were soft with tears. She whispered, "I am yours now, Tarl," she said. "You own me. You truly own me."
> "What is your name?" I asked.
> "Whatever Master wishes," she whispered.
> "I will call you Vella," I said.
> "I am Vella," she said, her head down.
> (John Norman, Tribesmen of Gor, 1976)

Gorean collaring ceremonies, even at their most formal, are typically conducted with the slave stripped naked and forced to assume traditional poses of submission. While many of the collaring ceremonies described in Norman's novels contain elements of humiliation and degradation, their inclusion in real world Gorean collaring ceremonies is *not* common.

> "Step before me naked," said Rask of Treve. I did so.
> We faced one another, not speaking, he with his blade, and in his leather, I with nothing, stripped at his command.
> "Submit," he said. I could not disobey him.
> I fell to my knees before him. Resting back on my heels, extending my arms to him, wrists crossed, as though for binding, my head lowered, between my arms.
> I spoke in a clear voice. "I, Miss Elinor Brinton, of New York City, to the Warrior, Rask, of the High City of Treve, herewith submit myself as a slave girl. At his hands I accept my life and my name, declaring myself his to do with as he pleases." Suddenly I felt my wrists lashed swiftly, rudely, together. I drew back my wrists in fear. They were already bound! They were bound with incredible tightness. I had been bound by a tarnsman. I looked up at him in fear, I saw him take an object from a warrior at his side. It was an opened, steel slave collar. He held it before me.
> "Read the collar," said Rask of Treve.
> "I cannot," I whispered. "I cannot read."

> "She is illiterate," said Ena.
> "Ignorant barbarian!" I heard more than one girl laugh.
> I felt so ashamed. I regarded the engraving on the collar, tiny, in neat, cursive script.
> I could not read it.
> "Read it to her," said Rask of Treve to Ena.
> "It says," said Ena, "I am the property of Rask of Treve."
> I said nothing.
> "Do you understand?" asked Ena.
> "Yes," I said. "Yes!"
> Now, with his two hands, he held the collar about my neck, but he did not yet close it. I was looking up at him. My throat was encircled by his collar, he was holding it, but the collar was not yet shut. My eyes met his. His eyes were fierce, amused, mine were frightened. My eyes pleaded for mercy. I would receive none. The collar snapped shut.
> There was a shout of pleasure from the men and girls about.
> I heard hands striking the left shoulder in Gorean applause.
> Among the warriors, the flat sword blades and blades of spears rang on shields. I closed my eyes, shuddering. I opened my eyes, I could not hold up my head. I saw before me the dirt, and the sandals of Rask of Treve.
> Then I remembered that I must speak one more line. I lifted my head, tears in my eyes. "I am yours, Master," I said.
> (John Norman, Captive of Gor, 1972)

As these passages illustrate, the Gorean collaring ceremony is typically just the *beginning* of a kajira's education. The riveting of a collar about her neck, whether it is done *brutishly or lovingly*, serves as an unforgettable initial lesson on the Master/slave relationship dynamic:

> "The collar," I said, touching it," is put on from without, but what it encircles, the slave, comes from within."
> "Master?" she asked.

> "Slavery," I told her, "true slavery, comes from within, and you, my lovely little red-haired beast, I assure you, as was evidenced by your behavior and performances this night, are a true slave. Do not fight your slavery. Allow it freely and spontaneously, candidly, sweetly and untrammeled, to manifest itself. It is what you are."
> Yes, Master," she said.
> "That, too," I said, "will save you many bouts with the lash."
> (John Norman, Savages of Gor, 1982)

Unfortunately - *or fortunately, depending upon your perspective* - here on Earth, *consent* is kind of a *big deal.* That pesky requirement that you obtain consent *before* you slap a steel collar and padlock around a woman's neck suggests that the traditional Gorean strategy of *"collar first, explain later"* may not be the optimal approach on *this* particular planet.

There are very few traditional Gorean traditions and practices that can be transplanted as-is, without some measure of adaptation, to a *real-world* Gorean lifestyle. I'm not saying it *can't be done.* I'm simply saying that it requires a relatively *thick skin*, the *proper mindset*, a great deal of *flexibility*, and a refusal to *take yourself too seriously*.

Gor in Real World Relationships

Contrary to popular belief, Gorean relationships not only *do* exist in real-life, they often thrive in relative obscurity there. The common misconception that there aren't many real-world Gorean relationships out there is based on a variety of factors, not the least of which is the general scorn with which such relationships are sometimes viewed by others.

Knowing that your relationship dynamic is likely to become the subject of insults, jokes, or dismissive commentary can have a chilling effect on how forthcoming you are in making it public. You might think that being part of the allegedly non-judgmental and tolerant fetish culture would preclude this from happening, but that's not always the case. In fact, it is ironic that the harmful misconceptions about Gorean relationships are far more common and negative *within* the BDSM lifestyle than they are among the general population, where an almost complete lack of awareness among the vanilla folk works to the Goreans' advantage.

While a significant percentage of real-life Master/slave relationships are Gorean *to some degree*, a *"Gorean lifestyle"* need not be defined solely by Master/slave relationships, nor *should* it be. As we noted at the beginning of this chapter, John Norman's thirty-two Gor novels painted a complex and fascinating portrait of an entire planet, complete with its own unique customs, traditions, and philosophies. Sex, slavery and submission may have been some of the more *interesting* and *titillating* aspects of Gorean culture as described by Norman, but they were by no means the primary focus of his books. Gor enthusiasts exist along a wide spectrum of fandom that ranges from the pitifully misinformed chat room role-players at one end, and the fanatically literal *triviacrats*, who will go so far as to speak *Gorean languages,* on the other. Somewhere, between those two extremes, you can find the *practical* real-life Goreans, quietly trying to live their lives and doing their best to stay under everyone else's radar.

A *practical* Gorean lifestyle typically involves adopting the mindset and philosophy of Gor, and then looking for ways to successfully *integrate* them into your day-to-day Earthly lives and intimate relationships. These Gorean teachings typically involve embracing the natural order of dominance vs. submission, being willing to swim against the tide of socially accepted norms, embracing the real differences between men and women, being honorable and accountable in all things, and the glorification of a warrior ethic.

A person living a practical Gorean lifestyle adopts and applies these philosophies *not* simply because he or she is a big fan of John Norman's novels or because it's an entertaining internet chat room activity. They do it because they *truly believe* in those ideals and *because they work* in their lives and in their relationships. This is not to say that the same ideals would work as effectively in *any one else's life.* Author Robert A. Heinlein once said, "One man's theology is another man's belly-laugh," and it is equally as true when it comes to philosophy and culture. Just as the *Buddhist* philosophy may work wonderfully for *some* people, but not for *others,* so it is with Gorean philosophy.

The Gorean way of life may not be your particular cup of tea, but for those who are happily ensconced in a delightfully fulfilling Gorean relationship, what matters most is not our opinion of them, but the joy that they share in their own little piece of Gor on Earth.

# # #

My Two Cents on Gor

I *admit* it. I've never really been a big fan of the Gorean lifestyle. Sure, I *loved* reading John Norman's *Gor* novels as a teen, but the *Gorean thing* always struck me as a little too *role-play* and not enough *real life,* and I've always fancied myself as a *real life* kind of guy. My initially negative bias was no doubt influenced by an endless parade of teen D&D geeks posing as Goreans in internet chat rooms. I have, however, learned a great deal more about the real world Gorean subculture since then, and become good friends with many who follow the Gorean way.

So, to all of my Gorean friends and associates, I would just like to say, I apologize for once believing that you were all self-deluded, pervy, sci-fi whack jobs. I now know how misguided I was in that belief. That description *probably* only applies to about *half of you.* Seriously though, I *do* believe that Gor, like D/s in general, is a *mindset* that can be expressed healthily in a *variety* of ways, but a Gorean friend probably said it best, when she wrote:

Dear friends and Future Friends,

Please don't lecture me about my lifestyle choices, one of which happens to be the Gorean lifestyle. Don't insult my intelligence by calling me misguided or naïve because you think I'm living in a "fantasy" world. The Gorean way isn't just a fantasy, it is a mindset and a philosophy. It is a belief in a natural order of things, which includes the inherent dominance of men over women. It is striving to learn how to freely surrender one's will to her Master, and belonging to him with all of my might, mind, and soul.

Yes, I *am* aware that Gor is a fictional planet, the subject of a pulp science fiction series by John Norman. It doesn't exist. I *know* this. I really am not the fool you apparently think I am. I not only exist right here on planet Earth, but I also happen to be a very capable, fully functioning member of society with a good job, a nice car, and an awesome Master, whom I refer to as my husband around the people who just don't *get it.*

It doesn't matter to me that they don't get it. It doesn't matter to me that you don't seem to, either. It doesn't matter that I haven't read all thirty-two of the Gor novels or consider myself some kind of whiz-bang expert on all things Gorean. I don't join all the Gor discussion forums, or register on Gorean web sites. It doesn't matter that I am a primal *and* a pet, as well as a kajira. It doesn't matter whether I adhere to all of the protocols of Gor. No, none of *that* stuff matters.

Only one thing matters and that is my heart and mindset, which governs my relationship with my Master. I am his, mind, body and soul, and it is this philosophy and way of life that makes it possible for me to feel this way. That's what matters, not some science fiction planet, not your silly protocols. We've made the Gorean lifestyle our own by molding it to fit our real-life down-to-earth needs and desires. We don't live our lives to satisfy your fantasy of how Goreans should conduct themselves on Gor, or even on planet Earth. We live our lives striving to be the best kajira and Master we can possibly be. And *that's* all that matters.

"The meeting of two personalities is like the contact of two chemical substances: if there is any reaction, both are transformed."

- - *Carl Jung*

CHAPTER 8: THE FIRST MEETING

Nothing strikes fear into our hearts like the prospect of meeting someone who is important to us for the very first time. The list of anxieties that can threaten to turn this event into a nightmare is practically *infinite*, the chief among them being: *What if I don't live up to his or her expectations?* Fear of the unknown, dreading the inevitable awkwardness, concerns for safety, and even uncertainty about the possibility of intimacy or sex can make any first meeting a harrowing experience, even for someone who has been through it many times previously. We may never be able to completely get rid of those butterflies in your stomach, but there *are* some things you can do to get them flying in formation long enough to survive that first meeting.

First meetings can be *particularly* tricky for Dominants and submissives, for the simple reason that it's often difficult to know just how much of your D/s side is appropriate for this get-together. You don't want to conceal what is undeniably an integral part of your core personality, but you also shouldn't want to exceed the boundaries of propriety, frighten the other person, or endanger yourself in any way. What you're left with is a delicate balancing act between *revealing who you* are, and *imposing yourself* upon the person you're meeting.

An *imposition* occurs when someone feels pressured or obligated to *act or make a hasty decision* based upon your revelations or behavior. To understand the difference between the two, consider how a Dominant might choose to conduct himself at a first meeting with a submissive. He can choose to *reveal himself* by his mannerisms or by discussing the fact that he is a Dominant, or he can *impose himself* on the other person by unwisely attempting to *dominate her* at this first encounter. The former is a *revelation*; the latter, an *imposition*. His date may be a submissive, *but she is not his submissive*. Even if a submissive is normally attracted to this sort of dominant behavior, she may not appreciate being placed in a position of *having to decide how to react* to his attempt at asserting himself in such a fashion this early in the process.

Feeling *imposed upon* may be an *uncomfortable feeling*, but it is of relatively *minor* consequence compared to the very real danger that *some* submissives may face in the event that a Dominant unwisely asserts himself in a way that oversteps the boundaries of everyday etiquette and lifestyle protocol. A submissive can sometimes find herself in a potentially dangerous first meeting scenario where her usual good judgment and survival instincts are swept aside when she is caught up in the overwhelming emotions of the moment.

How do you know if you are about to do something potentially stupid and dangerous? *Here's how:* If you're considering a mid-meeting *change to your original plan* for how things were supposed to go, then this would be a good time to take a couple of deep breaths, count to ten slowly, and remind yourself that there were some very good reasons for the original plan. One of those reasons was to protect you from your own emotionally compromised judgment and impulsivity. No matter how badly you may *want* to turn off your phone and follow him back to his hotel for a good spanking, odds are that if it wasn't part of the original plan, it's *probably not a good idea.* At times like that, it might be a good time to say, "I love you, but *not* in an *I-want-to-be-featured-on-an-Investigation-Discovery-episode* kind of way."

Types of First Meetings:

First meetings can come in a variety of flavors, and your strategies for surviving them depends a lot upon what kind of first meeting you're considering. By the way, when I say *surviving*, I generally mean *getting through the meeting with your dignity intact*, but we'll be discussing the other kind later in this chapter as well. First meetings typically fall into five categories: imaginary, serendipitous, acquainting, hook-up, and transitional.

The Imaginary First Meeting

The imaginary first meeting is a first meeting that never happens, for whatever reason. It is neither inherently a *good* thing, nor a *bad* thing. It is what it is. It is almost always idealized in our minds as the coming together of two souls in a perfect alignment of love, lust, libido, laughter and any other sexy, happy "L" words we can think of. The truth, however, is that the real thing *rarely* lives up to the fantasies that we've built up in our heads. Some people in certain circumstances should be willing to acknowledge the fact that an imaginary first meeting is all that they can realistically hope for. Others sometimes go through with a real-life first meeting only to find themselves wishing that they had kept things virtual or long-distance. And then, there are those who *attempt* to meet someone in real-life, but the encounter remains imaginary *despite* their best efforts. You may count me as someone who has found himself in *all* of these scenarios at one point or another, but the most interesting experience involved my attempt to arrange what I had hoped would be a *transitional* first meeting but, instead, ended up being mostly an *imaginary* one.

Her screen name was *Sensual*. Just *that*. There were none of the numbers, extraneous letters, or silly modifiers that are tacked on to a name these days to differentiate a person from the thousands of other people using the same or a similar name. We were among the earliest adopters of internet chat and for all I knew she may have been the very *first* Sensual. She was an intelligent and funny redheaded submissive with piercing blue eyes and the most adorable freckles. In other words, she had all the qualities that can effortlessly turn my legs to Jell-O. I didn't know much else about her at first, but we grew incredibly close over the course of the next several months as we went from text chats to trading photographs and spending hours on the telephone. That, in itself, was quickly becoming somewhat problematic, since she lived in Washington State and I was serving in the Army, stationed in Germany at the time. This was long before the era of cheap long-distance plans or the advent of internet voice calling and, as a result, I was beginning to see phone bills (which included a pricy data plan) from Deutsche Telekom in excess of a *thousand dollars per month.* Clearly, we wouldn't be able to keep doing that for much longer. We would either have to scale back our relationship or take it a step forward, and neither of us was willing to step back.

I started making plans for what would be our first meeting. Once we agreed upon a date, I got approved for two weeks of leave. On the first day of my leave, I drove two hours to Frankfurt's Rhein-Main Air Force Base (which today no longer exists) and hopped aboard an Air Force C-5A Galaxy headed for McChord Air Force Base (now known as Joint Base Lewis-McChord) which is near Tacoma, Washington. The flight, which was 5200 miles as the crow flies but *not*, apparently, as the Air Force flies was mind-numbingly long and excruciatingly uncomfortable.

I arrived in Washington State at mid-day, and took a taxi to my hotel in the center of the city. From the hotel room, I called *Sensual* (who lived fifteen minutes away) to let her know that I had arrived, and to inform her where I was staying. I explained that I needed a shower and a short nap, but would meet her for dinner downstairs, in the hotel's very nice restaurant at 7 PM. We lingered for another thirty minutes on the phone like the star-struck lovers we were, tittering in complete and utter disbelief at the notion that we were *finally* about to meet each other in real life. We had talked about this for *months*, and now it was really about to *happen*.

At the appointed hour, I went downstairs to the restaurant, where I lingered in the waiting area for twenty minutes before finally agreeing to be seated at a table. I told the waiter that I was expecting someone, and he responded a sly grin and a wink. It was an intimate little place, so I was fairly certain that I'd be able to spot her as soon as she arrived. Today, just about everyone has a cell phone, so it's hard to imagine just sitting alone in a restaurant for an hour waiting - *hoping* - that someone shows up, without trying to *do something about it*. But this was before cell phones were commonly available; there wasn't a whole lot I *could* do, other than drop a quarter into the lobby pay phone in an attempt to call her, which I eventually did. There was no answer, which only served to give me false hope that perhaps she'd been delayed, and was now on her way. Finally, after almost ninety minutes of waiting, I gave up hope and ordered a meal, which I consumed alone as I juggled equal portions of anger, concern and gloom.

I went back to my hotel room, frustrated and angry, and attempted to call her again. This time the phone was answered, and on the other end of the line, she was *sobbing.* My anger instantly melted away as she tearfully told me about driving to the hotel and experiencing a debilitating anxiety attack which made it impossible for her to get out of the car. After sitting in her vehicle in front of the hotel for close to an hour, she then circled the block several times before finally just returning home. She begged for my forgiveness, and promised to see me after she got off work the following day. Thinking that perhaps meeting in a *hotel* might have contributed to her anxiety, I suggested meeting at 7 PM at a nearby Irish pub which had caught my eye along the route from the airport to the hotel. She said she knew the place, and promised to be there *without fail*. I was cautiously hopeful once again.

I spent most of the day meandering through this strange new city, exploring its nooks and crannies and taking in the sights at its quaint, bustling harbor. As the sun sank into the sea, I treated myself to a light but tasty dinner at the Oyster House as I watched the fishing boats returning for the evening. I went back to my hotel to shower and prepare to go out again. As a final precaution, I called *Sensual* to confirm the time and place of our meeting, and to verify that she still intended to be there. *"I'll be there, my Love,"* she assured me, "*with bells on!"* I smiled, and my *cautious optimism* took an immediate turn towards *buoyant expectation.*

The Irish pub was, in a word, *amazing.* It oozed with Gaelic charm, boasting a huge selection of Irish brews, friendly barmaids, and even a talented musical trio that played lively Irish tunes throughout the evening. It might have been the perfect evening, if only my date had shown up. Fortunately, the cheery music and their selection of superb beers were sufficiently good to keep me from wallowing in self-pity for very long. Some five hours later, I staggered back to my hotel in a pretty decent mood, considering the fact that I'd used up my vacation time, spent a great deal of money, and flown over five thousand miles to be stood up, not just once, *but twice by the same woman.*

When I opened the door to my hotel room, the telephone was ringing. I answered, and once again, she was sobbing. This time around, I was far less inclined to be as sympathetic as I had been the previous evening. I knew better than to attempt to have any kind of a coherent conversation with her while I was both highly annoyed *and* drunk, so I stopped her in mid-explanation. I said, *"Hush.* Obviously, this trip was a *huge mistake*. I'm sorry things didn't work out, but *I'm done here.* I'll be flying out tomorrow on the 2 PM flight to Germany. Have a nice life." *Click.*

The following day, I checked out of the hotel and made my way back to the passenger terminal at McChord Air Force Base to check in for my return flight to Germany. I still had a few hours to kill before boarding time, and spent much of it in quiet contemplation of my own incredible stupidity. Eventually, an announcement was made that it was time to board the aircraft. I gathered my things, stuffed them into my carry-on bag and stood up, only to suddenly find myself standing face-to-face with the very woman I'd flown so far to meet. We stood like that, silently looking into each other's eyes for what seemed like an eternity before either of us uttered a single word.

"Hi," she said.

"Hi," I replied. I floundered for something remotely intelligent to say, but all I could seem to manage was, "You're... beautiful!" I took her hands in mine.

She blushed crimson red and dropped her eyes for a moment. She said, "I... was so afraid... that you would be disappointed with me. It *paralyzed* me. I am *so* sorry. I never meant to hurt you. I *do* love you."

I nodded. I told her, *"I love you too."*

A long and awkward silenced followed, during which neither of us knew what to say next. The final call for boarding was announced and I said, "I really have to go now."

She nodded. We kissed. I flew away. We never spoke again.

The Serendipitous First Meeting

The serendipitous first meeting is one that occurs without any prior thought or planning. That isn't to say that you may not have *wanted* it to happen; it just means that *you didn't expect it* to happen, or at the very least, you didn't expect it to happen *when, where or how* it happened. Frankly, this is a pretty *rare* occurrence. It happens *so rarely*, in fact, that it almost never fails to arouse *someone's* suspicion that it may not have been as random as it appears at first blush. Nevertheless, these things *do* happen, typically when the two individuals live in the same region or have the same circle of friends and associates. People who are part of the BDSM lifestyle tend to be a fairly small and insular group, even if it happens to be spread over a large geographical area. It isn't uncommon, therefore, to attend a lifestyle social or fetish event and serendipitously run into people there whom you've been dying to meet for quite some time. When you *do*, be sure to tell them that you've always wanted to meet them; even if they are *rock-stars.* It'll probably make their day.

If a serendipitous first meeting happens to you, you should treat it like the *priceless gift* that it truly is. After all, it isn't every day that you get to meet someone whom you've always wanted to meet, without having to put any real effort into making it happen, or even having to go through the pre-meeting anxieties that you'd typically have to endure. You need to decide fairly quickly whether you want to see this person again and, if so, how best to make it happen. This may turn out to be your one and only chance to not only make a good impression, but to lay the groundwork for a second meeting that is planned, rather than accidental, and better suited to getting further acquainted.

The Acquainting First Meeting

The acquainting first meeting is one that occurs when two people decide to meet in order to simply get to know one another a little better. It's one way of saying *I don't know you, and I'm not even sure I want to know you, but I'm certainly willing to meet you to explore the possibility.* The nice thing about the acquainting first meeting is expectations are typically kept low or nonexistent and, consequently, it usually isn't terribly hard to *exceed* them. This can be a *very good thing* for people whose anxieties are rooted in a fear of having to live up to someone else's expectations.

When it comes to the acquainting first meeting, it is important to remember that *you don't really know anything about the person* whom you are about to meet for the first time. That means if you happen to be considering a get-together of this sort, the safety precautions on the following pages are *especially for you.* True, the odds of that person being a psychopath are *extremely low* but, then again, you've probably bought lottery tickets on slimmer chances of winning. *Think* about that.

The keys to a executing a successful acquainting meeting are: keeping expectations realistic, avoiding misunderstandings, staying safe (which we'll discuss at length later in this chapter), having fun, and having a plan for success *as well* as failure. Keeping expectations realistic and avoiding misunderstandings go hand-in-hand. To that end, it may sometimes be necessary to explicitly spell things out for the person you're about to meet by saying, *"I just want to be sure that we both understand that this is just lunch. No pressure. It's not a hook-up."* The discomfort of having to say such a thing prior to the meeting is *minimal* compared to the discomfort you *could feel later* if it turns out that the two of you had differing notions concerning the purpose of the meeting.

You *might* think that the notion of *having fun* at this initial meeting would be something of a no-brainer. Unfortunately, it is often easier said than done. You should choose a *vanilla* venue that allows you to focus your attentions on one another or gives you something fun to *do* together. It is also usually a good idea to avoid fetish lifestyle events as a place to get acquainted, *particularly* if you don't really know what preconceptions your new friend may be bringing to the table. In the unlikely event that your first meeting *doesn't* go as swimmingly as you hope, it's probably a fair bet that having your entire munch group there to witness it *isn't* going to make you feel any better about it. Do yourself and your kinkster friends the favor of arranging this meeting elsewhere. It's also advisable to avoid venues that might force you to devote your attention and energy to distractions or other people. Generally speaking, you will probably be able to learn a lot more about each other over beer and pizza than you will sitting in the dark at your local movie theater.

Having fun often depends as much on the topics of discussion as the venue and activities. It is often all too easy for some people to forget that *no one* enjoys having to endure an unending stream of negative or depressing discussion on topics such as divorce, abuse, mental illness, medical problems, anger issues or self-destructive behavior. There's absolutely nothing wrong with *mentioning* such things but, if at the end of your first meeting you realize that it's *all you talked about*, it's probably not a good portent of things to come. Your chances of a *second* meeting with your new friend are directly proportional to the number of times the two of you laugh and smile during *this one*.

The final key to success when it comes to acquainting first meetings consists of having *contingency plans* for both success *and* failure. You should already know, *before this meeting*, what the next step should be, *regardless* of the outcome. If, by the end of this meeting, you discover that you have absolutely no interest in seeing this person again, it's always a good thing to have a way to *tactfully say so* ready for deployment. Having to come up with something on-the-fly rarely turns out well. The best way to say, "Gee, I'd love to see you again," is *not* "Well, it was nice meeting you. *Bye!*"

It definitely helps to have at least *some* notion of what might constitute a fun *second date* ready to toss out when the time is right.

The Hook-up First Meeting

The hook-up first meeting consists of meeting someone for the first time for the primary purpose of having a sexual encounter, which *may or may not* include BDSM activities. For a wide variety of reasons, most of which should be fairly obvious to anyone old enough to be reading this book, this kind of first encounter is *almost always a bad idea*. Nevertheless, *they happen* in this lifestyle, and it would be exceptionally foolish to pretend that they don't. If you are considering meeting someone for the first time for a sexual hook-up, I would frankly advise you to reconsider. Failing that, I would then advise you to take *plenty of safety precautions* and to keep your expectations *realistic*.

Unrealistic expectations are hard enough to manage in *any* first meeting. Just think of it as a giant, *lickalicious* double-decker ice cream cone. Adding a big scoop of *sex* to the already towering treat may seem like an *exciting idea*, but it comes at the price of making your cone increasingly difficult to manage. You might even be irresistibly tempted to top *those* three scoops off with an additional dollop of *whipped BDSM* and *sex-toy sprinkles.* That's usually when it all topples over into a gooey mess on the pavement and you're left holding an empty waffle cone.

You would be well-advised to *take things slowly.* Don't expect to be able to live out all of your fantasies in a couple of hours, or even over the course of just a few days. Allot yourselves plenty of time to *feel your way* through the process of getting *comfortable* with one another socially, physically, intimately *and kinkily,* even if you think you already know each other better than you've ever known anyone.

There are *always* surprises.

You should probably grab a highlighter right now and *highlight the crap* out of that last sentence.

The Transitional First Meeting

A transitional first meeting is one that is planned for the express purpose of taking an online relationship to the *next level.* It doesn't necessarily mean that a 24-7 life together under the same roof is about to commence immediately but, for many, it *does* constitute a necessary first step towards that goal. It is an acknowledgment that the nature of the relationship is about to change, and that you are both willing to accept a greater degree of risk in hopes of reaping greater rewards as a result.

A true *transitional* first meeting assumes that you already know each other quite well, and that you have discussed your mutual goals and possible plans for the future. Despite the fact that you are already well-acquainted and have a foundational relationship from which to work, your expectations for a meeting like this *still* need to be managed. The odds may be skewed more to your favor as a result of your preparation, but there is still a *lot* that can go wrong, particularly if you are expecting it to be all rainbows and unicorns.

Much of what we said earlier regarding hook-up first meetings applies equally to transitional first meetings. Be sure to give yourselves plenty of time to get comfortable with each other on a variety of levels, and expect to hit a few bumps in the road. Surprises, when they are met with the proper attitude and some degree of preparation, don't necessarily have to turn into show-stoppers. It certainly doesn't hurt to have a back-up plan ready, *just in case* things don't go according to the script.

Take, for example, the disheartening case of William and Suzanne, who meticulously planned their first week together *so* extensively and exclusively around the mind-blowing kinky sex that was supposed to occur, that when they hit their first minor bump in the road, it mushroomed to the height of *Mount Everest.* The two had been friends in high school, but had never actually *dated* and, during their college years, they lost touch completely. *Twenty years later* and newly divorced, Suzanne was contemplating a return to the dating scene when she got the notion of reconnecting with William. She did, and was thrilled to learn that he was still single. They lived 1500 miles apart, but that didn't discourage the torrid *online romance* that blossomed quickly between them in the next few months.

It was decided that they should meet. True, it wasn't technically their first meeting, since they had known each other in high school, but that was over *twenty-five years ago* and, for all intents and purposes, they had each matured into different people now. Suzanne made plans to fly from Texas, where she lived, to Florida, where she would spend an entire, glorious week with William at his beachfront home. As the date grew nearer, their anticipation and expectations grew exponentially with each passing hour.

Finally, the much awaited day arrived, and Suzanne stepped off a plane and leaped joyously into William's waiting embrace. They raced back to the house where, unfortunately, the mounting anticipation, stress and performance anxiety all combined to create a perfect storm of *erectile dysfunction* for William. As acutely embarrassing as that must have been for *him,* it was further compounded when Suzanne interpreted it as a confirmation of *her* worst fears - *that she was a disappointment to him.*

The next six days were agonizingly awkward and uncomfortable for the two of them. Neither was particularly interested in making another attempt at intimacy; they each just wanted the week to be *over,* so they could put this experience behind them. It had simply never occurred to *either* of them that actual events might *deviate* from the script in their heads. Sadly, their relationship never recovered from this blow. After Suzanne returned home to Texas, there were a few chats and phone calls, but they slowed to a trickle and then eventually stopped altogether. They are now back where they started; *no longer in touch.*

If there is one lesson to be learned from their story, it should be that it wasn't a case of erectile dysfunction that waylaid their plans; it was the *emotional reactions* based on their deep-seated *insecurities and fears* that magnified what should have been a simple speed-bump into a *mountain.* I typically refer to a minor mishap like this one as a *speed bump* for a reason. If you are *prepared* for it and drive across it *slowly and deliberately,* it's not a problem *at all.*

Hit it at fifty miles per hour, and it could just screw up your whole week.

Practical Considerations

There are plenty of factors which should be taken into consideration if you're planning a first meeting of any kind, and *especially* if your budding relationship falls outside the boundaries of what might be considered a *vanilla* connection. The most important, of course, should be *safety considerations*, and we'll cover them at length in the next section. Before we do that, let's discuss timing, expense, settings, distractions, and some of the other practical considerations you should include in your plan.

Timing, as they say, is *everything.* The timing of a first meeting should be commensurate with its *purpose.* It may *never* be too early for an acquainting first meeting, but a hook-up or transitional first meeting that happens too early in a relationship could be a disaster. There are other timing considerations that you might not think to include in your planning, but can definitely spell the difference between a successful meeting and an epic failure. Take, for example, the timing of a woman's *menstrual cycle.* By failing to take something like *that* into account while coordinating your kinky weekend together, you could inadvertently be throwing a monkey wrench into your well-laid plans.

Expense is one of those considerations that we don't really *like* to have to think about, but are *forced* to by the harsh realities of life. Factoring the expense of a meeting into your plan should go beyond simply deciding whether you can *afford* to do it or not. It's obviously not going to be an issue of any real significance if your meeting is *local* and can be accomplished at minimal or no expense. But if there's going to be any travel involved, things begin to get a little more complicated. You may be able to afford to do it, but the question that you should *really* be asking yourselves is, is this the best way to commit our resources? To better illustrate this point, consider this hypothetical question: Assuming you had the *money to do it,* would you spend two thousand dollars on meeting and spending a fun-filled *week* together *now,* if it meant that you'd have to wait an *additional six months* before *moving in together?* Finances are almost *always* a trade-off. Make sure you both fully understand what it is you're *sacrificing* in order to accomplish your plans.

The setting for a first meeting is another one of those considerations that we typically just don't think about until it's too late to do anything about it. A little contingency planning for any likely scenario can go a long way towards making your experience a good one.

Janet, a twenty-year-old submissive friend of mine who lives at home with her folks while attending a local college, told me about her plans for a transitional first meeting with her Dominant, Bradley. They were planning on spending *four days together* and were trying to decide on an affordable way to do it, since Bradley would have to travel quite some distance to come see her. For obvious reasons, spending four days together in her *parent's home* was *not* going to be a viable option. I suggested that they find a modestly priced hotel that was within walking distance of restaurants and entertainment. Instead, they chose to spend the most important four days of their relationship in the *guest room of a friend's home.* The friends were certainly gracious and hospitable enough, but their home had paper-thin walls, three small children, a noisy macaw, two cats and a dog, which Bradley just happened to be *allergic to.*

Potential distractions should certainly be high on your list of considerations for your first meeting. Having friends or relatives around while you're trying to focus on your new partner can be *incredibly* distracting, even in the best of circumstances. You not only run the risk of them *disliking* or *criticizing* your potential new partner before you've even gotten to know him, but the *alternative* can be just as bad. They *may* like your new partner so much that you *can't get rid of them.* Other potential distractions may include such things as cell phones that never stop ringing, frequent texting, or an addiction to social media such as Facebook, Twitter or Tumblr.

First Meetings: Sheila's Story

When it comes to safety precautions for a planned first meeting, *regardless of the type of meeting,* it is important to remember that sometimes, when it comes to our own affairs, we are absolutely the *worst judges* of what may or may not be a potentially dangerous encounter. Our good judgment quickly becomes clouded by emotion and hope and we start to make critical mistakes, one of which is to *seriously* underestimate the magnitude and possible consequences of those mistakes.

When I caution friends to be wary and to take precautions prior to a first meeting, I'm sometimes told, "Don't worry, *that won't be necessary.* I've been chatting with this guy for *months;* I think I know him pretty well." One very pretty but incredibly naïve nineteen-year-old friend cockily assured me, "Nothing *bad* is going to happen!" When I asked her *how* she knew, she replied, "I know how to tell a guy *no,* if I need to." And, I believe her; *she probably does.* Unfortunately, there may be times and circumstances when *that simply isn't going to be enough.*

Take, for example, the case of Sheila, who was a hard-working, intelligent forty-five-year-old widow who lived in Pueblo, Colorado with her twenty-one-year-old daughter, Debbie. Her husband had passed away eight years previously from cancer, and she missed his companionship. Her daughter Debbie was confined to a wheelchair due to a spinal condition called *spina bifida,* and Debbie's care requirements kept Sheila at home most nights with only her internet chat room friends for company. She had just moved to Pueblo a few months earlier from Fullerton, California and hadn't yet made many friends in Colorado.

Eventually, through a personal ad and subsequent online chats, she became acquainted with John, a successful fifty-year-old businessman in Kansas City, Missouri. John was a lifestyle Dominant who was also a scoutmaster, tee-ball coach, Sunday school teacher, and had even been a member of the board of directors of a charitable organization that helped the handicapped. As far as Sheila was concerned, the fact that he was knowledgeable and experienced in the BDSM lifestyle and *financially secure* were just icing on the cake.

It didn't take very long for Sheila to fall head-over-heels in love with John. He seemed to be everything she had ever wanted in a mate;

incredibly smart, funny, successful *and* kinky. He told Sheila he had a job lined up for her in Kansas City. He even promised to support Sheila and Debbie financially, take care of their mounting medical bills, and pay for Debbie's therapy if they would be willing to move in with him. Sheila didn't have to be asked twice. She jumped at his offer. The last eight years had been exceedingly difficult, struggling to survive on the $1,016 per month she received from Social Security. Sheila and Debbie immediately began making preparations to move to Kansas City.

Sheila told her friend Nancy about her plans, and got lectured about the dangers of running off to meet someone that she only knew through internet chats and phone calls. Sheila told her friend that her ship had finally come in; John was her *dream come true* and no one was going to dissuade her from following her dream of a happy and secure life with him. Nancy truly *wanted* to be happy for her friend, but she was still very much concerned, and begged her to take precautions. A few days later, in the middle of the night, John arrived in Pueblo to take Sheila and Debbie back with him to Kansas City. Nancy never saw nor heard from her friend Sheila Faith, ever again.

No one knows for certain exactly *where* or *when* it happened, but at some point after he picked them up in Colorado and took them to Kansas, John raped and tortured both Sheila and her daughter Debbie and then killed them both with hammer blows to the head. John Edward Robinson, *who lived with his wife and four children* and was known in internet chat rooms as *SlaveMaster,* then loaded the bodies into two fifty-five-gallon drums and deposited the drums in a storage facility in Raymore, Missouri. He performed this task quickly and routinely, a natural consequence of the fact that he'd done this several times previously. *For the next six years* John Edward Robinson collected and cashed Sheila Faith's monthly Social Security checks, while he continued committing similar rape-torture-murders until his arrest on June 2, 2000.

John Edward Robinson is *known* to have murdered *at least* eleven women, and some investigators believe the actual number may be significantly higher. Sheila's story really wasn't much different from the stories of any of the other women who became his victims, the one glaringly tragic difference being that Sheila's misjudgments led to her daughter's death, as well as her own. Robinson found many of his victims in internet BDSM chat rooms and used highly sophisticated deceptions to gain their trust, stoke their emotions, and compromise their judgment by promising them the world. Even when his victims were *warned* to take precautions by friends and family, those warnings were invariably *ignored.* John Edward Robinson has never offered a confession, explanation, or even expressed an ounce of contrition for the murders and the many other heinous crimes that he committed. He is currently awaiting execution on death row at El Dorado Correctional Facility in Kansas

Bottom line: Knowing how to tell a guy *"no"* is not considered to be a particularly effective method of preventing hammer blows to the skull.

Safety Precautions

Realistically, the odds of your date turning out to be a serial killer are *quite low* and for *that,* we should *all* be eternally thankful. It is a sobering thing to note, however, that *many* of us have gone out and bought *lottery tickets* with a *one-in-a-million chance* of being a winner, thinking that *those were pretty good odds.* You may not be able to do much to improve your odds of winning the *lottery,* but there *are* some things that you can do to improve your chances of not only *surviving* your first meeting, but of *enjoying* it.

How can taking *safety precautions* help you to *enjoy* your first meeting? You just might be surprised at all the ways! First, it can help to silence those nagging little voices of doubt in the back of your head that make you wonder if you're doing the right thing, or exercising proper judgment. Second, it will help to reassure your friends and family (assuming anyone has any idea what you're about to do) that you are *not* a complete *idiot.* While you may not particularly *care* what they think, overly concerned friends and family have sometimes been known to do *crazy things* to protect you from your own worst instincts. The *last* thing you probably need is some sort of whacky family *intervention* right in the middle of what might otherwise have been a perfect first meeting! Finally, the fact that *you* took safety precautions can make your *partner* feel better about *you.* After all, there are essentially two kinds of people who *don't* take safety precautions: *stupid people*, and *predators*. Whenever *I* meet someone for the first time, and she tells me that she *hasn't* taken any safety precautions, I think, *"Seriously? Maybe she isn't as smart as I thought she was."*

Here are some simple safety precautions that you can take prior to your first meeting. For the most part, there isn't anything terribly complicated or difficult to accomplish about any of them. You may not be able or willing to do *everything* on this list but *any one of them* could save your life or, at the very least, ensure that there will be a trail to follow in the event you simply *vanish.*

Know Who You're Meeting

The first of our safety precautions probably seems as if it should be absurdly obvious to anyone with a lick of sense; however, there really is a big difference between *thinking you know someone,* and *really* knowing someone. A harsh reality that we don't like to think about is, we rarely ever truly know *anyone*, even when *we interact with them every day* in real life. John Edward Robinson, aka *Slavemaster,* lived with his wife and four children, arranged to be named "Man of the Year" by a charitable service organization, and had even been featured on the cover of a national trade magazine all while methodically raping and murdering at least eleven women. Over the course of almost twenty years, Robinson skillfully avoided becoming a suspect in the murders, but he *wasn't* as successful in avoiding being convicted of *dozens of other crimes*, to include theft, embezzlement, fraud, and forgery.

Robinson's long and well-documented history of criminal activity *was a matter of public record* and he was even sent to prison a few times. In fact, it is widely believed that Robinson met and seduced his *fourth* murder victim *while incarcerated* and serving time for fraud at the Western Missouri Correctional Facility. Her name was Beverly Bonner, and she was the prison librarian. Upon Robinson's release from prison in 1993, Beverly Bonner divorced her husband and moved to Kansas to be with Robinson, who promptly murdered her and then cashed her alimony checks for the next seven years. In June of 2000, her body was found in a drum at the same storage facility as Sheila and Debbie Faith's.

Could any of Robinson's many victims have avoided their fate by doing a little bit of research on the man they loved and *literally* trusted with their lives? We'll never know for sure. But one thing *is* certain; it is *far easier today* to check someone out online than it was just ten or twenty years ago. Whatever information you *do* have about the person you're meeting, *Google it.* Even phony information can reveal a lot of *real information*. Google his name, email address, mailing address, and phone number. Google his job, business, friends and family members. *Reverse Google* any photographs. With the proper use of quotation marks in your searches, you could even Google his *poetry,* or other writings. *Google it all.* You may not be able to immediately differentiate between true information and phony information, but *you can usually spot inconsistencies pretty easily.*

Another way to know who you're meeting is to tactfully *ask for personal references* from others who purportedly know the individual in real life. *Everyone* knows *someone.* If someone tries to tell you that he has *no* friends, acquaintances, family members, associates, clients or coworkers who would be willing to vouch for the fact that he is a real person with real community ties and *not* an axe murderer, then that should serve as a warning flag. He *doesn't* have to reveal his kinky lifestyle to those people. All he has to tell them is, "I'm meeting someone for the first time, and I thought that maybe some personal references might reassure her that I'm not an axe murderer. Would you mind if I gave her your phone number?"

Finally, if *all else* fails, you could always resort to the tried-and-true strategy of *blaming somebody else:* "This is stupid, but my best friend is really worried and won't let me come meet you until she sees a photo of your driver's license first. I tried to tell her that I trust you *implicitly,* but she just isn't budging. I really don't want to lose her as a friend over this. Can we do this just to shut her up?" He may or may not agree to it, but *either way,* his response will tell you a *lot.*

Clarify Expectations

Clarifying expectations may not seem like much of a safety precaution at first glance, but it can make a *huge* difference in how your first meeting turns out. Even if you honestly believe that you both fully understand the purpose and limits of the planned meeting, it certainly doesn't hurt to *confirm* what you think you both know. You *may* feel a little foolish doing so *(see the section below on being willing to do just that)* but no one ever really dies of embarrassment. People *do,* however, sometimes die of *stupidity.*

The most common reason for misunderstandings which could potentially lead to trouble involves one person's naive anticipation of *sex,* when it is neither warranted nor planned. Even though you may have been *asked to lunch*, made the date for *lunch*, meticulously planned every detail of the *lunch*, and even *enjoyed the lunch* with your date, it's entirely possible that your date is thinking, *"Great lunch, but can we just get to the sex part now?"* Some people simply have to have it spelled out for them in no uncertain terms. Here's one example of how you can phrase it: "I'm really looking forward to meeting you! I just want to be *absolutely clear,* though. No matter how much I *like you* or how much I may *want to*, there is simply *no way* we're going to be having *sex* on this first date. If that is going to be a problem, you need to tell me so *now*."

On the other hand, if sex *is* mutually understood to be part of the plan for your first meeting, you may *still* need to clarify the fact that *consent can be withdrawn at any time by either party.* Just because you've *discussed* having sex, *planned* on it, *anticipated* it and have every intention of following through with your plan doesn't mean that you can't *change your mind,* even at the very last second. You need to not only *trust your gut* when it comes to such things, but you also need to be able to trust your partner to understand that *no means no,* even if you're naked and tied to a chair.

Meet In a Public Place

Meeting in a public place isn't always going to be appropriate or possible, but whenever you *can* make it part of your plan, *you should do it.* Do it *even* if the plan is to go immediately to a hotel room and get naked. That way, in the event of trouble, at least *someone* will have seen the two of you together at some point. It's even possible that the meeting will be captured on a business establishment's security camera, which could be very helpful to the police, if they need to conduct any kind of an investigation. Award yourself big bonus points for actually knowing *ahead of time* where security cameras may be located, making that part of your plan, and letting a trusted friend know what to tell the police, if necessary.

Make Sure Someone Knows

Not everyone has friends who can be trusted with all of the sordid details of their kinky sex lives. That shouldn't stop you from letting *someone* know *where* you plan to be, *who* you plan to meet, and most important of all, *when you plan on returning.* Serial killer John Edward Robinson actually sent *forged letters,* purportedly from the murdered women to their friends and families, which essentially said, "Don't worry about me; I have a new job overseas and may be out of touch for a while."

Again, there's *rarely* any need to reveal *everything* about what you're planning to do. It should be relatively simple to limit what you say to, "I'm meeting someone new this weekend, and expect to be back on Sunday. Please call the police if I am not." The person you tell *may* indeed be curious about your plans and *may* even pepper you with questions, but you are really under no obligation to answer any of their questions. The important thing is to ensure that *someone* knows when you should be back.

Just knowing that you're late returning from your encounter or missing altogether may not be enough to assist the police in finding you or in figuring out what might have happened to you. If you prefer not to entrust a friend or family member with the details of your plan or with any information about your new friend, you can *still* leave a bonanza of information in a sealed envelope somewhere in your home or office where it will be found, in the event that you disappear. Another novel approach might be to *mail the envelope to yourself.* While it might be tempting to simply leave something like that *locked in your vehicle*, you should be mindful of the fact that anyone who might be holding *you* captive will also have the keys to your home and car, *and* all of the information contained in your wallet or purse.

Leave a Paper-trail

When police investigators begin reconstructing the events surrounding a possible disappearance, one of the first things they look for is any evidence of a *paper trail.* By that, we mean such things as bank deposits or withdrawals, credit card receipts, and even records of phone calls or texts. One way to leave a trail of bread crumbs that will be easy to follow is to use a debit or credit card, if at all possible, to make some sort of a purchase *during your meeting.* Even the simple act of placing a call from your cell phone can help police investigators to pinpoint your last known location.

Have a Backup Plan

It isn't enough to simply know that your well-laid plans may not come to fruition; you need to have a back-up plan that can be implemented when things go seriously awry. Not all of the John Edward Robinson's victims ended up being murdered. At least two women travelled separately to Kansas to meet Robinson in a hotel room, where they were bound, brutally raped, severely battered, photographed against their will, robbed of their money and belongings, and then abandoned for several days with no cash and no way home.

In each instance, Robinson returned to the hotel room several days later and gave the women a small amount of cash so they could return home, and gave them instructions to put all their belongings in storage and return to Kansas. *Incredibly, one of the women actually did so,* only to have him repeat his earlier performance, which caused her to contact the police. How either of them avoided being brutally murdered by this man is a mystery, but it may have been due to the fact that each had left a trail of breadcrumbs that led right to him, *and he knew it.*

Your back-up plan doesn't necessarily have to be the answer to, "What should I do if my date turns out to be an axe-murder?" Your back-up plan simply needs to be there for you in the event that *anything* unexpected or inconvenient happens. Your back-up plan should, at the very least, include knowing some important phone numbers and having ready access to emergency cash.

Most of us have gotten so used to being able to store important phone numbers in our cell phones, that we rarely memorize even our most commonly called numbers, anymore. How many of us would know how to contact our friends or extended family members if our cell phones were lost or *taken away from us?* If you have a poor memory for such things, you might want to secrete a few important phone numbers somewhere that would be accessible and available to you in *any* emergency. While in the military, I actually knew a few people who had important numbers unobtrusively *tattooed* somewhere on their bodies.

Learning how to get ready access to emergency cash if your wallet or purse is lost or stolen can be *exceedingly difficult,* but it *is* possible. Some banks, for example, have pre-scanned your identification into their computer system and so may not require you to show ID in order to conduct a financial transaction. Tellers are able to just pull it up on their computer monitors. Find out if your bank has a similar system. Many credit card issuers have special programs that are designed to help you out in the event that your wallet and credit cards are stolen. Give this problem some thought *before* it becomes an *emergency.*

Have Someone Check On You

Having someone check on you is critical. By having a friend or associate place a phone call to you at some point during your meeting, you greatly increase the odds that (1) you'll be missed, should you disappear, (2) you'll get timely assistance, if you need it and (3) the person you're meeting will realize that there is someone out there watching out for you. This knowledge *could* make him think twice about any plans to harm you.

Your arrangement of a safety check phone call should also include plans for what is commonly referred to as a "duress signal." A duress signal is a code-word that only you and your friend know, which tells your friend that she should immediately contact the police. Duress signals are designed to be used when someone is forcing you to lie and claim that everything is okay. To arrange a safety check and duress signal, simply tell a friend, "I'm meeting someone for the first time this evening. Would you please do me a huge favor and call my cell phone at around 7 PM? If I say anything about my *dog*, then you know you should call the police, *since we both know I don't own a dog."*

If you are not fortunate enough to have a friend or family member who can be trusted to check on you with a phone call, the next best thing is to *simulate one.* This can be accomplished in a number of ways. Perhaps the easiest, if you have a smartphone, is to download and use a free application that *simulates* receiving a phone call, often complete with a phony caller ID. These applications are typically used as pranks or to give busy people a plausible reason to bail out of a boring meeting, but it can also be used to create the illusion that someone is checking up on you. That, in turn, could save your life someday.

Another way to create the *illusion* of receiving a check-up phone call is to use your smartphone to *call yourself* from an internet phone service such as Skype, AOL, Yahoo, or Google-Talk. Most of these services have the option to make calls to a landline or cell phone, and though those options may not always be free, they usually cost just a few cents per call.

There are also a lot of web sites where you can register to receive free *wake-up calls.* They are designed primarily for people who are traveling and want to be awakened to catch a flight, or to make an early meeting, but they work just as well when you are wide awake and simply need your phone to ring at a specified time. To learn more about these services, just Google "wake up calls."

There's another thing you really should know about your safety and phone calls. Depending on where you are, and your particular service provider, calling 911 from a cell phone *may not always work* the way it would if you were calling from a landline. FCC regulations require that all wireless carriers transmit mobile 911 calls to "a Public Safety Answering Point" (PSAP), but *doesn't* require that the agency be *local* or even associated with *emergency services.* Additionally, calling 911 from a landline typically provides the dispatcher with your *exact location*; calling 911 from a mobile phone provides them only with the location of the *nearest cell phone tower.* What that means is you need to know how to tell an emergency dispatcher *where you are* by providing an address, landmarks, or street intersections.

Finally, if you'll be traveling to another city for your first meeting, use Google to find the phone number for the local police dispatcher there, and program that number into your phone for quick reference.

Be Willing to Make a Fool of Yourself

There is a rule of thumb that I've tried to follow for most of my life, ever since reading an article about what it takes to survive crimes, accidents, and disasters. The article examined the differences between the people who *survived* life-threatening situations, such as muggings or plane crashes, and those who *didn't* survive. Somewhat surprisingly, the critical difference between the survivors and those who didn't survive turned out to be a *willingness to react as if their lives depended upon it.* In other words, the people who were more concerned with *staying alive* than they were with *looking foolish* tended to be the people who lived to talk about it. Consequently, my rule of thumb became: *When in doubt or in possible danger, be willing to make a fool of yourself.*

Trust your gut. Do whatever it takes to secure your safety. Don't agree to *anything* that doesn't feel right to you, no matter how much you may want to avoid being embarrassed or embarrassing the other person. Don't worry about looking foolish, or about making a scene. The attention you draw *just might determine whether you live or die.* When your instincts tell you that you are in danger, *do the unexpected.* Make some noise. Fight back. Throw something through a window. Disable your vehicle or strike another vehicle with your car if you're being forced to drive somewhere. If you want to increase your odds of surviving a life-threatening situation, then you need to be willing to put up a fight or, at the very least, *call some attention to yourself.* Looking foolish should be the *least of your worries*, at that point. No one ever *really* ever dies of *embarrassment.*

An Ounce of Insurance

No, you're not going to find an actual *insurance policy* that covers first meetings that go horribly wrong. You *can,* however, get a great deal more mileage out of some of the *other* safety precautions you've taken, if the person you're meeting is *aware* that you're taking precautions. You definitely don't want to reveal the details of every safety precaution planned, but there's certainly nothing wrong with casually informing your new friend that you *are* taking some. If your new friend truly has your best interests at heart, he will be *glad* that you're taking a smart and cautious approach. On the other hand, if he was hoping you'd be an easy target, *he now knows otherwise.* Think of it as a final bit of insurance that helps to *prevent* bad things from happening.

After The Meeting

After the meeting, assuming you both survived and perhaps even had a great time, you'll probably have some *decisions* to make. The first should be coming to a mutual understanding, if not agreement, in answering the question, *"What just happened?"* It can be awfully easy to simply assume that because *you* had a great time that your *partner did too*, or that because it seemed obvious to *you* that the two of you *didn't* click, that it was just as obvious to your partner.

Differing perspectives, needs, and desires sometimes have a way of spawning completely different *interpretations* of the same events. The key to doing this successfully is to be frank and to avoid simply telling your partner what he or she *wants to hear.* Considering the fact that what you say now could end up being the foundation of your future real-life relationship, this is definitely not a good time to start sugar-coating the truth.

If you are able to come to some measure of mutual understanding about *what just happened*, the next logical step is to figure out *what it means.* For *some* people, a successful meeting might mean that *everything changes.* For some, it may be interpreted as a signal that you've crossed a significant *threshold* in the development of your relationship. Still others may feel that *nothing* has changed as a result. Don't allow the *success* of your meeting lead to a *misunderstanding* that could undermine your relationship. Conversely, if the meeting *wasn't* successful, it probably won't be hard to figure out what *that* means.

You should also be aware of a well-documented psychological

phenomenon called *"buyer's remorse."* It typically occurs after someone has made a major *purchase,* and then immediately begins to wonder if he *made the right choice.* He worries that he could have gotten it cheaper elsewhere, whether it's the right model, color or size, and about whether or not he can really afford it. In short, the buyer is quite simply *overwhelmed with doubts* about the wisdom of his decision. The very same thing can happen *after even the most successful first meeting.* If it happens to you or to your partner, *don't panic.* It's *perfectly normal.* This storm of self-doubt usually passes relatively quickly and, until it does, you should try to avoid making any rash decisions.

A successful first meeting really *can* be the first major milestone in a long and fulfilling D/s relationship, as long as expectations and events are properly managed, safety precautions are taken, and you have a mutual understanding of where you want your relationship to go from there.

May *all* your first meetings be great ones!

# # #

My Two Cents on First Meetings

"Scrabble?" Dee was struggling to contain her incredulity. "You want me to bring *a Scrabble game* to our first real-life meeting? Don't get me wrong, Master... I really do love playing Scrabble with you, but... *seriously?"*

I nodded toward the webcam and monitor that connected us across the 1500 miles that separated us. "Seriously," I replied. I could see that she was fighting an almost irresistible urge to ask *why*, but her training vanquished the impulse, and she responded with a simple, *"Yes, Master."*

Three days later, I was on a flight from Texas to North Carolina to meet Dee for the very first time. We'd met online, and in the course of the following six months, developed an open and trusting D/s relationship. Now, it was time to take the next step – to see whether our *online* chemistry would be able to survive the transition to *the real world*. During a flight layover in Atlanta, I texted, "Wear a nice little sundress, *without panties.* Bring a bottle of your favorite wine. Once I get there, I'll call you to give you the name of the hotel and room number."

"Yes, Master," came her reply.

After the final leg of my flight and a short taxi ride, I was finally at my hotel. I dropped my luggage, and made the call. "I'm at the Holiday Inn, room 216. The phone number to the room is (555) 626-0216. Write that information down, and make an additional copy. One copy, you should bring with you, and the other, you should leave on your kitchen table before you leave the house.

I also want you to tell a trusted friend that you're meeting someone for the first time, and you'd like her to call your cell later this evening. Arrange a code word that only you two will know; something that means, *"Help, I'm in trouble, call the police."* Please *do not* tell me what that code word is."

"Is all that really necessary, Master?" she asked. "I trust you. I know you would never do anything to hurt me." I told her *yes*, it was *absolutely* necessary.

"Be here at 5 PM. Oh, and by the way," I added, "I'd like to try something that I think will be fun. There will be *no speaking* for our first hour together. *Not one word.* Think you can do that?" She chuckled, as if to say, *only you could come up with something as crazy as that.* Instead, she simply replied, *"Yes,* Master. *I think I can do that."*

Three days later, as we lay entangled in the sheets of the bed, Dee propped herself up on one elbow and asked, "Master, what made you decide that we should spend our first hour together playing *charades?"* I laughed and said, "Well, I don't know about you, but I really hate worrying about what to say when I meet someone for the first time. So I figured, *let's just not say anything at all!"*

She giggled at that, then said, "And you told me to bring Scrabble, but we never played!"

I nodded. "Oh, *that,"* I replied, "Actually, I never intended for us to play any Scrabble. That was just your *security blanket.* I knew you loved Scrabble, so I made it your imaginary emergency back-up plan. It gave you confidence, and allowed you to believe that the *worst* that could happen is we could end up enjoying a few days together playing Scrabble."

"I once bought my kids a set of batteries for Christmas, with a note on it saying, toys not included."

- - *Bernard Manning*

CHAPTER 9: BDSM TOYS AND SAFETY

Typically, when *most* people think of BDSM, the first things that come to mind are the *awesome toys.* There is an infinite variety of implements that can be used in the many different kinds of BDSM play, with new concepts, designs and technology being added every day. In this chapter, we'll examine some of the basic types and examples of BDSM toys, equipment and furnishings, and discuss how they can be used *safely.*

Toy Tips

There are a few things that I think are important to touch upon before we get too wrapped up *(pun semi-intended)* in our examination of the *joys of kinky toys.* The first would be this one: As *exciting and wonderful* as these toys can be, they can't replace the human touch and they are piss-poor substitutes for real *relationships.* Perhaps my personal bias towards *meaningful D/s relationships* is showing here, but I *truly* believe that, *ideally,* these toys and their related activities are *best enjoyed with someone you love.* If *that* isn't possible, the next best thing is to enjoy them with a *good friend.* I'm not saying you shouldn't or wouldn't enjoy using them with *strangers*; *I'm just telling you where you'll get the best bang for your buck.*

The second tip I'd like to give you is this: Avoid becoming so focused on your *toys* that you begin to see *people* as *accessories.* A person with a *healthy* perspective thinks, "I love being with my girl; I can't wait to try out some of these news toys with her!" Conversely, someone with a *toy-focused* perspective thinks, "I love my new violet wand; I can't wait to try it out on *whomever."* It is, of course, perfectly *natural* to be excited about your new toys. But do try to remember that your toys should exist to please your partner; your partners don't exist to justify your toys.

The third word of advice concerns an unfortunate tendency among many in the BDSM lifestyle to equate sophisticated or expensive fetish equipment with *experience and judgment.* It's natural to believe that because people have the latest gadgets or top of the line fetish equipment, *that they know what they're doing.* But that *isn't* always the case. Be careful about assuming *anything* about potential play partners based simply on their toys. *They may not have a clue.* It is not uncommon for *some* people - typically people who have more money than common sense and who are relatively new to BDSM - to attempt to *purchase credibility* through their toys and equipment. They may not have any *experience* to speak of, but at least they can boast that they have the *best toys in town.* Just as some *vanilla folks* may use expensive cars and fine jewelry to *bolster or flaunt their social status*, there are a few BDSM folks who do the same with fetish toys and equipment. Owning a Rolls Royce doesn't necessarily make someone a good driver, and owning cool or expensive BDSM gear doesn't necessarily make him a good Top, either.

Fourth, and finally, you should understand the need to *fluid bond* certain types of fetish toys to specific individuals. *Fluid bonding* is the practice of ensuring that toys or equipment which come into contact with *bodily fluids* are reserved for the exclusive use of a *single person,* and *no one else.* Most of us instinctively understand this concept when it comes to things that are *designed* to come into contact with bodily fluids, such as vibrators, dildos and butt plugs. But how many of us can *truly say* that we know where a flogger, or riding crop, or even a length of rope has been? The problem is further complicated by the fact that porous materials, such as leather, wood and hemp, can be practically *impossible* to sanitize effectively.

This leaves us with two unpalatable options; one of them outrageously expensive, and the other absurdly unrealistic. The first option is to *always assume* that toys will come into contact with bodily fluids and to *fluid bond* certain toys to certain individuals. The logical consequence of this is you'll end up purchasing new equipment *each time you play with a new partner,* which can quickly get prohibitively expensive. The other option involves going to ridiculous lengths to *ensure* that your equipment doesn't *ever* come into contact with *anyone's* bodily fluids, under *any* circumstances. The only conceivable way to accomplish such a thing would be to play only with *fully-clothed individuals.* I don't know about *you,* but the realistic odds of that being *my* plan are pretty low.

So, what do *most* people do, when faced with these two dreadful choices? Most simply *do a little of each,* picking and choosing which toys will become fluid bonded and which will not, and taking extra care with the non-bonded toys to avoid bodily fluids of any kind, or to sanitize them as best they can when it becomes unavoidable. Is it a perfect solution? Not by a long shot. But for *most,* it's the only *practical* one.

Types of BDSM Toys & Equipment

We could *easily* fill several volumes discussing the many different kinds of BDSM toys that are available and how they can be used to best effect. Every day, new and exciting items are introduced, and it can be an exhausting task just trying to keep up with the latest technology and lifestyle trends. What follows is an admittedly *cursory* treatment, intended only to introduce the novice to the fascinating world of BDSM *hardware.* Readers who already have a great deal of experience with BDSM toys and equipment may find this section a bit tedious, and are invited to skip ahead to the next section.

For the sake of simplicity, we'll classify all BDSM toys and equipment into seven general categories: bondage, impact, piercing, sensation/sensory deprivation, torture, role-play accessories, and furnishings.

Bondage Gear

Bondage gear is primarily designed to restrict a person's mobility or functionality. The most *common* use for bondage gear is to restrain the arms and legs, however, it can also be used to immobilize or reduce the functionality of the head, neck, torso, hands, feet, and even *genitalia.* The quality of this kind of gear can range from *absolute junk* at the low end to *exquisitely crafted works of art* at the high end. Generally speaking, the comfort, durability and functionality of bondage gear purchased from *novelty stores* are usually *quite low*, since those establishments cater primarily to *vanilla* purchasers who are looking to *experiment.* For higher-end, better constructed bondage gear, your best bet is to patronize the specialty retailers that cater exclusively to a BDSM clientele.

The following is a list of some of the most common types of bondage gear you may encounter, in no particular order, with descriptions, purchasing tips and some observations on their safe use. Some types of *generic sex toys* are *not* listed here, so we can better focus on *BDSM-specific* items.

Wrist and Ankle Cuffs

Wrist and ankle cuffs are probably the first items that most novices think of and purchase when they begin experimenting with bondage toys. They come in a wide range of styles, designs and materials and can range in cost and quality from *"pretty, but completely non-functional"* to *"made-to-order awesomeness."* Typical wrist or ankle cuff designs consist of quality heavy-duty leather, stainless steel buckles for adjustments, and one or more D-rings to facilitate attachments. Some of the signs of an inferior product are poor leather quality, the use of non-colorfast dyes in the leather or other materials, flimsy or sloppy construction with sharp or rough edges, plastic or coated aluminum D-rings, or any disclaimer that states the product is *"for novelty use only."* That's *marketing-weasel-speak* which, in plain English means, *"you shouldn't expect this product to actually function."*

We should also include in this category a large assortment of handcuffs, thigh cuffs, thumb cuffs, shackles and even zip-ties. In addition to the obvious *psychological* impact of their use, all cuffs are designed to keep a person's limbs immobilized or dysfunctional, and they can *all* become a safety concern if not used correctly. Any time you use wrist or ankle cuffs *of any kind*, you should maintain *continuous supervision* of the bound person and make periodic checks of his or her extremities for loss of feeling, poor circulation, or unnecessary chafing, pinching or cutting. You should also be aware that the use of wrist and ankle cuffs can sometimes force a person's *body* into a position that causes difficulty in breathing, or *postural asphyxiation* - another good reason for maintaining that continuous supervision. Finally, it is *extremely rare* for wrist or ankle cuffs to be designed to bear any significant portion of a person's *body weight.* While it might be a wonderful *fantasy* to suspend a person by their wrists or ankles, *it is almost always a very, very bad idea to attempt to do so in reality.* Most wrist and ankle cuffs are *not* designed to support that kind of weight and frankly, *neither are most wrists and ankles.*

Collars

Collars, aside from their aesthetic and *symbolic value*, can also be an extremely erotic and versatile piece of bondage gear. When we are referring to a collar that is used primarily for *bondage* purposes, as opposed to *other uses*, we typically will refer to it as a *play collar.* The most common use for play collars is to immobilize the neck and often, by extension, the torso and head. Through the use of D-rings or other connectors, a collar can easily be attached to furnishings and equipment, or even to a person's own limbs in such a fashion that it forces the Bottom to assume a posture or position desired by the Top.

As for design and product quality, many of the same considerations we discussed in relation to wrist and ankle cuffs apply equally to collars. *Safety* considerations, however, deserve significantly *more* attention when it comes to collars, since the human *neck* is *particularly* vulnerable and the potential consequences of a mistake can be absolutely *catastrophic.* Continuous supervision is *absolutely* a must. Not only is *postural asphyxiation* always a danger, but *strangulation* can occur in the event of a mishap or poor product design. Collars should *never, ever,* be expected to support *any body weight at all* under any circumstances. In fact, it is *extraordinarily dangerous* to attach a collar to *anything* in such a way that an unforeseen event could cause the collar to choke or injure the wearer. The *last* thing you want is for a failed suspension or collapsing piece of fetish furniture to result in *a broken neck.*

Bondage Tape

Bondage tape is one of those relatively new developments utilizing technology that didn't even exist twenty years ago. This high-tech polymer tape, *which sticks only to itself and not to skin or hair*, was originally developed in the early-nineties as a *veterinary bandage,* since putting a traditional bandages on an animal's limbs or other body parts covered with *fur* could be somewhat *problematic.* Recently, in a stroke of *marketing genius*, the very same *veterinary products* have been rebranded, repackaged, marked-up in price 500%, and sold to the fetish community as *"bondage tape."* Only in America! I don't know about you, but success-stories like that *bring a tear to my eye.*

Bondage tape can be used to bind, gag, blindfold, or even mummify a person. It truly is one of those products that has a million and one uses, and is sure to bring out the *MacGuyver* in you. Most brands also have that glossy latex look that can add a bit of pizazz to just about any occasion.

One of the really nice things about bondage tape, aside from the fact that it *doesn't hurt* when you remove it, is its ability to *attach people to things* without leaving a sticky residue on *either,* and without pulling the paint or finish off of your cherished furnishings. Imagine, for example, being able to secure your Bottom's arms to the arms of your priceless antique armchair *without* having to worry about what the tape may do to the chair's finish. Anyone who has ever regretted using *duct tape* on his furniture knows *exactly* what I'm talking about here.

Bondage tape is also *reusable,* though the utility of reusable tape is directly proportional to your willingness and ability to *reroll it.* Another great advantage to using bondage tape is the fact that, for all intents and purposes, it looks exactly like any *other* big roll of tape. You may not consider this much of an advantage *now,* but just wait until the luggage screeners at the *airport* start pulling sex toys out of your suitcase in front of a crowd of strangers or, *worse,* in front of the *coworkers or associates you're traveling with.*

Bondage tape is a relatively safe product to use, as long as you adhere *(sorry, I just couldn't help myself)* to the safety guidelines we've discussed previously. There is, however, one unique aspect of using bondage tape that can sometimes be problematic. Some users are tempted, because the tape is somewhat *stretchy and elastic,* to apply it too tightly, which can restrict blood circulation. It should also go without saying that bondage tape should never be wrapped around a person's *neck,* or placed over his face in a way that might restrict his ability to breathe.

Sleeves

A BDSM sleeve is typically a long tube, constructed of soft leather, canvas or other heavy material, sewn closed at one end, and sporting one or more buckles or straps along its length. It is designed for the insertion and immobilization of one or both of a Bottom's arms, typically *behind the back.* Single-arm sleeves are most often used in *pairs*, with straps, buckles or D-rings used to attach one sleeve to the other. Dual-arm sleeves may consist of two separate arm-tubes permanently attached to one another, or a single large sleeve that is wider at the top and tapers toward the end where the Bottom's hands meet behind the back. Extra touches may include shoulder or chest straps to hold the sleeves up, wrist straps to secure the hands tightly, decorative lacing or buckles, and extra reinforcement of the sleeve for rigidity.

The odds of finding BDSM sleeves in your typical sex novelty store are pretty low. They tend to be available only from specialty retailers that cater to the fetish crowd, and can be somewhat pricy, ranging anywhere from $150 to $400, depending on the materials and quality of construction.

There are some real advantages to using sleeves. First, sleeves immobilize the arms in a way that wrist cuffs simply cannot. Wrist cuffs may be good at keeping a person's wrists *together,* but a flexible person will always still have plenty of room for movement. Second, sleeves take a great deal of stress off the wrists themselves, transferring and distributing most of the stress to the entire length of the arms, instead. This greatly reduces the chances of unintended pain or injury to the wrists. Third, sleeves with multiple straps, D-rings or other attachment points along their lengths provide a *multitude* of ways to integrate the immobilization of the arms into your overall bondage scene, and gives you more control of a Bottom's posture and positioning. Finally, sleeves have a unique aesthetic quality that ranks right up there with *Shibari* when it comes to artistic impact. In other words, *they look cool as hell.*

The potential safety concerns related to the use of sleeves include all that we've previously said about the need for continuous supervision and monitoring blood circulation and breathing. There are two additional concerns when it comes to the use of BDSM sleeves. The first is the fact that the hands are often *hidden from view*, which makes it harder to see if a person's fingertips are turning purple or blue from poor circulation. This can be further complicated by numbness in the extremities, which means the Bottom *may not realize that it is happening.* The Top should periodically squeeze the Bottom's fingers through the sleeve and ask about numbness or pain in the hands.

The second concern relates to the stress placed on the Bottom's shoulders, or as the medical geeks might describe it, where the *humerus* bone meets the *scapula* at the *glenohumeral joint.* Raising the attached arms too high behind the back, or placing too much stress on them can cause a dislocation or a partial dislocation, which is ironically called a *subluxation.* This is extremely rare, however, some individuals who have experienced dislocations before maybe particularly susceptible to reoccurrences. A Top should ask about any past history of shoulder dislocations before putting someone in a sleeve.

Mitts

BDSM *mitts* are pretty much exactly what you'd expect them to be: *mitts.* Think *oven mitt*, or *baseball mitt*, only a whole lot *kinkier.* BDSM mitts are typically made of leather or other heavy-duty materials, and are used to prevent a Bottom from using his or her hands and, most commonly, *to prevent masturbation.* Other common uses include immobilizing the wrists and hands by attaching them to other bondage gear, hobbling someone to make an assigned task near-impossible to accomplish, or for disciplinary or humiliation purposes.

You're not likely to find BDSM mitts in a typical sex shop or novelty store. You will probably have to get them from an online specialty BDSM retailer, where you can expect to pay between $100 and $200 for a pair, depending upon the workmanship and quality. Mitt designs can range from extremely simple to complex and multifunctional. Some come with inner liners, some don't. Some come with buckles, straps, zippers or locks, and some don't. D-rings are a common feature on most mitt designs, but some are designed to be load-bearing while others are not. Your best strategy in purchasing BDSM mitts is to have a clear notion of how you may want to use them in the future and to seek out the specific features that support that plan.

Safety considerations for the use of BDSM mitts are similar to those for cuffs and sleeves, though mitts may make it much more difficult to check a Bottom's fingertips to ensure proper circulation and feeling. Additionally, a very serious safety concern arises if someone is left alone at home for any length of time with *mitts locked onto her hands.* In the event of a real emergency, she could find herself unable to dial the phone, bandage a wound or even open the front door in order to escape smoke or fire.

Harnesses

A BDSM harness is a fairly generic term for just about anything that is worn about the torso, and to which you attach *other things.* A simple example would be a *dildo harness,* which is usually *(but not always)* worn around the hips and groin and is designed to hold a dildo in place for *pegging.* Other common types of harnesses include cock and ball torture harnesses, chastity harnesses, purely decorative body harnesses, and specialty bondage harnesses. Some harnesses are designed to be used *only* with other types of equipment, fetish furniture, frames, hoists, swings or devices. In short, a harness can refer to *damn near anything* that attaches your body to *something else.*

Straitjackets

Straitjackets have come a long, long way in the past few decades. The boring but classic beige canvas straitjacket that most of us have seen only in the movies has recently been joined by a wide assortment of new straitjacket designs in all-new materials and hot new colors. The classic straitjacket consists of a canvas garment top that closes in the back and has overly long sleeves which, when worn, are crossed over the chest and then tied or buckled in the back, which prevents the wearer from using his arms and hands.

The *newer* designs, which are more appropriate for *recreational* users, rather than *criminally insane* ones, are typically made with leather, latex rubber, PVC or a combination of those materials. Minor variations in their design can include arms that cross in the back instead of across the chest, the addition of wrist or crotch straps, breast-access zippers, built-in toy harnesses, built-in chastity belts, and sturdy closures or fasteners that will accommodate padlocks. Straitjackets make wonderful conversation pieces, and can always serve as the punch line to any joke questioning your sanity. They also happen to be one of the few forms of bondage that even vanilla people will line up to try at a party.

Straitjackets tend to fall into two general price categories: expensive, and *ridiculously* expensive. An authentic, old-fashioned heavy-canvas straitjacket will set you back roughly $200, but a latex rubber or PVC straitjacket can cost anywhere from $700 to $2,000 depending on the quality of workmanship and your selection of bells and whistles in the design.

As far as safety goes, straitjackets should be worn loosely enough to permit some movement and allow for proper blood circulation in the arms. If a straitjacket is worn for long periods of time, it can result in numbness in the arms or the pooling of blood and swelling in the elbows. When straitjacket-related injuries *do* occur they are, more often than not, the result of the wearer falling or striking nearby furniture while thrashing around in an attempt to *escape from it.*

Rope, Straps & Chain

What good are all those collars, cuffs and sleeves, if you can't *attach* them to anything? *That's* where the rope, straps and chains come into play. We can categorized them all by *functionality* as *connectors*, but that's pretty much where the similarities end.

Let's start with rope. When it comes to bondage, rope isn't always used strictly for simple bondage or just as a connector; it can also be used in the more advanced stand-alone bondage art commonly referred to as *shibari or kinbaku.* Both are Japanese terms which came into general usage in the West in the 1990s. *Shibari* refers to the generic art of *intricate knot-tying*, while *kinbaku* refers to the *erotic application* of the same skill. The types of rope traditionally used in shibari and kinbaku are jute (made from cellulose and lignin fibers), hemp (derived from cannabis plant fibers), and linen (which is woven from flax and sometimes cotton fibers), and various new synthetic fibers.

The type of rope you purchase for your BDSM activities should depend on what you plan to do with it. For most simple bondage play, solid nylon or cotton braid rope that is 3/8" or 7/16" in thickness is usually a good choice. Solid braid cord is often preferred over twisted braid for its ability to hold its shape when twisted into complex or twisted shapes. It also eliminates the need to remove the core from a twisted braid, since leaving the core can make it more difficult to tie secure knots; a 3/8" twisted braid rope with the core removed becomes a 1/4" *hollow tube.* For more advanced rope play, to include kinbaku and suspensions, jute or hemp is typically the preferred type of rope. A simple rope kit for novices should include two pairs of 10-foot lengths, one pair of 30-foot lengths, and at least one 50 to 60-foot length of rope. Rope pricing will vary widely, depending on the type of rope, braid, length, color, and any other unique properties. Rope that is specifically produced and sold for shibari purposes can be quite pricy.

Straps are often used in lieu of rope in some kinds of BDSM bondage play. Since straps are difficult to *knot*, they are used primarily as connectors or restraining devices. For most types of bondage play, the same kinds of nylon or canvas cargo straps that you would purchase from any hardware store to secure items to your car or truck will work just fine. They come in a variety of utilitarian styles, which include ratcheting straps, flexible rubber straps and straps with built-in D-rings or O-rings. You *can* get specialty straps designed specifically for BDSM play from many fetish retailers but, for the most part, they offer no significant advantages over the hardware store variety and tend to be far more expensive.

Chain, like the *riding crop*, is an iconic symbol of BDSM with a reputation which *may or may* not be entirely well-deserved. It is exceptionally good at supporting heavy loads, has great aesthetic qualities, and the *psychological* impact of chain is undeniable. On the *other* hand, chain can be heavy, unwieldy, and difficult to lug from place to place. Additionally, chain can oxidize or rust over time, which means it should be stored appropriately and lubricated at regular intervals. Adjusting the length of a chain typically requires heavy tools, and connecting a chain to *anything else* usually involves the use of hooks, shackles, pin-anchors, clevises, lock-links, snap links, carabiners, or padlocks.

For very short lengths of chain which can be used creatively in a wide variety of ways, consider purchasing several lengths of stainless steel or chrome-plated *dog choker chains* from your local pet store or big-box retailer. These herringbone-style chains typically range in length from 8” to 28” and have strong O-rings suitable for snap-links at each end. They’re very affordable, lightweight, attractive, and extremely useful in all sorts of ways, particularly as connectors between cuffs and equipment or furniture. For more traditional types of chain, simply decide on the lengths and number of segments you’ll need and visit your local hardware store to talk to a salesperson about how to cut the spooled chain to the lengths you want to purchase.

Ropes, straps and chains each have their own unique safety concerns that are the natural consequence of their design and utilization. Ropes, for example, are far more likely to be wound around portions of the body than straps or chains, and therefore pose a greater risk of impeding a person's circulation or causing strangulation.

Straps, on the other hand, may have hardware attached such as ratcheting gears that enable a strap to be tightened down very securely. A securing strap that is ratcheted down just a little too tight could easily suffocate a person through postural asphyxiation. It certainly doesn't help that some of these ratcheting devices can be exceptionally difficult to release or loosen once there is a lot of tension on the strap. Always be sure to test out any strap-ratcheting mechanism - especially the *quick release*, if there is one - on an inanimate object before tightening one down on a live person.

Chain presents us with a completely different set of concerns. Some types of chain can have an annoying tendency to *pinch the skin* under certain circumstances and, depending upon the degree of force applied, those pinches can sometimes turn into *cuts and lacerations*. Chain can also sometimes unexpectedly kink or bind in ways that alter the length of the chain in unforeseen ways. Obviously, if a length of chain that you were counting on to be a three-foot segment suddenly kinks up and turns into a two-foot length, it could be a potential problem. Chain is also incredibly *unforgiving.* There's absolutely no flexibility in a length of chain, and rarely any padding to cushion or protect vulnerable parts of the body such as wrist joints, ankle joints, hip bones, tail bones, or ribs from harm. You should always closely monitor the spots where the chain comes into contact with bare skin, keeping a close watch for binding, bruising, pinching or any other *unintentional* discomfort.

Another tip to keep in mind when using chain: some people can be *very sensitive* or even *allergic* to certain types of *metal* that come into contact with their skin. This sensitivity is common in women who are unable to wear *jewelry* that is made from anything but *gold.* In rare cases, even *gold of low purity* will trigger a skin reaction or infection; those women can only wear 18k or 24k gold jewelry. Try to imagine how the skin of someone *who can't even wear pure silver jewelry* might react when it comes into contact with a chain made from a *mystery metal* alloy and coated with unknown chemical compounds used to deter rust in some backwater third-world nation.

Spreader Bars

Spreader bars are BDSM bondage devices which are designed to do one thing and one thing *only:* keep a Bottom's legs spread wide apart to provide easy access to his or her *naughty-bits*. Spreader bars can range in design and quality from the homemade variety at one end of the spectrum to expensive, yet wonderfully functional *works of art* at the other end of the spectrum. The one thing they all have in common is their basic design; a spreader bar is essentially just a stick with rings at each end, to which *ankle (or sometimes, wrist) cuffs* may be attached.

Lots of do-it-yourself kinksters construct their own homemade spreader bars simply by cutting a wooden broomstick or garden tool handle to the proper length, screwing sturdy eye-bolts into each end, and sanding down or covering any rough edges. Homemade spreader bars may not win any *art awards* but, for the most part, they work just like the *high-end* variety. If, on the other hand, you prefer *not* being reminded of your spreader bar's previous life as a *kitchen mop* each time you use it, then you might want to consider shelling out $50 to $150 on one from an online specialty retailer.

Top-of-the-line spreader bars often come with a variety of ingenious features that you probably won't see on your typical mop-handle models. Those features and accessories may include the ability to adjust the length of the spreader bar as needed, swivel connectors at each end, designs that allow for disassembly into a very small package, built-in cuffs or shackles, customized locks, or the ability to attach other bondage accessories or parts of the body along its length. Spreader bars are typically constructed with steel or aluminum pipe, but can also be made from any sturdy material, such as wood or PVC pipe.

There are few safety concerns, to speak of, that are specific only to spreader bars, other than a recommendation that you check your subject's toes periodically for adequate blood circulation and numbness.

Chastity Belts

Chastity belts have been around for a very long time, although there is quite a bit of disagreement about *how* long and whether their *actual use* was consistent with the common myths about them that have persisted through the ages. Since none of that is really pertinent to our discussion here, we'll just *skip* the *history* lesson and go straight to the good stuff. It is probably worth noting, however, that chastity belts have been and continue to be used for *non-BDSM purposes* in various parts of the world. In 1998, race riots in West Java compelled a significant number of ethnic Chinese women to wear chastity belts fitted with combination locks in public in order to avoid being raped by roving gangs of thugs. In 2007, the Asian Human Rights Commission published a study claiming that some women were being forced to wear chastity belts in rural parts of India. And in 2008 in Batu, Indonesia, women who were employed in massage parlors were required by local authorities to wear locked chastity belts to prevent them from engaging in prostitution.

The modern chastity belts which are used in *BDSM play* come in both male and female versions and in a wide range of styles. They can be designed for a variety of purposes, which may include preventing sexual intercourse, oral sex, stimulation or masturbation, preventing the removal of *other* devices or attachments, preventing or controlling urination or defecation, preventing an erection, or as a harness to restrict a person's movements. They are commonly constructed from leather, PVC, or steel and can range in price from $50 to *thousands* of dollars. In 2002, a manufacturer in Cape Town, South Africa sold a *gold* chastity belt decorated with *diamonds and pearls* to an English customer for the equivalent of $16,000 USD.

One of the more popular types of chastity belts used in BDSM play is the kind that serves as a *reverse dildo harness.* Unlike a traditional dildo harness, which holds a dildo in place to facilitate *pegging a partner,* these chastity belts are designed to hold the dildo, vibrator or butt plug in place *inside the wearer* of the device, and prevents it from being removed. Another popular type of chastity belt is designed primarily for the prevention of masturbation, and is used by some D/s couples as a form of discipline or in *orgasm control play.*

When purchasing a chastity belt, you should always pay particular interest to what materials are used in its construction, and whether any attachments or accessories such as locks, links, wrist cuffs, dildos, plugs, or liners are included in the purchase price. Some designs will *only* function with additional equipment, such as *padlocks,* which may or may not be part of the deal. I know of at least one design that can't be worn *at all* without using *six additional padlocks.* Something like that could easily add $50 to $150 to the price of your chastity belt purchase.

Chastity belts have some very *unique* safety concerns which you should definitely be aware of before purchasing or using one. First, a chastity belt - regardless of whether it is a male or female version - is designed to come into contact with *bodily fluids.* It should, therefore, be *fluid-bonded* to a single individual, if at all possible. Keep in mind the fact that, if it is constructed of anything other than *stainless steel,* it will be near-impossible to adequately sterilize between uses. A chastity belt that is designed to hold dildos or butt plugs may also be susceptible to *cross-contamination* from the toys that it comes into contact with. Not only can this be a problem when it comes to chastity belt being used by more than one individual, but it can *also* be a potential concern for a *single user* if it allows harmful bacteria to be transferred from the anus to her vagina.

A second potential safety concern involves the *prolonged* wear of chastity belts. Typically, chastity belts are used for short periods of BDSM play or discipline. Unfortunately, there's always *someone* who pushes the limits of good sense and tries to keep his sub, slave or bottom in a chastity belt for extended periods of time. *This is almost always a very bad idea*. While it's true that a chastity belt *can be* very good at keeping penises, hands and toys *out* of the wearer's crotch, it can also be very good at *keeping harmful bacteria in* and creating the perfect environment for serious bacterial infections. There are no hard and fast rules for *how long is too long* when it comes to wearing chastity belts, but it's generally a good rule of thumb to ensure that it doesn't interfere with the wearer's routine personal hygiene.

The third and final tip is not so much a *safety* concern as it is a *personal dignity* concern. Never forget that it can sometimes be harder to *unlock* a lock, than it is to *lock it.* People sometimes do stupid or malevolent things. Keys get lost, jammed or broken off in the keyhole. Combinations get forgotten. Locks can malfunction. When something like that happens to you *while wearing a chastity belt,* it can add a whole new dimension to your predicament, depending upon where you are, who you're with, and whether you have ready access to a heavy-duty set of bolt-cutters. One woman found herself wishing she had thought of that when her steel chastity belt, which her husband had padlocked onto her just before she left for the airport, set off security alarms as she passed through the metal detectors in December, 2003. She explained to the authorities that her husband had put her into the device because he was convinced she intended to have an extra-marital affair. Eventually, she was allowed to board the flight while still wearing her steel chastity belt, but if she thought her embarrassment would be over at the end of her travel itinerary, she was wrong. Six weeks later, she was mortified to learn that the incident had been reported in USA Today to the bemusement of millions of readers.

Miscellaneous Household Items

Invariably, when people first discover the joys of bondage, they begin to see ordinary household items in *a whole new light.* Suddenly, that dog chain is no longer just a *pet accessory*; it's *bondage gear.* It becomes hard to look at a mop handle without thinking: *spreader bar.* And, of course, all of those tools and gadgets in the garage offer up *endless possibilities.* If such thoughts are dancing through your head *right now,* you can rest assured that it's a *perfectly normal thing*; we've *all* been there. That doesn't necessarily make it *safe,* however.

The biggest danger in converting ordinary household items to BDSM use comes from subjecting items to stresses and conditions for which they were never designed. A dog leash that was designed to prevent a Yorkshire terrier from running into traffic simply isn't meant to support the weight of an adult human being. Attempting to use it in that fashion can result in serious injury. Twine is designed to wrap packages, *not* for binding wrists and ankles. Using twine for bondage can lead to painful cuts and blocked circulation. Belts are designed to *look good* and *hold up your pants*. They make *lousy* bondage accessories.

Just to be clear, I don't believe there's anything wrong with improvising your own BDSM bondage gear from ordinary household items. For example, I happen to be a huge fan of using ordinary *Saran Wrap* for an entertaining, playful and eminently *affordable* bondage scene. I would simply caution you, however, to be fully aware of the limitations of the items and materials that you are using, and to take proper precautions. *When in doubt, rule it out.*

Impact Gear

BDSM *impact gear* is used in kink activities that involve striking the body with an implement of some sort, *usually - but not always* - to cause *pain.* People also engage in impact play for a variety of other reasons. Those reasons may include role-play, humiliation, discipline, sensation play, the marks that they leave, the sounds that they make, and even for *therapeutic* reasons! Each type of impact toy has its own unique qualities and the impact sensations associated with their use can often be adjusted in intensity along a scale ranging from *painless* at one end to *extremely painful* at the other. For me, the truly fascinating thing about impact gear is that sometimes, an item can *look a whole lot scarier than it really is* while, other times, an item can actually *be a lot more painful than it looks.* Appearances can *definitely* be deceiving, when it comes to impact toys.

Floggers

A flogger typically consists of a short-handled whip with multiple tails or strips of leather, which are called "falls." A flogger may also sometimes be referred to as a lash, scourge, or cat o' nine tails. The most common designs are made from high-quality leather, but they can literally be made from just about *anything.* I have seen floggers constructed from a wide variety of animal hides, including elk, elephant, stingray, kangaroo, sharkskin, bison and Russian boar. In addition to common and exotic hides, some flogger designers create their falls from fur strips, chain-mail, horse hair, strings of beads, and other unusual materials.

The quality and workmanship of floggers available commercially can range from *novelty trash* to exquisitely priceless *one-of-a-kind items.* At the extreme *low end*, you can find *novelty floggers* in most neighborhood adult novelty shops. These items are typically mass-produced imported novelties designed more for their *comic value* than for their *functionality;* their durability is often so bad, they fall apart the first time you actually attempt to use them. If you decide to purchase a novelty flogger of this sort, you'll likely be *wasting* $20 to $70 of your hard-earned money. At the *other* end of the spectrum, you can find unique and beautiful works of art, each constructed lovingly by hand by skilled craftsmen from a variety exotic materials. A flogger like *that* can *easily* set you back $400 to $1500. *Most* of us, at least for our *first few* flogger purchases, will typically settle for something *between* those two extremes.

The type of flogger you purchase should be commensurate with the type of sensations you want the flogger to deliver. The impact sensations of being flogged can range from *"thuddy"* at the low-end of the pain scale, to *"thwappy"* or *"slappy"* in the middle, and on to *"stinging"* or *"biting"* at the high end of the scale. The sensations can also be varied a great deal by adjusting the distance from the subject, changing the way the flogger is swung, and increasing or decreasing the amount of force of the swing. Generally speaking, the closer to the subject you stand, the *thuddier* the strikes will be. The further from the subject you are, the more *stinging* the strikes will be.

One of the most common misconceptions about floggers is the assumption that being struck with one will always be a painful experience. In actuality, most people describe the experience of being flogged as a pleasant or even *therapeutic* sensation, often equating it with a low-impact *massage*. Of course, a flogging can *always* easily be delivered in a painful way, if that is your personal preference. Floggers tend to be one of those BDSM items which *look* a lot scarier than they really *are* and, for that reason, are valued as much for their *psychological* impact as for their *physical* impact.

The use of a flogger doesn't typically raise many safety concerns, aside from the obvious ones. Have a safe word. Avoid breaking the skin. Watch for sharp or rough edges or foreign objects entangled in your flogger's falls. Give yourself plenty of room to swing the flogger, and be particularly mindful of overhead lighting which, if struck accidentally, could shower you in broken glass. If a flogger is going to be used on a subject's genitals, his or her bodily fluids *will* come into contact with the falls, which can be difficult, if not impossible, to properly sanitize. If doing so is a *conscious decision* and your plan is to fluid-bond the flogger to that individual, *that's fine.* But if it happens *inadvertently* or without much thought for the consequences, then you may end up having to purchase another flogger or, at the very least, with an unpleasant ethical dilemma on your hands.

Paddles

The types of paddles used in BDSM impact play, like many of the other items we've discussed, can range in style and workmanship from *novelties* to sophisticated instruments of pain and intimidation. The design of most paddles is pretty simple and straight-forward, consisting generally of a short plank of wood or other rigid material, wide at one end to form the *blade*, and narrower at the other end to form the *handle*. Wood is the most commonly used material in the construction of paddles, but they can also be made from metal, bamboo, plastic, carbon-fiber composites, and other synthetic materials. Design variations may include altering the size and shape of the paddle, adding holes to enhance the swing speed and strike of the paddle, cutting shapes or letters into the blade so that it leaves a unique pattern on the subjects skin, and using special or rare types of wood to enhance the weight, strength or beauty of the paddle. Paddles may be designed to be held in one hand, or swung with *both* hands.

When purchasing a paddle, personal preferences will typically dictate most of your choices, since the *functionality* of a paddle is rarely called into question. It is for that reason that a paddle's aesthetics and appearance often take on greater importance in the buying decision. Certain types of wood can lend a certain elegance and beauty to a paddle that otherwise appear very ordinary. Some of the more unique and attractive woods used in the construction of paddles include oak, bamboo, maple, black walnut, hickory, mahogany, teak, South American monterillo, Bolivian rosewood, African padauk, and African bubinga.

It's interesting that, for such a commonly used and simply constructed item, the safety concerns regarding paddles could probably fill an entire chapter. You might think that some of these safety tips are simply a matter of *common sense* but, unfortunately these days, there's nothing common about common sense.

When using a paddle, always strike using the flat side of the paddle blade, *never* with the edge. Striking with the blade perfectly parallel to the skin surface ensures that the force of the strike is evenly distributed across the full length and breadth of the paddle blade. If there is even the *slightest angle* which deviates from the parallel, the strike could be far more painful than intended, and might even cause serious or permanent damage. A full-force *edge strike* from a paddle could easily break a bone or sever nerves and tendons.

It's also very important to focus your paddle strikes to the muscled or fatty tissues of the body. By that, we mean the buttocks, thighs, breasts, shoulder blades and certain portions of the torso. Avoid bony areas, such as the arms, shoulders, shins, hips, hands and feet, and critically vulnerable areas like the spinal column, kidneys, neck and head. The most common targets for paddle play are the buttocks and the backs of the thighs, and it is not uncommon for people to simply *assume* that those will be your targets. If your plan involves striking *other* parts of the body, then it's extremely important that you discuss those plans with the person who'll be on the receiving end of the paddling.

Even well-padded areas of the body, such as the buttocks, can become problematic under certain circumstances. Certain body positions can sometimes pull the body tissues taut, reducing the amount of soft tissue providing natural padding, making bone and nerve tissues more vulnerable. If the sciatic nerve, which runs from the lower spine *through the buttocks* and down the legs, becomes irritated or compressed, it can lead to an *extremely painful* condition called *sciatica.*

Paddling the breasts, if it is done at all, should be done with a lighter instrument. Prior to engaging in any breast paddling, a discussion should take place with the bottom to determine whether she has a personal or family history of fibroids in the breasts. There have been studies published which seem to establish a connection between impact play to the breasts and the growth of fibroids in the breast tissue. Fibroids are not inherently dangerous to a woman's health, but they can result in false positives in mammograms and may affect the aesthetic appearance of the breasts.

Any impact play focused on the *genitals - male or female* - should be approached with a *great deal of caution,* not to mention forewarning and frank negotiation. Even if a bottom agrees to or even *craves* it does *not* necessarily mean it's *a good idea.* Impact play aimed at the genitals can not only be *extremely painful*, it can sometimes result in irreversible damage to a person's reproductive organs.

Whatever type of paddle you use there will *always* be a possibility of damage to the bottom's *skin.* Some paddles are constructed with holes in the blade to reduce air-drag and increase the speed and force of the blows, which can increase the probability of skin damage, as well. Beginners are sometimes quite surprised to see that a freshly paddled part of the body which appears to be harmlessly red *immediately after* the paddling can turn alarmingly *purple, black and blue within a few hours.* In other rare cases, large water blisters or blood blisters may appear, and skin may simply peel away or slough off. Every individual has a uniquely different skin type and impact tolerance, and the skin's durability may even differ widely from place to place on the same body. Obviously, the skin on the soles of your feet can take a lot more abuse than the skin on your *inner thighs.*

Our skin is the largest organ of the human body, and damaging it can interfere with a number of important functions that are critical to your health. Some of these functions include *sensation, heating or cooling* of the body through blood circulation or perspiration, and protecting the underlying tissue from infection. Damage to the skin - even if it isn't serious or permanent damage - can interfere with these and other critical functions which, in turn, can lead to serious health issues. For example, many people are tempted to discount the severity of blistering or skin sloughing by thinking, *"No problem; it will grow back."* But the issue isn't *whether it will grow back*; of course it will. The real issue is whether serious infection will gain a toehold in the body, and whether there will be scarring or long-term nerve damage.

Finally, if a paddle has ever caused a bottom's skin to become raw to the point where it appears that the pores of the skin are oozing tiny droplets of blood, then your paddle has come into contact with bodily fluids and should be thoroughly sanitized or fluid-bonded to that individual. Fortunately, paddles are typically a lot easier to sanitize than many other types of BDSM toys.

Whips

A whip can sometimes refer to a very wide range of BDSM toys, including floggers, lashes, cats-o'-nine-tails, and crops. Since we discuss each of those variations separately elsewhere in this section, we'll confine our discussion here exclusively to *single-tail whips,* which come in three basic styles. They are *stock whips, bullwhips, and snake whips.*

A *stock whip* is characterized by a long rigid handle that is not integrated into the lash, but is instead connected to the lash by a leather swivel-joint called a *keeper.* Many *buggy whips* and *horse whips* also fall into this category. Generally speaking, stock whips have a short rigid handle, and a lash that can range from three to ten feet in length. The Australian stock whip is a variation on this style, and has a longer handle and a lash made exclusively from kangaroo hide. A stock whip is used primarily for the noise that it makes; it is the easiest type of whip for creating the classic *"crack of the whip"* sound that many of us associate with whips in general. The sad reality is it can actually be quite difficult to replicate; it may look easy in the movies, but that's because it is almost always *a sound effect added later.* Stock whips are easy to use and make a wonderful sound, but are the *least accurate* type of single-tail.

The bullwhip is the type of whip that most people associate with *Indiana Jones.* The handle is generally short and integrated by braiding into the lash, which can be up to twenty feet long. At the end of the lash, you may also have a small strip of leather that serves as the *fall,* or business end of the whip. The *fall* is the part of the whip that is expected to actually strike the target. There may also be a small strip of cord or string called a *cracker or popper,* which is designed solely for the purpose of making it easier to produce the whip crack sound. The bullwhip is probably one of the *best-known* and iconic types of single-tail whip, but it is also one of the most difficult to learn to use effectively and accurately.

A snake whip is a whip with no rigid handle, which means the entire whip can be coiled up like a snake, hence the name. The most commonly used type of snake whip in the BDSM culture is the blacksnake whip, which is characterized by a heavy weighted handle or butt-end of the whip filled with lead ball shot or ball bearings. The weighted interior can sometimes extend as far as three-quarters down the length of the entire whip. Because of the weighted butt of the whip, that end can also be used as a blackjack or flexible club.

Purchasing a quality whip can be a daunting task for anyone who may be doing so for the first time. Novices are usually advised to start with a four or five-foot bullwhip, and plan to move to a longer one once their skills improve.

The advantages to starting with a shorter whip include lower cost, greater throw control and accuracy, it's less fatiguing to use during practice, and it requires less clearance space to use it safely. The skills and techniques that you perfect with a shorter whip can easily be applied to a longer whip later on.

Like any other leather implements, whips can vary widely in quality and workmanship. Beware of purchasing certain cheap *imitation* whips that are produced primarily in Mexico for the *tourist trade.* Many of them may *look* pretty *bad-ass*, but they are produced for *decorative purposes only,* and will likely not *work* like the real thing, nor *last* much beyond their first use. If it's being sold out of a souvenir store, that should be your first clue that it's just *tourist junk*. To purchase a *quality* whip, consider online specialty retailers that cater to those in the BDSM lifestyle and are *reputable.* A decent four-foot bullwhip will set you back $100 to $300.

The safety considerations related to the use of whips are similar to the ones previously discussed for floggers and paddles, with a few additional ones that are unique to single-tail whips. The longer the whip is, the less accurate it is going to be. That means you're going to strike places that you didn't intend to strike, which can be far more problematic with a whip than it would be with a flogger or paddle. You should never forget a whip makes a cracking sound *because its tip is breaking the sound barrier.* When something moving *that fast* hits a person where it shouldn't, *bad things can happen.* A whip is capable of producing more than just a *painful impact;* it can sometimes *cut like a knife.*

If you are learning to use a single tail whip, I recommend that you wear safety glasses or goggles, a wide brim hat, and a long-sleeve shirt. You *will* end up striking *yourself,* probably more than a few times. If you protect nothing else, *protect your eyes.* Being struck in the eye by a piece of leather traveling in excess of 340 mph *will blind you.*

You should also be mindful of any small, loose objects which may be lying about anywhere within the reach of the tip of your whip. A piece of gravel or any other small object can instantly be transformed into a dangerous projectile if it is struck by the fall of your whip.

A fast-moving whip can cause a lot of damage if you're not careful. While practicing, always clear a circle around you with a radius equal to the length of your whip *and then some,* and remember that you'll need the same amount of clearance *over your head, as well.* Forgetting to extend that safety zone *vertically* as well as horizontally can result in damage to ceilings or overhead light fixtures.

While you are still working on perfecting your skills, try to resist the temptation to make a *real live person* your target or, for that matter, placing *anyone* anywhere *near* your targets. Even after your accuracy has greatly improved, you may still want to have your partner wear eye protection and other protective clothing as appropriate until you can guarantee that an errant throw isn't going to take out an eye.

Crops

Crops, which are sometimes referred to as riding crops or horse whips, typically consist of a long, slender and flexible shaft which is thicker and reinforced at one end to form a handle and has, at the other end, a tongue of leather, neoprene or cord called the *keeper.* The traditional shape of the keeper can be a square, rectangle, circle, half-circle, fiddle, or half-fiddle. Keepers can also come in a variety of novelty shapes, as well. The flexible shaft adds leverage and speed to the strike, while the keeper is designed to come into contact with the target. Occasionally, you'll encounter a *split keeper*, which consists of *two* strips of leather designed to maximize the *sound* of the keeper's impact upon your subject's skin, or a *looped keeper*, which delivers a less painful strike. The traditional riding crop has long been favored as a practical fashion accessory by Dominatrices and used extensively in BDSM *pony play*, but it also makes a versatile play accessory for just about anyone interested in rounding out their impact toy collection.

Most crops are produced and sold primarily for the purpose of *horse training*, and are readily available in a variety of styles at most ranch and farm supply stores. Quite often, the very same crops that are offered there for $10 to $15 are purchased in bulk by kink toy retailers and resold at twice or even three times the original retail price. By the same token, there *are* plenty of craftsmen who produce similar products specifically for a BDSM clientele, and those crops are often enhanced with extra touches or unique materials not found in the local feed & tack stores. Some crops even come with a collapsible shaft for easy transport or storage. For a crop crafted specifically for BDSM use, you can expect to pay between $35 and $100.

The versatility of a crop has always been one of its major selling points. It's both fashionable *and* functional, can be used to deliver both playful *and* painful strikes, and is the most accurate of all the whip types. Some crops come with interchangeable *keepers*, which allow users to vary how the crop is utilized. Crops are most commonly used to deliver stinging or glancing strikes against particularly sensitive areas of the body such as the genitals or nipples, but they can be used practically anywhere on the body with varying techniques and levels of force. Crops are also good for caressing, flicking or sensitizing the skin through repeated small slaps to the same area. The appeal of the crop is rooted as much in its *psychological connotations* as its functional versatility. It's often viewed as a symbol of absolute authority or severe discipline, and those connotations can be used to effectively enhance a scene, role play activity, photography or a person's public image.

Safety concerns about the use of crops are few; the same basic rules for impact play in general apply equally to crops. There are only a few additional caveats. Always ensure that the keeper remains firmly attached to the end of the flexible shaft. If it should come loose or detach, the bare end of the shaft could cause some injury. Second, even with a keeper *attached*, the business end of a crop has the potential to cause serious eye injury if it is inadvertently poked into someone's eye, or if someone walks into the tip. It's usually a good idea to keep the tip pointed downwards when you're not actually using the crop, and to avoid ever intentionally pointing it into a person's face. Finally, since crops are often used to strike or tease the genital area, and because the keepers are usually made of leather, precautions regarding bodily fluids will sometimes need to be taken.

Slappers

A *slapper* is typically a *semi-rigid or flexible* paddle which is often slender in appearance and made from stiff leather which may or may not be reinforced by an inner metal shaft. Slappers are used on farms and ranches all over the country to control livestock, and are usually referred to as *pig slappers*. Like riding crops, basic leather pig slappers can be purchased quite affordably from just about any ranch and farm supply store for a fraction of the cost of similar items from a specialty BDSM retailer.

The slappers that are purchased from stores specializing in BDSM gear usually cost between $40 and $100 and will be made from higher quality leather, come in a wider selection of styles, and may have interesting features that you won't find on your typical farm-quality *pig slapper.* Some of those features may include custom textures, shaped cut-outs, noise-enhancing designs, inner reinforcement, and wrist retaining straps to ensure that the slapper doesn't become a missile when it slips out of your hand in mid-stroke. Human kinksters usually find the wide selection of styles, shapes and colors *exciting* but, obviously, on a farm, they'd probably be considered *pearls before swine.*

I happen to be partial to slappers; they are fun to use and every bit as *intimidating* as paddles, yet tend to be a *lot* more versatile. Depending upon their design, you can use slappers on parts of the body that simply wouldn't be appropriate for paddles, and for purposes that couldn't be accomplished with anything heavier *or* lighter. In many ways, slappers incorporate many of the best qualities of paddles, whips *and* crops.

To use a slapper safely, observe the safety tips we've discussed for all of the preceding impact toys, paying particular attention to the potential for skin and nerve damage. Slappers can be a *great deal of fun,* and for that reason, it can be *incredibly* easy to forget that it may *hours* before you see the full extent of the effects upon your subject's skin.

Canes & Switches

When most *Americans* think of a *cane,* they see a mental image of a rigid wooden walking stick with either a curved or ornamental handle. It's understandable, therefore, that when you mention the practice of *caning* to some BDSM novices, they typically imagine a scene vaguely reminiscent of being clubbed like a baby seal by hungry Eskimos. *Fortunately,* this misconception is simply the result of one of those subtle differences between *American* English and *British* English. To a *Brit,* a cane is a long, thin rattan rod used for corporal punishment, and it is *this* type of cane that is used in BDSM caning play. For all intents and purposes, the cane used in corporal punishment is virtually indistinguishable from the iconic *"switch"* that certain rural parents may have sent their kids outside to find, prior to applying discipline to their back-sides.

The rattan canes used for centuries in Great Britain for corporal punishment in schools, the military and the courts never really caught on in American institutions, possibly because rattan was harder to obtain in the Americas. As a result, Americans tended to substitute *hickory switches* and paddles to accomplish the same results. Today, rattan canes are not only more readily available in the United States, but they have managed to make a comeback as implements used almost exclusively in the fetish culture.

Canes are pretty simple in design. They typically range in length from 21" to 36", and may have a straight or curved handle. Some variations may have a tassel at the end, which allows the user to apply different striking styles. Most modern cane designs draw on a variety of materials besides the traditional rattan, to include wood, fiberglass, nylon, plastic, aluminum, bamboo and carbon composites. Purchasers generally choose the materials for their strength, flexibility and durability. Rattan switches can usually be purchased for $10 to $15, and are often so inexpensive that retailers offer them in sets of three or more. Canes constructed from high-tech or unusual materials can be priced *significantly* higher, ranging easily from $25 to $100.

Despite their elegant simplicity, the proper use of a cane can require a great deal of nuance and skill. Cane strikes, which are more accurately referred to as *strokes or cuts,* will almost always *sting,* but the degree of pain and nature of the effects upon the subject can easily be controlled through proper technique and by striking with different parts of the cane. Some users like to employ an unpredictable mix of painless taps and stinging strokes to intensify the bottom's sensations. A significant part of the caning experience is *psychological,* and so varying the strength, location, timing, or grouping of strokes can spell the difference between an *erotically stimulating* caning scene and an *inept beating.*

For most caning aficionados, the *sweet spot* - or target to which cane strokes are delivered for best effect - is the lower half of the buttocks. Canes strokes can, however, be targeted at just about any non-bony part of the body, save the face and genitals. Common targets include the backs of the thighs and calves, the fleshy part of the back or shoulders, palms of the hands, and the soles of the feet.

The safe use of canes can be summed up pretty well in a single sentence: It's a long, slender, pointy stick that is a lot of fun to swing around, could easily poke an eye out, and is perfectly capable of turning human skin into something resembling *raw hamburger.* And, as always, you should exercise caution in the event that a caning results in open wounds or bleeding.

Evil Sticks & Evil Wands

Evil sticks and *evil wands* are two relatively fresh types of BDSM toys made possible by new technology and materials. An evil stick is essentially a *tiny cane*, usually measuring between 8" and 16", and made from an ultra-strong carbon fiber composite. The way it is used is to hold the handle firmly in one hand while flexing the tip back with the other and releasing it to strike the subject's skin. The high tensile strength of the carbon fiber rod produces an excruciatingly painful strike that invariably leaves a distinct mark. Depending on the force of the strike and the location on the body, the mark can last anywhere from a few hours to *three weeks.* As a result, evil sticks can be purchased in a variety of styles, some of which feature beads or custom shapes at the business end of the stick designed to leave simple designs imprinted on the skin. Masochists may love the *pain-infliction* capabilities of the evil stick, but its ability to imprint a *BDSM badge of honor* on the skin makes it extremely popular even with non-masochists, as well. Evil sticks can typically be purchased from specialty BDSM retailers for $15 to $40.

Evil wands are basically identical to evil sticks, *except longer.* They typically range in length from 14" to 20" and, as a result, are much more *flexible*. Just as an evil stick is essentially a *tiny cane*, the evil wand is basically a *tiny crop or mini single-tail whip* which makes a very intimidating sound as it is swung, and leaves beautiful red stripes wherever it lands. Evil wands are less common and finding retailers that carry them can be difficult, but when you do, they usually range in price from $20 to $50.

Even though evil sticks and wands are really just high-tech miniature versions of canes and whips, their size and versatility can make them the perfect *pocket impact toy*. There are even versions available that can be disguised as innocuous household objects or items that can be worn in public, such as hair accessories. An evil stick can be used in tight spaces where you might not have the space to throw a whip or swing a cane or crop, and its pinpoint accuracy and small impact zone make it ideal for parts of the body that you wouldn't *dream* of targeting safely with anything else.

More often than not, an evil stick is used for a single impact against the skin, either to demonstrate its *pure evilness*, or to literally *make an impression* on someone. When used in this fashion, and as long as the impact is targeted to a fleshy part of the body, there should be very few safety concerns. On the other hand, even a single strike targeting a joint or bony protrusion such as a wrist bone *could* ruin someone's entire week. Of even greater concern would be the temptation to use an evil stick or wand repeatedly or perhaps even *continuously* on the same part of the body. As is also the case with other types of impact play, the effects of your strikes upon a person's skin may not be evident right away. If you are engaging in impact play with someone for the *first time*, it is usually a good idea to test the skin's resilience and tolerance for this type of play by limiting the number and intensity of your strikes until you have a better feel for *how much may be too much* for that individual.

Piercing, Scarification & Branding

Any BDSM activity involving needles, pins, nails or hooks which pierce the skin requires meticulous care to prevent serious infections or the spread of communicable diseases. Even so, as long as it is done by a trained, experienced person who observes proper *sanitation* protocols, it doesn't have to be *dangerous.*

Needles

BDSM needle play can take many forms, most of which it involve piercing the skin with hypodermic or acupuncture needles. Strictly speaking, needles aren't inherently *painful* by themselves, but the obvious and often palpable *psychological effects* of needle play can make it interesting *indeed.* Some people have reported *endorphin highs* and even *orgasms* from needle play, but how much of that is *physical,* versus *psychological*, is debatable.

The most common forms of needle play usually consist of placing acupuncture needles into various fleshy parts of the body to induce or reduce fear, create aesthetically pleasing patterns or designs, stimulate the nervous system, cause or reduce pain, and for other therapeutic reasons. Acupuncture needles may be inserted into the flesh *perpendicular* to the skin or at a *secant*, where the needle is pushed through a fold of skin in such a way that the tip emerges again, leaving only the center part of the needle shaft below the skin. This aesthetic mode of needle play has recently become quite popular as a way to anchor *decorative corset lacing* to a person's back or chest.

Hypodermic needles are also used in BDSM needle play, though less often than acupuncture needles, for fairly obvious reasons. Hypodermic needles are *hollow*, and designed to inject or sample fluids from the body; that means the needle has to be *thicker* and will usually produce a slightly more painful poke. Some studies have shown that roughly 10% of the population suffers from *trypanophobia*, which is the fear of hypodermic needles. Whether that statistic holds up in the *kink* population is anyone's guess, but the most common form of fetish-related hypodermic needle play occurs in BDSM *medical role-play scenes.*

Both acupuncture and hypodermic needles can be purchased from any local or online medical supply retailer. Hypodermic needles are typically sold separately from the syringe portion, and range in size from 6 to 32 gauge. The higher the gauge, the smaller the diameter of the needle will be. For intradermal injections, use a 26 to 28 gauge needle that is 3/8" to 3/4" in length. For intramuscular use, a 26 to 30 gauge needle 7/8" to 1-1/2" long is appropriate. For subcutaneous injections, use a 19 to 27 gauge needle ½" to 5/8" long. A box of 100 hypodermic needles without the syringes will typically cost $20 to $30 at a medical supply store.

Acupuncture needles are constructed very differently from hypodermic needles. Since they aren't hollow, they can be made much, much *thinner.* They also typically have either a thicker end or thin plastic handle, and sometimes they come with a small knob, loop or bead at the handle end. The needles are *extremely* flexible, which is why many are sold with a coil, tube or sleeve which makes handling and inserting the needles much easier. Acupuncture needles usually range from 12mm to 25mm in thickness, and from 1" to 2" in length. Retailers typically market them in quantities of 100, 500 or 1000, with an average price of about $15 for a package of 100.

Safety, as you may well imagine, is a *big deal* when it comes to needle play.

Never engage in needle play with someone whose experience and skill level is unknown to you. Do *not* simply take someone's word on whether or not they know what they're doing. The best way to judge a Top's credibility when it comes to needle play is to observe him at it, and to speak to people who have scened with him previously.

Needle play should *only* be done with *brand new, sterile, medical grade needles*, and *never* with sewing needles or anything else that isn't specifically designed for this kind of use. Never re-use a needle, even on the same person. Needle tips degrade significantly with each use which not only make them more painful, but creates a larger and more ragged wound which increases the chances of an infection.

Always dispose of used needles by placing them into a *hard receptacle*, such as an empty soda bottle, detergent bottle, or jar. That way, they won't *stab* someone who inadvertently grabs or brushes up against a *trash bag* full of *needles.* When possible and practical, *label* the container with the word *"biohazard."*

Before engaging in needle play, always wash your hands with a strong anti-bacterial soap, and use a fingernail brush to get under the nails. Disinfecting the bottom's skin at the puncture site won't accomplish much if you are just going to touch it again with dirty fingers. Swab the site with alcohol just prior to play to ensure that pathogens on the surface of the skin aren't transported into the bloodstream by the needle.

When piercing the skin on a *secant* (where both ends of the needle are exposed to the air) always swab the exposed end of the needle with alcohol *again* before removing them. Otherwise, when you pull the tip (which has been exposed to the air and possibly to other materials) through the skin while *removing it*, it can pull pathogens into the bloodstream.

After the needles are removed, the puncture site should be disinfected immediately, and perhaps again in a few hours. Needle punctures may not look like wounds, particularly if there is no blood, *but they are,* and can result in nasty infections if they aren't properly cared for. Despite all of these dire warnings, the truth of the matter is, you probably have more to worry about - at least, in terms of *infection* - from being scratched by your family pet.

When engaging in needle play with someone for the first time, you should always ask if the person has (or has *ever* had) hemophilia, thrombus, blood clots, a stroke or heart condition, and whether they are taking prescription blood thinners or have taken any aspirin within the past five days. For individuals who fall into those categories, even a tiny needle prick can be a problem. Someone who is prone to blood clots should *not* engage in needle play, which could result in clots forming in the blood stream or a reduction of capillary blood flow to some areas. Additionally, people with certain types of heart conditions can be very susceptible to *infections of the heart*, and often have to take *antibiotics* before any procedure that might introduce pathogens into their blood stream - even a visit to the dentist for a *teeth cleaning.* Needless to say, if a *teeth cleaning* can pose a potential hazard to someone with a heart condition, it's a pretty safe bet that being poked with dozens of *needles* probably will, *too.*

Take care to avoid bony areas such as joints, sternum, hands, wrists, feet or the spine. Stay away from nerve clusters, sensitive organs, and major blood vessels. Obviously, you should always steer clear of the *eyes,* or for that matter, the face in general. Certain parts of a person's genitalia and nipples *can* be pierced in nipple play, but it will usually be *exceedingly painful,* and should be approached with *extreme caution* due to the high density of blood vessels and organs susceptible to damage in those areas.

Needle play, when done *properly* by an experienced and knowledgeable Top using the right equipment in sanitary conditions, is a *relatively safe activity.* Anything that *doesn't* meet those standards *isn't.*

Nails, Pins & Staples

One of the first things a person learns in the fetish lifestyle is that there are always people who enjoy pushing the limits, not only of their own pain endurance or social norms, *but of good sense.* Perhaps *some* of that is the legitimate result of a person truly wanting to explore the boundaries of his or her own fear, strengths, capabilities and senses.

Other times, unfortunately, it can be the result of someone who views the fetish culture as *competition to be won.* For *those* individuals, it isn't about relationships, sexual turn-ons, or even *having kinky fun.* It's all about *scoring points and one-upsmanship.* This is *not* a healthy approach to the BDSM lifestyle.

I believe that BDSM piercing play that involves common hardware such as nails, pins and staples should be *highly discouraged.* It may be tempting for some people to view it as just another form of *edge-play,* but I believe it is an extremely dangerous activity - *particularly for novices* - and only serves to perpetuate and enflame the gross misconceptions among the general public about what goes on in the fetish lifestyle. It's relatively simple to find extreme S&M photography online that depicts this sort of play in an erotic way, but what you *never* see is the massive infections, gangrenous body parts, or massive medical bills that followed.

Each safety concern that we discussed in the needle play section applies *ten-fold* to nails, pins and staples. While needle play *could potentially* lead to infection, it's almost *certain* that the use of common nails, pins and staples *will* lead to serious and perhaps even life-threatening infections. As if that weren't enough, this kind of play can also cause tissue scarring, nerve damage, loss of sensation or motor control, and even blood poisoning. Trust me; it simply isn't worth losing a body part, your health or potentially even your life to score points in a non-existent game of masochistic one-upsmanship that you *can't win.*

Pinwheels

The Wartenburg neurological pinwheel (also sometimes called a *neurowheel*) was originally designed to be used by medical professionals to test a person's sensitivity to pinpricks. It is a handheld instrument about eight inches in length, consisting of a simple slender handle and a small pinwheel of sharp spikes at the end. Pinwheels are typically constructed of stainless steel, but there are also disposable plastic versions available on the market. They are used in a lot of different ways, but primarily to cause the sensation of being pricked or to induce a feeling of apprehension or fear, particularly in people who are apprehensive about needles and similar devices. They are readily available from online retailers for $5 to $10.

These devices have been around for a long time and have always been very popular with the BDSM crowd, but have fallen out of favor due to their tendency to break the skin. Many readers may not be old enough to remember that there was ever a time when *HIV/AIDS* did not exist and therefore wasn't a concern, but the advent of the *age of AIDS* in the '80s and '90s literally *changed everything*, when it came to BDSM. Even so, pinwheels are still a relatively common and popular item in the BDSM lifestyle, and are generally safe as long as they are *fluid-bonded* to specific individuals, or thoroughly *sterilized* between uses. Fluid-bonding is the preferred option, since it's always difficult to know for certain whether an instrument has been properly sterilized, and especially considering their low cost.

Cell Popping and Branding Gear

Cell popping is a form of micro-branding that typically utilizes a very hot, thin metal rod or needle to burn a series of tiny dots into the skin to achieve a temporary design, which can often last several weeks. The designs can be quite intricate, and often involve the application of hundreds, or even thousands, of tiny burns which, *theoretically*, are confined each to a single skin pore or epidermal cell which can *sizzle and pop* while the hot metal is applied for about one second - *hence the name.* Since the artist has only two colors to work with - *burned and unburned* - designs requiring areas of darker shading will usually involve a denser dot-matrix to achieve the illusion of shading or coloration.

The equipment needed for cell popping is relatively simple, and readily available from your local hardware store. It typically includes a propane torch nozzle, propane canisters, a sturdy torch holder of the sort used by jewelers and crafters, a small rack or stand designed to hold your needles when not in use, and the thin metal rods or needles that will be used to mark the skin. Most people prefer to use the long, straight *teasing needles* that come as part of a medical dissection kit, and to have two or three available, so one can be heating while the other is being used. Some folks use canned *sterno* or chafing dish fuel as an inexpensive alternative to a propane torch.

A propane torch kit that includes a nozzle, igniter and one canister of propane will cost about $25. A torch holder isn't absolutely necessary, but it certainly frees up one of your hands to do other things, and removes any worries about a lit propane torch being bumped or knocked over and causing problems. A torch holder can cost anywhere from $20 to $50, or you can affordably make one of your own, using any kind of sturdy frame and some spring-loaded craft clamps. Your needle stand can be constructed easily from a simple block of wood with some holes drilled into it. Dissection needles are available inexpensively in a variety of lengths and styles; you might want to purchase a few different kinds, so you can decide on your personal preference. Do keep in mind that *shorter* dissection needles with *plastic* handles may be problematic, since the handles can melt when the needle is heated. On the other hand, dissection needles without heat-resistant handles may become uncomfortably hot or difficult to handle over the long periods of time that may be required for a complex design. Thick metal or wooden grips are usually the best solution. The only way to know what works best *for you* is to try them out. They're usually quite affordable, at $1 to $5 each.

Prior to a cell popping session, shave the area of any hair, and disinfect the area with alcohol or a topical disinfectant. Wash your hands thoroughly with an anti-bacterial soap. Position all of your equipment for easy access, and in a way that precludes anything from being bumped or knocked over. If you have an intricate design planned, you may want to mark the skin or transfer your design to it in order to ensure that your marks are on target. After all, there's no way to *erase* any mistake that might occur! You *can't,* however, burn directly *through* a paper design template, because that will cool the tip and it won't have the desired effect on the skin.

Novices may be a little startled at first by the sizzle-pop sound that can accompany the application of the needle tip to the skin; it is simply the result of moisture on or in the skin cell being converted instantly to *steam.* Warning: the procedure *will* be accompanied by the odor of *burning flesh.* Under normal circumstances, it shouldn't be *overpowering*, and it *will* differ from person to person, but if you or your subject happens to be someone who abhors or is sensitive to the smell, it could be a problem.

The needle tip is hot enough when it is glowing bright red, and you should be able to get three to five dots out of each hot needle before it cools. If you position your needle rack and torch holder well, you can heat one needle tip while using another, which will save time waiting while a tip is heating. The process *can* be *quite* painful, depending upon the location and complexity of the design, but most people claim that it is no more painful than getting a *tattoo.* It will, however, *continue* to hurt for longer than your typical tattoo.

The skin will typically appear *white* at the spot where the needle was applied, with redness surrounding each dot, and will appear quite *unimpressive* at this stage. Putting *lotions or creams* on the marks at this point will only delay the scabbing process, and could cause the marks to fade altogether. If you feel compelled to put *anything at all* on the marks, spray some *Bactine* or another first-aid spray that disinfects, dulls the pain, and *dries quickly* without *moisturizing* the wounds. Within a day or two, the dots will scab up and, about a week later, they will fall off, leaving a residual dark spot on the skin. During that time, the subject should do whatever it takes to resist the temptation to *scratch* the area or pick at the scabs. If desired, repeated applications to the same spots over time can result in a *permanent* design. Otherwise, the effects can typically be expected to last one to three months.

An alternative form of cell popping involves the use of a *violet wand* electrode at a high setting, and left stationary over a specific spot long enough to actually burn the skin. This method is generally less accurate, more time-consuming, and the end results can be somewhat inconsistent. On the *bright side*, it can be highly entertaining, it requires less equipment, doesn't smell as bad, and won't burn down your house.

Branding consists of essentially the same process, except on a *larger scale* and imprinting continuous lines or patterns into the skin with hot metal, instead of tiny dots. The process is far more *painful,* the marks are more likely to be *permanent*, and there is a significantly greater risk of infection.

Safety concerns for both cell popping and branding include the risk of fire, accidental burns from the instruments or the torch itself, deep tissue damage from pressing the needle too deeply into the skin, and the risk of subsequent infections.

Scarification Gear

Scarification is the process of marking the body *permanently with scars*. While a traditional *branding* is certainly one very effective method of doing so, there are plenty of other ways to accomplish it, as well.

These methods may include:

- *cauterization* with self-heating instruments
- *cold branding* with dry ice or liquid nitrogen
- *chemical burns* produced by applying caustic substances to the skin
- *abrasion* of the skin caused by grinding or sanding tools or materials
- *simple cutting* of the skin with a blade
- *complex cutting* of the skin, such as in *cross-hatch patterns*
- *removal* of patches or swaths of skin by cutting it away with a blade
- *packing open cuts with a foreign substance* such as clay or ashes (sometimes, even the *ashes of a deceased relative)*

Obviously, with so many different kinds of scarification methods and procedures available, there really isn't anything that should be considered *"standard"* scarification gear except, perhaps, a good *surgical scalpel.*

Generally speaking, the key to getting the skin to form a visible scar is to prolong the healing process for as long as possible, or to use substances on the wound that are known to cause more pronounced scarring. Some people deliberately irritate the wound with caustic chemicals or other substances to delay or prolong the healing process and to promote the formation of scar tissue. Others apply *tincture of iodine,* a common antiseptic which has fallen out of favor in recent years because it has been shown to promote scarring.

Scarification of *any sort* should only be attempted by trained and experienced individuals using the proper tools and materials, and observing strict protocols of hygiene. Cutting, abrading or burning the skin can also send potentially harmful pathogens from the subject *airborne*, so the Top should always wear a surgical mask when engaging in this sort of activity. For the *subject*, not only can the possibility of subsequent infections be quite high, but there is significant risk of other complications, such as uncontrolled bleeding, nerve damage, blood poisoning, or organ failure. To literally add *insult to injury*, larger scars may have a tendency to travel, lengthen, widen or spread into unintended areas, which can make the intended original design *practically undecipherable.*

Sensation Play & Sensory Deprivation

Sensation and sensory deprivation play are just two sides of the very same coin; one seeks to enhance or *stimulate* the senses, while the other seeks to *nullify* them. The many subcategories of this sort of BDSM activity could easily fill an entire book but, for the sake of brevity, we'll limit ourselves to about a dozen of the most commonly practiced forms of sensation and sensory deprivation play that you might encounter or have an interest in.

Blindfolds & Gags

The use of blindfolds and gags is probably the most pervasive form of sensory deprivation play in the world, both in the BDSM lifestyle, *and* outside of it. The relative ease with which a blindfold or gag can be fashioned or crafted from simple and readily available household materials makes this sort of kinky experimentation easy and exciting, even for *vanilla* couples.

Simple, ready-made blindfolds can be purchased from just about any fetish retailer, though the prices may be somewhat inflated, compared to similar products designed for and marketed to insomniacs and travelers. Some features to look for may include: shapes that conform to the contours of the face, a durable and adjustable securing strap, quality materials and stitching, and the use of color-fast dyes. You can expect to pay $7 to $25 for a blindfold from a fetish retailer.

Blindfolds can definitely be a great addition to your fetish toy box. When used with skill, they can alter or heighten a bottom's *psychological and physiological* responses to other stimuli significantly. Introducing an element of the unknown - not knowing *what* is happening, *how* it is happening, or even *who* might be in the room watching or participating - can make even a mundane scene a *lot* more interesting. The blindfold doesn't necessary even have to be used just to *deny* the bottom's ability to visually confirm what is actually going on around her. A blindfold can also be used to stoke the imagination or create the *impression* of things occurring when they are *not.* For example, the two of you may not be ready or willing to *actually* invite a third person into your bedroom for a *threesome*, but the use of a blindfold can make the *role-play scenario seem much more real*, creating the impression that there is someone else in the room with you. Serving up treats for the *other senses* can also enhance the imagined scenario by adding theatrical touches, such as a mysterious knock at the door, the distant presence of an unfamiliar voice, the nearby scent of a strange cologne, or being touched in an unfamiliar way.

There are few safety issues to be concerned with, when it comes to blindfolds. Just be careful to apply a blindfold to your bottom while he or she is stationary and, preferably, *immobile.* Attempting to move about with a blindfold on is not only awkward and dangerous, but difficult to explain at the local emergency room. Additionally, the use of a blindfold places the entire burden of consent and propriety fully upon the shoulders of the Top, since the bottom cannot see what is about to happen and, therefore, presumably does not have a chance to voice potential concerns or safe word out *before* it occurs. For that reason, a detailed discussion or scene negotiation should take place beforehand.

Gags, like blindfolds, are simple and affordable kink toys that lend themselves easily to experimentation by vanilla and fetish folk alike. Gags can consist of just about anything placed in or over the mouth (OTM) or even over the nose (OTN) as well. They can include such things as an unpretentious strip of cloth, a wide strip of duct tape, a wooden rod, a ball-gag, open-mouth bracing, or even a pony bit. While it may be tempting to create your own gags from common household items, some of those materials may be laced with noxious chemicals or be unsuitable for being held in the mouth for any length of time. When in doubt, stick with materials specifically designed to be placed in or over the mouth. The most commonly available types of gags are ball gags, open mouth gags, and bit gags. Less common gags include various types of medical or dental gags, inflatable gags, muzzle gags, funnel gags, forniphilic gags (which are used to humiliate or objectify the wearer by turning the gag into items like toilet plungers or dildos), and *novelty gags*, which I sometimes refer to as *gag* gags.

Ball gags are comprised of a small ball made of rubber or silicone which fits into the mouth and attached to a securing strap. The ball may vary in size, shape, color and materials, and may even have breathing holes or other unique features. The strap is typically an adjustable leather one, but sometimes can be elastic. While the *superficial* purpose of a ball gag is to prevent a person from *speaking,* the *true* value of a ball gag lies in its *psychological effects*, creating a palpable sense of helplessness, futility or humiliation in the bottom, and appealing to a wide range of motivations, aesthetics or fetishes for the Top.

An *open mouth gag,* like the ball gag, also prevents the bottom from speaking, but does so by keeping the mouth propped wide open in much the same way that a dentist does to get a better look at your teeth. These are sometimes called ring gags, spider gags (ring gags with hooks or braces to prevent slipping or turning), Whitehead dental gags (what your dentist uses), or blowjob gags. Again, the *ostensible purpose* of an open mouth gag is to allow the insertion of a penis, fingers, dildo or other toys into the bottom's open mouth or to permit the Top to ejaculate or urinate into the mouth, however, the *psychological* effects are always of significant importance. A typical open mouth gag will cost between $15 and $100.

A bit gag is designed to resemble and function like a *horse's bit,* and is often used in BDSM pony play. It typically consists of a short slender rod which is placed between the teeth, with straps attached at each end which can be secured around a person's head to hold it in place. The rod is usually straight; however there are bit gag designs that are curved or contoured to a person's face. Some bit gags are extremely rigid, having a steel or aluminum inner core with a softer layer of rubber or silicone surrounding it to protect the teeth from damage, while others may be constructed entirely of solid rubber, silicone, PVC or other synthetic materials. The quality of a bit gag purchased from retailers can *vary widely*, so it's always a good idea to check the product reviews for feedback before purchasing one. Due to the relative simplicity of a bit gag's design, some unscrupulous retailers will charge $15 to $30 for *"bit gags"* that are nothing more than a short length of PVC pipe with holes drilled into the ends for O-rings and a thin leather strap, all of which can be purchased in any hardware store for about $2. A *well-built* bit gag will be constructed for serious and/or regular use, rather than as a *novelty*, and will be made from *quality materials*. It typically should *not* be uncomfortable or painful to wear for short periods of time, and it should protect the teeth from damage.

Any type of gag can be dangerous if it restricts a person's breathing in any way, *including psychological causes*. It is extremely important to monitor the bottom's condition and respiration *continuously*, since the situation can change very quickly without notice, *even if nothing has physically changed.* A person wearing a gag may be able to *breathe perfectly* one moment and *not at all* the next, possibly due to allergic reactions, panic attacks, hyperventilation, discomfort, sudden illness, vomiting, or choking on his or her own saliva. For obvious reasons, it can be quite difficult for a gagged bottom to *tell* you what is happening, so I *highly recommend* that you arrange a *non-verbal* safe word or emergency signal that can be communicated to the Top, *whether or not the wrists or hands are restrained.*

Masks & Hoods

BDSM masks and hoods come in all shapes, sizes, materials and functional forms. *Generally speaking*, a mask is designed to give the wearer *anonymity*, while a hood is designed to limit or prevent the wearer from *seeing*. *Both*, however, can be used to perform a variety of other nifty functions as well, and there is a lot of interchangeability in the terms among users and retailers. To reduce confusion and for the sake of simplicity, we'll refer henceforth to them all simply as *hoods.*

Hoods, unlike *blindfolds*, are typically fitted over the *entire head.* They are commonly constructed from cotton, silk, spandex, leather, rubber, PVC, nylon or other synthetic fabrics. There is such a wide spectrum of products that fit into this category it's difficult to make *any* generalizations which would apply across the board. Some hoods come with straps, flaps, and holes; others *may not*. Some are designed to keep people from seeing out; others are designed to keep people from seeing in. Most hoods function to limit a person's *vision;* others may be uniquely constructed to limit a person's ability to speak, hear, breathe, *or all of the above.* Hoods may be simple or devious, sensual or cruel, loose-fitting or elastic, and they may be secured in place by laces, zippers, snaps, buttons, straps, or Velcro. In fact, since many of the hoods used in BDSM play are *custom-made* for their owners, it would not be much of an exaggeration to say that there are practically as many different kinds of BDSM hoods out there as there are *people who enjoy using them.*

When shopping for hoods, you should expect the price that you pay to be a direct reflection of the materials, features, and quality of workmanship of the product. A simple cotton hood will average $5 to $20. A nylon or spandex hood will be a bit pricier, at $15 to $40. Rubber, PVC or latex hoods generally range from $20 to $70. Leather hoods can start at $25 or cost as much as $200, depending on the quality, complexity, and unique features included in the design. If you are unable to locate the type of hood you're looking for, you should have no trouble at all finding skilled kink apparel crafters online who'll be glad to customize a hood to your tastes and specifications.

The safety concerns related to hoods are virtually identical to those for *blindfolds* when they block the wearer's vision and to *gags* when they cover the mouth and potentially limit the wearer's ability to speak or breathe. Additionally, since some hood designs require the hood to be secured below the wearer's chin or around his neck, there could be some risk of accidental strangulation. As always, continuously monitoring the wearer's well-being and psychological state will serve to minimize the risks.

Vibration & Oscillation

Vibration and oscillation toys can basically be summed up in a single word: *vibrators.* The various types of vibrators used in BDSM play do not differ in any significant way from the ones used in vanilla sex play. Generally speaking, the only real difference will be *in the ways that they are used.* When you add bondage, discipline, and sadomasochism to the mix, even *simple vibrators* can start looking *pretty scary.*

Rather than slog through the thousands of types of portable vibrators of both the battery-operated and corded varieties readily available in the marketplace, we'll focus instead on just two of the more interesting retail products, the Hitachi Magic Wand and the Abco Sybian, and some ideas for a couple of *home-made* oscillation toys.

The Hitachi Magic Wand, for many, has become the holy grail of hand-held personal vibrators since being introduced in the U.S. in the mid-1970s. It is a corded device which is marketed primarily as a *"massager"*, but has become so closely associated with its popular use for masturbation that Hitachi has begun a subtle rebranding effort to de-emphasize or remove its corporate name from the product's promotional materials. The Magic Wand is extremely popular with both vanilla *and* kink users, and it can be seen with increasing frequency in BDSM photography and porn, most often in bondage or forced orgasm scenes. It's powerful motor, rubberized head, adjustable speeds, and sleek design not only puts it at the top of the list in terms of *functionality*, but it can be used in hands-free mode by sitting on it or by integrating it into your bondage, and it is generally considered to be almost as good at inducing orgasms for men as it is for women. Comedienne Roseanne Barr is reported to have once quipped, "Hitachi makes such good vibrators, I think I'll buy one of their TVs!" The Hitachi Magic Wand retails for $50 to $70.

The Abco Sybian, often referred to simply as a *Sybian* or *Sybian Saddle,* is a patented and trademarked product of Abco Research Associates in Monticello, Illinois. In other words, if your device wasn't manufactured by Abco, it isn't a Sybian; it's just another vibrating saddle. The Sybian was invented in 1985 by a dance instructor named Dave Lampert, who felt that the key to helping a woman achieve orgasm was to simulate what occurs when a woman is sitting atop a reclining male during sexual intercourse. If you have never *seen* a Sybian, you can familiarize yourself with its appearance and functionality by visiting practically any porn site on the web and simply typing the word *Sybian* into the search box. Interestingly enough, Abco also produces a high-end *male* penis-pump type of masturbation device called the Venus 2000. The Sybian, like the Hitachi Magic Wand, is popular among both vanilla *and* fetish folk, however its hefty price tag ($1300-$1600) generally keeps it beyond the reach of casual or experimental users. On the other hand, if you're a professional Dominant, sex worker or fetish photographer, you may be able to claim it as a tax-deductible business expense. Is this a *great country*, or what?

You don't have to spend a lot of money to enjoy sensation-play that utilizes vibration or oscillation effectively. In fact, you may not have to spend anything *at all*, if you already have the right items sitting around in your home. Take, for example, the simple hand-held, battery-operated *electric toothbrush.* They can be purchased for a pittance ($3 to $10) at just about any drugstore, and most can be turned into *very effective sensation-play toys* with little or no effort. Simply remove the brush-tip if it is removable, or cut it off with a sturdy set of kitchen shears if it isn't. What you are left with is typically a stainless steel metal rod that extends a few inches from the handle. Turn the device on, and you'll see the metal rod *oscillating* very quickly and intensely, which - *if you're as pervy as I think you are* - should easily conjure up *infinite possibilities* for sensation play. The slender metal rod may or may not have a bulbous or rounded tip, but if it doesn't you can file it down a bit so there are no sharp edges. The oscillating bare metal rod tip can be an *incredibly intense* and effective way to stimulate or torture any part of the body, particularly the most sensitive ones. Additionally, various kinds of items can be permanently or temporarily attached to the rod tip to achieve different effects. Such items may include small rubber or plastic balls, small dildo or finger-shaped items, or even a variety of *ticklers.*

Another household item, which you are probably less likely to have sitting around but may be tempted to procure once you read this, is the *Waterpik*. If you're unfamiliar with the Waterpik, a product patented, trademarked and marketed by Waterpik Inc., it can be best described as a *high-pressure water-jet flosser or oral irrigator.* There are several different models available, which range in price from $35 to $115, but they all essentially consist of a reservoir which holds the water, a powerful compressor that forces the water in rapid high-pressure pulses through a small flexible hose to a variety of interchangeable nozzle-tips. Most models allow you to adjust the water pressure to your liking, and there are even models which are entirely hand-held, self-contained, portable, and battery operated. They are, for all intents and purposes, just like the pulsing high-pressure water nozzles you see at your local coin-operated self-service car wash, *except smaller, and for your teeth.* Or, if you're an adventurous and creative kinkster, for your *nipples, clit, cock and anus.* Of course, now that you've read this, *whether or not* you ever use a Waterpik in this fashion, you'll probably never be able to look at the *coin-op car wash* the same way, *ever again.*

Vibrating and oscillating toys are generally quite safe to use, as long as a minimal amount of common sense is applied. Obviously, you should *always* avoid using a *corded electrical device* anywhere where it might become submerged in water. Make sure that any vibrating attachments or, for that matter, *anything* that is inserted into a body cavity can be easily *retrieved.* And *do* keep in mind that too much of a good thing - *even good vibrations* - can sometimes be a bad thing. The continuous or excessive application of a vibrating implement *of any kind* to a single spot on the body *may* result in localized numbness, loss of motor control, or residual tingling.

Violet Wand

It can sometimes be difficult to describe a *violet wand* to someone who has never seen one before. I usually do it thusly: Remember visiting Spencer's Gifts in the mall and seeing those little glass globes crackling with purple lightning on display? Did you ever touch one and watch how the electricity sizzled, tickled, and followed your fingertips wherever they went on the surface of the globe? Now imagine the same thing, only smaller, safer, designed to be hand-held, and with a wide variety of kinky attachments.

Violet wands have recently become quite popular in the fetish culture, so it's easy to see how some people might be surprised to learn that these things have been around, in one form or another, for close to a *hundred years.* In the 1920s, they were called *"violet rays"* and used by medical quacks to treat a variety of physical, psychological, and sexual maladies. Eventually, the courts and the FDA forbade the manufacture and sale of violet rays for *medical* use after finding the makers' claims of medical efficacy to be completely groundless. Violet rays *were* allowed to be sold as skin and scalp treatments, neon light gas-leak detectors, and for purely aesthetic purposes, however. Sales of violet rays diminished significantly and most of the companies that sold them either went out of business or focused their efforts on supporting the WWII manufacturing challenge. Several more decades would pass before they were rediscovered in the 1990s by the fetish community, adapted for kink play, and rechristened *"violet wands."* By the way, if you're at all interested, I've included at the end of this chapter the tale of how I serendipitously became the proud owner of an authentic 1922 Parco Super High Frequency Generator & Violet Ray.

Modern violet wands aren't really much different from their violet ray predecessors. The major differences include safer and more reliable electrical components, the use of acrylics or safety glass, a wider and kinkier variety of electrode attachments, and the ability to plug them into a wall socket. Most violet rays were manufactured long before electrical wall sockets became common in homes, therefore, users had to connect them to ceiling *light fixtures* to power them. When wall sockets became more universal, most existing violet ray owners clumsily spliced standard wall plugs onto their power cords, which also explains why the power cords on most antique units that are still around tend to look like the dog ate them.

If you are in the market for a modern violet wand, here are a few things to be on the look-out for. The first should be the components included in the package that you're considering. Some violet wands are sold in such a way that you must purchase all of the components *individually.* Components may include the wand itself, standard or specialty electrodes, adapters or attachments, holsters, kits, and cases. Other times, you may be offered *starter kits,* complete with a handy-dandy case and/or an assortment of electrodes and attachments. Either way is *fine,* as long as you understand what you're getting for the price. Just be sure to read the fine print. It can be pretty frustrating to receive your brand new violet wand in the mail, only to learn that you can't try it out because the *electrodes weren't included in the purchase price.*

Pay close attention to the interchangeability of electrodes and attachments. There are several violet wand manufacturers, with new ones popping up all the time. Most violet wand electrodes and accessories are interchangeable and compatible with one another but you should always check, to be sure. The standard electrode socket size in the United States is 7/16". You might also want to take note of the type of plug at the end of the device's power cord. Some violet wands use a grounded three-prong plug, others a simple two-prong plug. It probably won't matter much to you, either way, until you can't plug your three-prong plug into a two-prong socket or extension cord.

Prices on violet wands can vary widely, but you should expect to pay $100 to $300 for the wand, and $10 to $100 for most common types of electrodes or attachments. Rare or custom-made violet wand attachments can, of course, be much more expensive. For *those* accessories, you may want to consider the old maxim, *"If you have to ask the price, you probably can't afford it."*

Violet wands are used in many different ways. *Direct use* refers to the direct application of an electrode and current to the subject's skin, which arcs to the subject because he or she is grounded. *Indirect use* refers to the practice of the wand user touching or holding an electrode, and allowing the current to pass through his or her own body before passing it to a grounded subject, either by touch or through an electrically conductive object. *Reverse use* typically involves attaching an electrode or accessory to an ungrounded subject and applying current in such a fashion that the current will arc from the subject to anything or anyone that is grounded. Permanent and semi-permanent *branding* can also be done with a violet wand, with proper training and the right attachments.

The most common uses for a violet wand are for *sensation or tickle play* at lower settings, *torture and branding* at higher settings, as an igniter for fire play, and for the general *amusement and aesthetics* of playing with *electricity.* Once you own a violet wand, you'll find yourself classifying everything in your house as either *electrically conductive or non-conductive.* Trips to the local crafts store or hobby shop take on *new meaning,* as you pore over their selection of supplies and wonder about their electrical conductivity. Suddenly, tinsel and garlands *aren't just for Christmas, anymore!*

The sparks that you feel from a violet wand are, for all intents and purposes, just like the static electricity spark that you get from touching a doorknob, only *continuously.* Unlike most of the electrical appliances and devices in your home, a violet wand converts potentially deadly household electrical current into one that is extremely low *amperage,* but high *frequency and voltage*. When *used correctly,* a violet wand is an extremely safe kink toy; when used *incorrectly* or by the wrong people, *not so much.*

The safety concerns for violet wands are often confused with those for TENS units, which we'll discuss in the next section. The bottom line up front is, a violet wand is safer to use than a TENS unit, and has an entirely different set of safety precautions to be aware of. Contrary to popular belief, violet wands *are* safe to use above the chest and on the head and face, as long as they're kept away from the eyes. Even though the wand is kept far from the eyes, contact lenses and metal-framed eyeglasses should be removed as a precaution. Violet wands should *not* be used on anyone who has implanted electronic devices such as pacemakers, insulin pumps, or chemo-therapy pumps. Additionally, the wand should be kept away from any *metal in the body*, such as replacement knee joints, orthopedic pins and braces, or dental braces. Long ago, these types of devices were sold as ultraviolet (UV) light and ozone generators, but the amounts of UV light and ozone produced by a violet wand are insignificant and should not be a concern to users.

Never use a violet wand around liquids. This includes not only showers, tubs, and sinks, but *any* nearby liquid, including drinks which could spill and become electrical conductors. If a violet wand gets wet, the full force of the household electrical current could travel along the wet exterior of the wand and deliver a potentially lethal shock.

Do not use the violet wand anywhere near flammable fumes, as the open spark will ignite them, and could cause a fire or explosion. Flammable fumes may include hair spray, rubbing alcohol, hand sanitizer, fresh paint fumes, lubricants, and fuels for household lamps or air fresheners.

Many people wonder if a violet wand can be used *internally* in the mouth, vagina or ass. The answer is *yes,* you *can,* as long as the device you're using is a true violet wand and you are using an electrode that is *specifically designed for such use.* As a general rule, internal electrodes are built more ruggedly and have a larger, sturdier plug than the standard 7/16" to prevent the electrode from snapping off under pressure. In other words, if you're interested in using a violet wand for internal play, you're going to have to buy one that will accept the larger-sized plugs on internal electrodes.

Despite taking every other possible precaution, there will always be a *miniscule* chance of an electrical malfunction of some sort that could cause unfiltered household current to travel through the violet wand. This risk may increase somewhat if the wiring in your house is getting old or if you've had electrical problems in the past. If that worries you, you should consider purchasing an inexpensive portable Ground Fault Circuit Interrupter (GFCI) at any hardware store or electronics shop for

$20 to $40. When it senses the type of electrical surge that could cause a problem, it automatically breaks the connection the same way that your computer's surge protector does.

All things considered, a violet wand is actually much safer than it might seem at first blush. Obviously, if you notice that someone is particularly sensitive to the effects of a violet wand, you should reevaluate their suitability for this sort of play. If your subject continues to experience tingling or numbness after a few days in affected areas, that should definitely be considered a big red flag. As is the case with just about any BDSM toy, the greatest risks associated with the use of a violet wand are usually the result of careless or inappropriate use.

TENS and EMS Units

Electrical BDSM play can take many forms. As we've just learned, violet wands are primarily used to stimulate the *skin.* TENS units are designed to stimulate the *nervous system*, while the purpose of EMS units is to stimulate *muscle.* TENS and EMS devices may appear superficially similar; both typically consist of a control console, long wires or leads, and dermal adhesive electrodes, but that's pretty much where the similarities end.

TENS stands for *Transcutaneous Electrical Nerve Stimulation.* In medicine, it's a somewhat controversial treatment for chronic pain that's been around since the early 1970s, though the idea of using electricity to dull pain is not particularly new. Ancient Romans wrote of alleviating pain by touching live electric eels and in the 18th century, Ben Franklin tinkered with the use of electricity as a treatment for pain and a cure for various ailments. Today, in addition to its questionable efficacy as a medical treatment, it is used by many *fetishistas* for *BDSM electrical play*. To some, it may seem counter-intuitive that a device designed as a *pain reliever* is used by sadomasochists for *pleasure.* While its real effectiveness as a pain reliever is highly doubtful, the tingling or ticklish sensations that it produces are *anything but.* A portable TENS unit will typically cost between $30 and $100.

EMS stands for *Electrical Muscle Stimulation.* EMS units are typically used in medicine, sports training, cosmetic treatments, and in therapy to produce repeated muscle contractions through electrical stimulation. EMS devices range in quality and complexity from the very intricate and expensive machines used by medical and sports professionals to the simpler, less expensive devices marketed to the flabby masses via late-night infomercials. The odd experience of having your muscles stimulated electrically to *involuntarily* contract and release in rapid succession makes the EMS unit an interesting option for BDSM sensation play. An EMS unit can usually be purchased for $30 to $250. The higher price range for the EMS, versus the TENS, is probably a reflection of the fact that EMS units are often marketed to an increasingly chunky and gullible public as *weight loss and muscle toning devices.*

Both TENS and EMS units must be FDA approved for sale in the U.S. and must meet certain industry safety guidelines. Most of the safety practices applicable for violet wands are also recommended for TENS and EMS devices, along with the following exceptions and additional recommendations

Neither device should ever be used by anyone with a heart condition, epilepsy, blood circulation problems, any sort of malignancy, or may be pregnant. People with pacemakers, metal implants, and internal pumps or monitors should avoid them as well. *Never place electrodes on open wounds, directly on the spinal column, on either side of the head, near the eyes and sinuses, on the neck near the carotid artery, or near the front of the throat, as it could cause a vasovagal reflex or laryngospasm. (Translation: choking, gagging, turning blue, and flopping around on the floor like a tuna on a boat deck.)*

Clamps, Clips, & Vices

BDSM sensation play just wouldn't be the same without all of the little *squeezy* devices that can be used to apply exquisite *pressure* to those sensitive parts of the body. There are an infinite number of different types of clamps, clips and vices that can be used in BDSM play; the most common are nipple clamps, clit clips, ball crushers, and other cock-and-ball torture (CBT) devices. Rather than get bogged down in trying to discuss *all* of them, we'll focus instead on just a few of the more common or interesting.

Nipple clamps are probably the most commonly purchased and well-known pressure sensation play toys available. They are popular both in and outside the fetish culture, and are typically one of the first kink toys purchased by couples who are just beginning to explore the wonderful world of kink. Their popularity is certainly helped by the fact that they're usually inexpensive, simple to understand, and non-threatening to novices. Unlike many of the other BDSM toys there are to choose from, you don't need the cooperation of a *partner* to experiment with nipple clamps; all you really need is *nipples.*

Nipple clamps are typically either spring operated (like clothes pins) or screw operated (like thumbscrews or a C-clamps) or employ a combination of the two, which allows users to adjust the spring tension to their personal comfort level. If purchasing a pair of spring operated nipple clamps, you should test the strength of the tension spring before purchasing, if at all possible. Nipple clamps are usually packaged in a way that makes it almost impossible, but you might want to ask a sales person if you can open the package before purchasing it or, barring that, open it immediately *after* purchasing and before you've left the store. Of course, if they have a strict no-return policy, even that will probably be fruitless. It's actually quite common, especially in the budget-priced varieties, for the spring tension to be *so severe* that *no one* would ever consider actually *using them.* Apparently, either the third-world nipple clamp manufacturers have never bothered to try out their own products, or they have some *gnarly-tough nipples.*

Nipple toys can also take the form of *clips.* The most common form of nipple clip is the *tweezer clip,* which is typically nothing more than a small device which resembles a pair of household tweezers, medical hemostat, cotter-pin, or large bobby-pin. At the open end, there may be a metal loop, elastic band, or bead which holds the loose ends of the clip together, preferably after a nipple has been firmly wedged between the two strips of metal. Nipple clips are simple and inexpensive to buy, typically costing under $10 for a pair. In a pinch *(sorry, couldn't resist)* you can easily fashion your own home-made nipple clips from a few short lengths of wood or metal, and a couple of rubber bands. The next time you order *Chinese take-out,* be sure to have them toss some disposable nipple clips - *chopsticks* - into the bag.

Sometimes, clip and clamps are designed to combine pressure sensation play with *other* forms of play. Take, for example, *bi-polar electrical stimulation clamps,* which incorporate the fun features of a TENS or EMS unit to create an electrical circuit which flows *from one side of the same clamp to the other.* When a bi-polar electrical stimulation clamp is attached to a nipple or any other body part the electrical current flows *directly through the tissue.* This focuses the electrical effects on a very small area, and eliminates the need to create a ground circuit. Rather than having to attach two separate electrodes to the subject's body, both electrodes are contained in the *same clamp,* which makes it perfect for intensely focused nipple, labial, clit, or cock stimulation.

The word *vice* isn't commonly used in reference to BDSM toys, but that's basically *what some of them are* - devices that often look and function exactly like the *workbench vice* that may be sitting in your garage right now. Vice-like BDSM toys generally fall into three categories: tit crushers, cock crushers, and ball crushers. They all work in essentially the same fashion - using the incredible power of *screw mechanisms* to tighten two rigid plates together while a sensitive part of your body is wedged *between them.*

Tit crushers are typically custom-designed and constructed for their owners, though you should be able to find a few commercially available products on the market, if you look hard enough. The cost and complexity of any tit crusher device will naturally vary widely, depending upon its design and materials. Some tit crushers are stand-alone items intended to be attached to the breasts by the pressure that they exert. Others are designed to be attached to a larger mechanism or piece of bondage furniture, which makes the device non-portable and immobilizes the bottom. Most tit crushers operate in exactly the same way: Place the breasts between the two rigid plates, and then screw the plates down to flatten them. *Easy-peasy booby squeezies.*

Cock and ball crushers operate on the same basic principle as tit crushers, only on a smaller scale. There are many different product designs for cock and ball crushers, but most are based on one of two simple approaches: two plates squeezed together by thumbscrews, or a metal tube which is narrowed in diameter by thumbscrews. Practically all of the other permutations can be attributed to aesthetics, construction materials, and whether the device is designed to accommodate just the penis, just the testicles, *or both.*

Obviously, when the name of your BDSM toy includes any mention of the word *"crusher,"* there are probably going to be some safety concerns to be aware of, and these toys are not going to be the exception to that rule. When using tit crushers, it is important to perform continuous monitoring of the breasts and of the overall condition of your subject. Once the breasts become discolored, blue or purple, that's a sign that blood flow to the breast tissue has been severely restricted, which means the clock is ticking and you only have a short time before you must reestablish proper blood flow to avoid causing serious or permanent damage. Bondage photography often depicts models with tortured breasts in this state; however, what you *don't* know is *how long* they were allowed to *remain* so. Most professional bondage photography requires very short windows of opportunity to get the best shots; being kept in the equipment or pose any longer can be hazardous to the model's health.

If you plan on combining tit crushing with any form of impact play, you should use a low-impact toy that will not break the skin. When the breast tissue is highly compressed, the taut skin is thinner and under a great deal more pressure than usual. The effect is not unlike that of a balloon which is inflated almost to the point of bursting. It may be difficult to pop an *underinflated* balloon, but an *overinflated* one will pop at the mere suggestion of a pointy object.

Finally, as is the case with most other forms of breast torture, you should be aware that some studies have shown that habitually rough treatment of the breasts can result in the growth of fibroids in the breast tissue. Fibroids are not inherently dangerous to a woman's health, but can result in false positive readings on mammograms, and may negatively affect the breast's aesthetics.

Cock and ball crushers present us with an all new and very scary set of safety concerns. The first and probably most common, aside from the obvious risk of blocked blood circulation, is cuts, bruises or abrasions. Placing pressure on the penis or testicles stretches the skin thin, making it much more susceptible to punctures, tears and other injuries. It also greatly increases the risk of *edema.* Edema is abnormal swelling caused by an excessive buildup of interstitial fluids beneath the skin or in body cavities. The rupturing of blood vessels can cause hematomas, which are the collection of blood outside of the blood vessels. The most common form of hematoma is *bruising.* Crushing the testicles can also result in spermatoceles, which are a type of cyst that can occur in the scrotum. Spermatoceles are generally painless and relatively harmless, but have the potential to cause some alarm and become problematic.

Far more serious is the risk of testicular rupture and torsion injuries. A testicular rupture is a tear in the *tunica albuginea,* which is the fibrous membrane covering the testes within the scrotum. When a testicular rupture occurs, the contents of the testes spill out into the scrotum. This is a very serious kind of trauma which usually requires surgery to save the testicle. Testicular torsion is another serious risk that should be checked out immediately when suspected. Testicular torsion occurs when the spermatic cord (which suspends the testes) becomes twisted and cuts off the blood supply to the testes. The result is typically immediate and severe pain; if testicular torsion is suspected, you should seek *immediate medical treatment.* In cases where testicular torsion is the diagnosis, prompt surgery is usually the only way to save the testes. Interestingly, testicular torsion is sometimes referred to as "winter syndrome," due to the fact that it occurs more frequently in low temperatures. That's something you might want to keep in mind when playing in cool environments.

Weights & Stretching

The use of weights is a form of sensation play or torture that is most commonly applied to a woman's nipples or labia, or to a man's scrotum. The weights themselves can take any form, from common heavy household items to commercially produced training weights. The focus of weight play is typically less on the weights, themselves, but on how the weights are attached to the sensitive body parts in question. The methods employed usually consist of clamps or alligator clips when it comes to the labia or nipples. Rings, testicle cuffs and parachutes are commonly used on the scrotum.

Suspending a heavy weight from a woman's nipples or labia can often be far more difficult than it looks. The difficulty arises when a suspended mass becomes heavy enough to force the clamp or clip to slip off of its *moorings.* To combat this unfortunate tendency, it often becomes necessary to use clamps or clips with *non-slip gripping surfaces*, which usually means *teeth* or something similar. This, of course, creates a whole *new* set of potential problems involving the triple-threat combination of great weight, sharp teeth, and sensitive body parts, which can result in ripping, tearing or lacerations.

When it comes to males, the natural silhouette of the scrotum makes hanging things from them a little *simpler*, if not *safer*. Rings and testicle cuffs made of metal, rubber, PVC or leather are often used for this purpose, but the CBT (cock and ball torture) toy that is specifically designed for suspending weights from the scrotum is called a *parachute.* A parachute is a small, conically-shaped device, typically made of leather, which attaches around the scrotum. Around its hem, there are usually short lengths of chain dangling, which gives it the appearance of a *tiny leather parachute,* and hence its name. There are many variations available on the market, including some designed and marketed specifically as *ball-stretchers.*

The safety concerns previously mentioned for clamps, clips and vices apply equally, if not more so, to any play involving the suspension of heavy weights to the nipples, labia, scrotum or any other vulnerable body part.

Heat & Cold

Sensation play involving heat or cold rarely requires any specialized toys or equipment. The most common forms of play in this category consist of ice-cube play, ice dildo play, ice water torture, hot water torture, hot surface torture and, to a lesser extent, fire play. Its appeal has little or nothing to do with heat.

Heat and cold in small amounts and for short periods of time are relatively harmless. It is only when your activities cross the boundaries of common sense that they can become problematic and potentially lethal. Running an ice cube over someone's nipples or clit? *Good.* Leaving a nine-inch ice dildo in someone's ass? *Bad.* A little ice water on sensitive body parts? *Good.* A chunk of *dry ice* on sensitive body parts? *Bad.* Water hot enough to give the skin a nice rosy hue? *Good.* Water that is hot enough to scald and cause blistering? *Bad.* A little common sense goes a *long way* when it comes to this kind of play.

You should always be cognizant of the signs of *hypothermia* (low core body temperature, shivering, mental confusion), as well as *hyperthermia* (high core body temperature, hot dry skin, nausea, vomiting, headache, dizziness). Both conditions are potentially life-threatening, and can develop relatively quickly and easily under artificially cold or hot conditions. Additionally, some of the normal functions of our bodies can be severely disrupted by being exposed to abnormal temperature ranges for more than a very short span of time. For example, an ice cube in the rectum may be relatively harmless, but an ice dildo left too long in there can cause a week of severe pain, cramping, diarrhea, and rectal bleeding.

Abrasion

Abrasion play is relatively uncommon in the BDSM lifestyle, though it has enjoyed a small surge in popularity as people seek out new and unique tactile experiences. Abrasion play consists of using rough-textured objects or surfaces to rub or abrade the skin in such a way that it produces desired sensations in the subject. Anyone who has ever gotten a skinned knee as a child knows that even a small abrasion can create some *pretty intense sensations.* Abrasion play generally falls into two basic categories. There's abrasion play that is done purely for the sake of producing *pain or sensitivity* in a localized region, and there's the kind of abrasion play that is *pleasurable or even therapeutic.* Of course, most masochists would argue that pain and sensitivity are *the very definition* of pleasurable and therapeutic.

Similarly to heat and cold sensation play, abrasion play requires little or no specialized equipment or toys. For the most part, the only thing needed is an adequately rough surface to rub against your subject's skin. Examples can include sandpaper, steel wool, pot scrubbers, cleaning brushes, toothbrushes, Emory boards, nail files, rasps, or even your own fingernails. The concept is really quite simple: rub, rasp or scratch the subject's skin until it becomes sensitive, raw, or painful. This can be an end in itself, or a means to other ends, such as serving as a precursor to impact play, violet wand play, or other activities.

A *therapeutic* form of abrasion play that I happen to enjoy is one that is practiced widely in Asia to treat aches and pains, chills, and various minor illnesses. Since the practice lacks an English-language name that I'm aware of, I simply refer to it as *"coin striping."* It typically consists of having a subject lie on his or her stomach, disrobed from the waist up. The Top takes a quarter, and applies a small dab of mentholated oil or muscle rub *(such as Ben Gay or Icy Hot)* to either the coin or to a spot on the subject's back. Then, gripping the coin firmly, he rubs the dab of liniment into the skin using the corrugated edge of the quarter. The quarter is drawn repeatedly in a long steady motion across the skin *in one direction only*, along the same path in such a way that, after about a dozen passes, a *bright red line* begins to appear on the skin. Stop abrading that line when it's glowing red, but *before* it begins to rupture the skin. Choose another spot about an inch from the first line, and repeat the process, creating another parallel red stripe across the back in the same fashion. Continue until the entire back is covered in glowing red stripes. The visual effect of the stripes can last anywhere from one to four days, depending on the subject's skin type and resiliency.

Some people enjoy creating intricate and attractive patterns in this fashion. The edge of the quarter forces the mentholated oils through the skin, and each stripe produces a *hot* sensation that lasts several hours. When the entire back is covered in coin stripes, the subject will usually feel toasty warm all night long, which can be particularly soothing for anyone with chills, aches, or pains. In many parts of Asia, people pay for professional treatments of this sort in much the same way they go for massages, acupuncture, or cupping. The procedure is rare enough in the U.S. that the sight of your red stripes may elicit some concerned reactions from some people. After all, it *looks* as if a scurvy pirate has tied you to the ship's mainsail mast and given you fifty lashes. I usually recommend that anyone who will be going to see a doctor within the next few days delay their abrasion play until after their appointment!

The safety concerns related to abrasion play are minimal, with the main worry being infection. The wider the area of skin that is rubbed raw, the greater the possibility will be of harmful bacteria passing through the distressed skin and into the bloodstream. The Top should always wash his hands thoroughly with a strong antibacterial soap and sanitize the bottom's back with an alcohol or peroxide wipe prior to the procedure. Any stripes that result in breaks in the skin should be treated as open wounds to prevent the transmission of disease or infection and to promote healing.

Irritants

Irritant play isn't something you *hear* about very often and, even when you do, it's rarely referred to as such. Even so, it's a fairly common form of sadomasochistic play which usually involves creating pain or discomfort to sensitive parts of the body by applying substances like Tabasco sauce, toothpaste, hot peppers, wasabi, chili powder, ginger root, peppermint oil, clove oil, citrus oil, witch hazel, and other irritants.

Sometimes, a specific substance develops a wide following and gets a name all its own. One example is *figging*, which is the practice of inserting a freshly peeled *ginger root* into the anus or vagina. The ginger is typically carved into a dildo or butt-plug shape and, when inserted, produces a tingly warm sensation which gradually grows in intensity until it becomes painful. Figging can also be combined in various ways with other forms of play to intensify the sensations. Any activity that causes involuntary constrictions or spasms of the vagina or anus (such as occurs during orgasm) will squeeze the ginger, producing a rush or heat, tingling or pain. The sensations associated with figging typically last 15-20 minutes before they begin to fade.

When it comes to safety, irritants can be as safe or as dangerous as their potential for misuse. You should attempt to differentiate between the water-soluble substances and the oil-based irritants. That way, you know best how to *remove* them if they become excessively painful or begin to cause tissue damage. Certain oils, such as pepper oil, cinnamon oil, clove oil, and mentholated oil can cause significant damage to sensitive tissues if used in concentrated form or left on for too long. When using an irritant for play for the first time, you should test it out in diluted form, preferably first on normal healthy skin, then abraded or sensitive skin, and lastly on exterior then interior mucous membranes. Many irritants have a specific counter-agent that *immediately* counteracts its effects. One example is using *boric acid* to immediate counteract the effects of hot peppers. Do a little research to learn if the irritant you plan on using has a counteracting agent. For the ones that don't, it might be a good idea to keep some soapy lukewarm water and a washcloth nearby, just in case the irritant needs to be removed very quickly. No one who is screaming her safe word along with, *"Get it off me now!"* wants to hear you say, "I *might* have a bucket somewhere in the garage, *let me go see."*

Speaking of soap and water, I highly recommend that you wash your hands thoroughly after handling irritants like hot peppers, wasabi or Tabasco sauce. It's terribly easy to forget where those fingers have been before absent-mindedly wiping your eyes with them; a mistake that would not only be an *epic buzzkill,* but could seriously undermine any credibility as a Top that you might have had.

Finally, you should be cognizant of any *allergies* your bottom might have, including *food allergies.* It might be tempting, for example, to assume that a food allergy would only be a problem if the substance is *eaten;* however an allergic reaction can often be triggered by exposure of the substance to the mucous membranes.

Cupping

Cupping, like *coin-striping and acupuncture,* is another Asian therapeutic practice that has recently been adopted by the BDSM culture and become immensely popular. The practice, which has been around for thousands of years, involves the use of *cups* in which a partial vacuum is produced by heat, flame, or suction in order to draw a ball of the subject's flesh up into the cup. The procedure is most often performed on the subject's back; however, it can be done to just about any fleshy part of the body. Quite often, the subject's entire back will be covered with these "suction cups", which are typically made of glass.

The two basic types of cupping are *dry cupping* and *wet cupping*. Dry cupping, or cupping that doesn't involve any breaks in the skin, is practiced throughout Asia and parts of Europe for its relaxing, therapeutic sensations, which are similar to getting a deep-tissue massage. Wet cupping, or cupping that involves blood-letting, is practiced in many cultures as a way of "drawing toxins" out of the body, a dubious medical claim at best. Due to increasing concerns and awareness of the risks of blood-borne diseases and infections, wet cupping has seen a marked decrease in popularity in the BDSM culture. Dry cupping, at the same time, has seen an almost geometric surge in popularity.

The mechanics of cupping are typically achieved in one of three ways: heat, fire, and suction. The heat and fire methods rely upon this simple principle of physics: hot air *expands* in volume and cooler air tends to *contract*. Placing a cup full of *hot air* on the skin produces a curious phenomenon - the air rapidly cools, and creates a volume of low pressure or a partial vacuum. That, in turn, draws a suddenly purple ball of the subject's flesh *up into the cup,* where it will stay until the vacuum seal at the edge of the cup is broken. This suctioned ball of flesh includes muscle tissue which is pulled and stretched in ways that cannot be accomplished through ordinary massage. If the back is coated with a thin sheen of *oil,* the cups can be *moved around* while still suctioned to the skin, making it even more like a deep-tissue massage and spreading the therapeutic effects over a *wider area.*

Fire cupping isn't really any different from any other kind of heat-based cupping procedure, except for the fact that it is much more efficient at heating *the air inside the cup* without significantly heating *the cup itself.* A *hot cup on your skin* can introduce an element of *pain* to a procedure which is usually not associated with being a painful activity. It's somewhat ironic that the introduction of *flame* to the cupping procedure makes it more *frightening* to some, while simultaneously making it *safer and less painful* than placing hot cups on the skin.

When performing fire cupping, the Top simply swabs the interior of the cup with a flammable liquid, tips the cup edge on the subject's skin, ignites the cup interior with a spark igniter, long-tipped lighter, or violet wand, and immediately seals the cup to the skin. The best type of swab to use is usually an extra-large cotton swab on a wooden stick, similar in appearance to a Q-tip, but several times larger. These can be purchased in any medical supply store, many pharmacies, or online. You can also easily improvise a swab by putting a cotton ball or make-up removal pad into a long pair of tension tweezers or locked medical hemostat. The swab is actually more important than one might think, at first blush. The ability to *control* the amount of flammable liquid used to coat the cup interior is critical. Too much, and it could drip onto your subject's skin and perhaps even ignite any oils that may be there. Too little, and cup interior won't ignite *at all.*

The flammable fluids used most commonly in fire cupping are isopropyl alcohol and mentholated oil. Isopropyl alcohol is sold in varying proofs, so you'll want to ensure that the rubbing alcohol you purchase is at least 91% strength; anything lower will not burn. Mentholated oils are sold in Asian pharmacies and online for use in cupping, acupuncture, coin-striping, and other therapeutic procedures. Some of the advantages of using mentholated oil are: its cooling effects on the skin, it is less harsh on the skin, and many people find the scent soothing. The disadvantages are: it's harder to find, not as affordable to purchase, and *not everyone* likes the scent of eucalyptus.

The cups used in fire cupping (or *any* sort of cupping, really) don't have to be particularly special in any way, other than being *structurally sound* and without any *sharp edges.* The size should allow for a good-sized ball of flesh to be drawn into it, but is mostly a matter of personal preference. The average size is about the size of a standard juice glass or what a bartender calls a *"rocks" glass.* The glasses that are specifically produced for cupping are often distinguishable by their rounded bottoms, indicating that they aren't meant to sit on anything but their *open end*. In cupping, as in so many other things, *round bottoms are a good thing.*

The third method of cupping involves *mechanical suction.* Cupping sets which are specifically designed for mechanical suction are typically comprised of glass or plastic cups of various sizes and styles, each with a tiny one-way air valve at its top, and a vacuum gun, which usually resembles a large toy squirt gun. The difference is, instead of being designed like a squirt gun to *shoot water out* of its barrel, the vacuum gun is designed to *suck air into its barrel* with each squeeze of the trigger. The barrel of the vacuum gun is placed on the tiny valve at the top of each cup, and the air is swiftly sucked out of the cup with a few quick squeezes of the trigger.

The advantages of using a vacuum gun for cupping are: no need for flammable liquids and swabs, there's no risk of a mishap or injury due to flame, and some sets come with cup inserts that have specialized functions, such as poking or imprinting the skin or serving as electrodes for electrical play. The disadvantages are: lost or broken cups may be difficult to replace, malfunctioning air valves are usually impossible to repair, and the rubber seals for the valves deteriorate over time.

Once in place, the cups can be left on the subject's back for up to thirty minutes, depending on the circumstances, the appearance and resilience of the subject's skin, and his or her comfort level. Cupping should not *necessarily* be a painful experience, so if your subject reports unintended pain, that should be interpreted as a sign that *something* is not right.

For the benefit of our *masochist* friends, there are *plenty* of ways that cupping *can* be done in ways that *are* painful. Cups can be placed on a *dry* back and then *mercilessly twisted* to create some incredibly intense sensations. Cups on an *oiled* back can be moved in ways that can be uncomfortable or even painful. Cup *inserts* specifically designed for use with violet wands or other electrical devices can add a whole new dimension of sensations to the cupping experience, to include painful ones, if desired. Cupping can also easily be combined with other types of BDSM play, such as bondage, suspensions, CBT, sensory deprivation, or even impact play.

Cupping is a relatively safe activity to engage in, as long as common sense is employed. When flammable liquids are being used, the container should be secured in a location that precludes it from being knocked over or spilled. When the swab is being used to coat the interior of the cup, a minimal amount of fluid should be used. If the fluid can drip from the cup when it is inverted, *you're using too much.* A drop of flaming fluid falling onto a person's oil slathered back could easily ruin his or her entire week.

It's usually a good idea to apply a few test cups prior to a full treatment in order to gauge how well the subject's skin tolerates cupping. Most people will have no problems, whatsoever. In rare cases, some people may have very fragile or thin skin that isn't suitable for cupping. Cupping should not be done on the neck, face, or directly atop the spine.

Cupping should be avoided by people with infectious skin disorders, heart disease, circulation problems, blood clots, history of stroke, autoimmune disorders, or who are unusually susceptible to bruising. There is always a possibility of breaks in the skin; therefore, your subject should be asked about any blood-borne disease or infection, and proper precautions should be taken regarding contact with blood.

Some cupping practitioners strongly recommend that a subject should be well-hydrated at least several hours prior to a cupping session to ensure that there are enough fluids in the body to facilitate the proper circulation of blood and the body's ability to handle capillary ruptures, bruising and minor clotting that can occur during and after the procedure.

Knife Play

Knife or blade play is one of those activities which could properly be placed in a number of different categories of fetish play; however, after giving it a great deal of thought, I have decided - at least for the purposes of this chapter - to categorize it as a form of *sensation play.* After all, it is not just the sensation of a blade against the skin that makes knife play so interesting, but the associated *sensation of fear.* Knife play typically involves various kinds of knives, daggers, razors, swords, cutters, shears, and scissors.

Knife play scenes can consist of blades being used to create fear, shave pubic or body hair, cut or scrape the skin, cut away clothing, scrape hardened wax off the skin, or to *poke* the subject. Blades may range in sharpness from very dull to razor sharp, and sometimes two identical blades (one sharp, the other dull) are used to first create the impression of a dangerously sharp instrument before switching to the dull blade in subsequent play to reduce the risk of injury. The critical ingredient in any knife play is always the psychological aspect of the scene. The proper cultivation and exploitation of anticipation, intimidation, anxiety, and fear is every bit as important as the blade you use, and the manner in which you wield it.

Safety concerns regarding knife play are, as one might imagine, a *big deal.* Knife play is generally considered a form of *edge play*; it pushes the boundaries of what most people consider to be safe. (Contrary to popular belief, *edge play* refers to the *edginess of the play*, rather than the edge of a blade.) The prime directive of knife play is: *Try not to cut anyone unintentionally.*

While accidental cuts are usually the primary fear and focus of those engaging in knife play, cuts themselves are typically not terribly dangerous unless you sever a major blood vessel, rupture a critical organ, or slice something off that should have stayed where it was. More concerning should be the risk of serious infection to the subject from a non-sterile blade or the risk of transmission of blood-borne disease or infection from the subject to others, if any bleeding occurs.

To reduce the risk of infection, the subject should shower prior to the knife play scene, and the Top should wash his hands thoroughly with a strong antibacterial soap. Knife blades should be disinfected with isopropyl alcohol or hydrogen peroxide, rather than with boiling water. Putting a knife in boiling water can warp the construction of the knife and will hasten the oxidation (rusting) of the blade.

One particularly useful rule of thumb is to treat all blades as if they are dangerously sharp. That way, a momentary lapse of concentration or mix up in blades won't result in a trip to the E.R. It is rarely the sharp knife that causes a mishap; it's the *one that you thought was dull.*

Always anticipate sudden or seemingly irrational fear reactions. It's always tempting to toss out the worn-out saying, *"expect the unexpected,"* but the truth is, fear should be expected and when people are afraid, they can do incredibly crazy things. *You should expect that,* and plan accordingly. Flinching, jumping, jerking, and pitching forward or backward may not be entirely *rational* things to do when someone is holding a knife to your throat, but the Top should always *anticipate* it, nevertheless.

If you do not have a *fully stocked* first aid kit nearby, I *highly* recommend that you postpone your knife play scene until you *do.* And by *fully stocked,* I mean that there are enough sterile bandages (*not band-aids,* but real cloth *bandages*) and gauze pads to properly dress a wound with a standard first aid dressing or - in the event of *very* heavy bleeding - a pressure bandage. If you *don't* know basic first aid, I would suggest that you have absolutely no business engaging in BDSM knife play.

Finally, I would be remiss if I didn't address what is - *at least for the Top* - quite possibly the most dangerous aspect of BDSM knife play. Cutting your subject's *clothing,* without first getting permission to do so, is almost always going to end up being *hazardous to your health.*

Hot Wax

Hot wax play isn't just for *kinksters* anymore; it's become increasingly *mainstream* in its appeal as both an erotic *and* artistic pastime. Wax play generally consists of dripping or pouring molten candle wax onto someone's skin to produce erotic *sensations*, for *aesthetic* purposes, or *both*. The types of candle wax used for erotic wax play *typically* fall into two categories: *paraffin* (a man-made, petroleum-based compound) and *beeswax* (which is secreted by the wax glands of worker bees). There are many other varieties of wax that can be used, but they all generally fall into these two categories, differing only in the various additives that are combined with the waxes to change its properties, such as its burn characteristics, melting point, plasticity, or effects upon the skin. Of those four factors, the most important consideration for wax play should always be the wax's *melting point.*

Pain tolerance naturally varies from person to person but, on average, the wax will feel *hot* on the skin at around 110° F., and *painfully hot* between 120° and 125° F. Anything *above* that may cause second-degree burns, blistering, and perhaps even permanent scarring. Pure paraffin wax has an average melting point between 115° and 154° F. Unadulterated beeswax has an average melting point of about 145° F. Wax and candle manufacturers routinely add substances to the wax to change its properties and some of those additives *will* raise or lower the melting point of the wax in unpredictable ways. For that reason, store-bought candles can vary widely in terms of their melting points. Candles that come in glass jars typically have a melting point of about 120° F. Standalone pillar-type candles usually have a melting point of 140° F. Elegant taper candles of the sort that may grace your dinner table at a fine restaurant are the most dangerous of all, with an average melting point of 160°. The *wild card* in all of this is the unfortunate fact that candle manufacturers *rarely* label their products *in any way* that indicates the type of wax or additives, *much less it's melting point.* That's why most people who are serious about hot wax play *make their own* candles; so they'll positively *know what's in them.*

Crock pots, double boilers, and fondue sets are a convenient way to melt paraffin for making your own candles or for wax play itself. Do keep in mind, however, that just because you adjust the temperature of your crock pot, that doesn't necessarily change the temperature of your *molten wax.* You should also be sure to regularly *stir* your molten wax, as the temperature of the wax can vary widely in different parts of the same pot. You should be able to obtain all the materials you'll need for candle-making at your local hobby store, to include paraffin, wicks, dyes (crayons work beautifully), molds and *thermometers.*

There *are* several safety concerns you should be aware of, when it comes to wax play. First and foremost, you should always be aware of the temperature of the molten wax you are using. This includes knowing how different factors can affect that temperature. Molten wax will cool as it falls through the air onto the skin, for example. The closer you hold a candle to your subject, the hotter the wax will be when it reaches the skin. Molten wax that *pools or puddles* in low areas, cracks, and crevices will retain more heat and will have a higher risk of causing burns or unintended pain. That could be *especially* problematic if those *cracks and crevices* just happen to be where you keep your *naughty-bits.*

All types of wax have a *flashpoint,* which is the temperature at which the wax will burst into flame. Under normal conditions your wax will never get that hot in the course of a wax play scene, but accidents *do* happen. Keep your molten wax away from hot objects, heating elements, or open flames and remove unnecessary objects which are flammable from your play area. Want to know what's worse than molten wax that has reached its flashpoint and has burst into flames? *This:* molten wax that bursts into flames and *startles you into dropping it,* and is now spreading flames across your floor towards the curtains. On a somewhat related note, it's usually a good idea to keep a portable fire extinguisher handy.

The one thing that some people sometimes find exasperating about wax play is the *mess.* A little forethought can go a long way towards avoiding those kinds of frustrations. Avoid getting wax in your bottom's hair. It can be exceedingly difficult to remove, once there. Some folks have had luck using nit-combs to remove hardened wax from their hair. Wear expendable clothing, and cover your furnishings or carpet with a plastic drop cloth to protect them from drips and spills. When accidents happen, use a hot iron and a paper towel or old t-shirt to blot the wax out of whatever it's gotten into. Be sure to keep the iron's temperature set low enough that it doesn't melt the material, particularly if it's a synthetic. Depending on the situation and material, a hot blow-dryer may work even better. To remove hardened wax from your bottom's skin more easily, consider a light coat of oil massaged into the skin prior to the hot wax session.

Wax play can be a *great* way to introduce someone to sensation play, express your artistic talents, or just enjoy a slow, sensual evening of eroticism with your partner. It can also be a fun learning experience for a small gathering of intimate friends or munch groups. It's safe, sexy, fun, and artistic. What's not to like?

Role Play Accessories

Role play accessories may or may not technically qualify as BDSM toys in the strictest sense, since *one* person's role play accessory may simply be a regular part of another person's daily wardrobe. We've already covered quite a few of the items that can be used in role play, such as impact toys and bondage gear. Given the breadth and scope of all the other items which *could* be considered role play accessories, I've chosen just a few of the possibilities to illustrate a couple of the more interesting types of fetish play, and perhaps give you some ideas for accessorizing on your *own.*

Pony Tack and Accessories

The ancient Greek philosopher Aristotle (384 BC - 322 BC) is well-known for his writings on physics, politics, ethics, and logic, but few people are aware of the fact that he purportedly enjoyed being ridden like a horse. Today we call it pony play, and it is an increasingly popular form of BDSM animal role play. *Ponyboys* and *ponygirls* generally fall into three categories: cart ponies, riding ponies, and show ponies. There *can* be, and often is, a great deal of overlap between the three groups. The role play accessories related to pony play are highly specialized, both in the sense that they are not typically used in any other kind of scene or activity *outside* of pony play, and also in the sense that each category of pony play requires specific kinds of gear or *tack,* as it is referred to by pony play enthusiasts. Tack that is fairly common to *all* three categories of ponies includes a crop, bit or bit gag, collars, butt-plug or harness pony tail, wrist and/or ankle cuffs, bridles, reigns, plumes, harnesses, spurs, and hoof-mitts or hoof-boots. Less common, but still applicable to all forms of pony play are items such as blinders, breast reigns, masks, horse-head hoods, hobbles (which limit leg movement), martingales (which minimize head-tossing), polos (wraps for a pony's legs), tongue-ties or tongue-ports (for securing the tongue), and specialized leather, latex or PVC body suits. This list *barely scratches the surface* when it comes to the incredibly wide assortment of available pony play toys, tack, and accessories.

Cart ponies will naturally require a cart, carriage, chariot, sleigh, sulky, or wagon. As pony play accessories go, these items can be among the most expensive. *Carts and sulkies* are typically lightweight two-wheeled vehicles similar in appearance to Chinese *rickshaws* which are pulled behind the pony. *Chariots* are similar to carts and sulkies in construction, being a lightweight two-wheeled vehicle; however the rider remains *standing* as the chariot is pulled. A *wagon* is a four-wheeled vehicle that is designed to be pulled by a single pony or a pair of ponies. Replace the four wheels with runners designed for use on ice, snow, or grass, and it becomes a *sleigh.* Finally, a carriage is considered the largest of the pony conveyances; it can be designed to be pulled by as many as *six ponies.* Pony carts can be quite expensive to purchase, which is why some pony enthusiasts acquire the necessary skills to construct their own. In addition to a *cart*, cart ponies usually require *long reigns*, and specialized *belts or harnesses* to which the cart can be attached. This helps to reduce the strain on the pony's arms, and allows the arms to be posed or bound behind the back for aesthetic or postural purposes.

Riding ponies don't pull their owners behind them; they *carry them* and, therefore, typically will require a *saddle*. Saddles may be the kind made for *real horses*, or designed specifically for humans who like pony play. Of the latter variety, there are saddles specifically constructed for *two-legged* and for *four-legged* human ponies. Since the human back is not really designed to support the full weight of an adult rider (particularly in the four-legged configuration) riders often support the bulk of their own weight with their *own legs.* Even so, the right saddle fitted and used appropriately can make the ride far more pleasant for *both* the pony and rider.

Show ponies are ponies who are specifically trained to compete in shows. They wear very elaborate tack, such as ornamental plumes, harnesses, bridles, boots, tails, and learn various skills. These skills may include a variety of gaits, jumps, dances, or *dressage* techniques. The highly ornamental tack worn by show ponies is usually unique or custom-made, so there are few generalizations that can be made about it other than to say it's fancy, fascinating, and fabulously *fetish.*

Pet Play Accessories

While *pony play* is technically just another form of *pet play*, the need for highly specialized tack and accessories in pony play puts it in a *toy category* all its own. Pet play *in general,* however, is usually far less complicated or expensive. Pony play *aside*, pet play typically falls into three categories: puppy play, kitten play, and miscellaneous or generic pet play. As you might imagine, the toys and accessories used in pet play are relatively simple, inexpensive, and may even already be sitting unused, somewhere in your house. For puppy play, you might consider a muzzle, mittens, butt-plug tail, collar and leash, a simulated doggy bed, pet cage, dog food bowls, and chew toys. For kitten play, kitty ears, butt plug tail, cat collar, cat toys, scratching post, and simulated catnip might be more appropriate. The third general category of miscellaneous pets can consist of anything from aardvarks to zebras, and their associated accessories. I know of at least one couple that enjoys role playing as penguins. I would assume that, beyond the occasional dead fish and a lot of ice, it's a role that should be fairly easy to accessorize.

Age Play Accessories

Age play accessories fall into that classification of toys that is so broad and nonspecific that it becomes practically meaningless. There are, however, some *exceptions* which we'll take note of here. First, we should probably clarify that *age play* refers to a *wide variety* of activities that aren't just limited to *Daddy Dom/babygirl* kinds of role play. Age play is widely enjoyed by people of all ages, genders, and sexual orientations, and can be sexual or *nonsexual* in nature. Age play involves at least one of the people in a scene assuming the mannerisms, appearance, and/or attitudes of a person whose age differs significantly from his or her own *actual chronological age* and at least one other person interacting with him or her *age-appropriately,* if not *societal-norms appropriately*. It doesn't *always* have to be about role playing the part of someone *younger,* even though that is most often the case.

Adult babies and diaper lovers (AB/DL) enjoy activities that involve at least one of the partners assuming the role of a baby or toddler still in diapers. Obviously then, *diapers* should probably be at the top of any AB/DL's list of must-have accessories. Diapers in adult sizes come in a huge variety of styles, including the old-fashioned cloth diapers and the new-fangled disposable ones. The disposable variety is also available in a wide selection of printed cartoon character and other fun designs. In place of, or to supplement the adult diapers, you can also find adult-sized pull-ups, plastic diaper covers, nappy pants, and diaper-doublers, which are pads which make a diaper more absorbent. Some of the other accessories that can enhance AB/DL play include adult-sized onesies, twosies, pajamas, changing mats, safety-pins, bibs, pacifiers, baby bottles, cribs, baby beds, and play pens. Oh, and *whatever you do,* don't forget the *plushy toys.*

Age play, apart from *AB/DL play,* tends to fall into four general age divisions: prepubescent, pubescent, teen, and *senior age play*, which is relatively rare. The toys, accessories, and clothing appropriate for each type of age play is entirely a matter of personal kink, preference, and taste. Obviously, they will differ *significantly* based on not only the role play age assumed, but by whether the activity is *sexual or nonsexual,* whether it involves *other types of play* such as spanking, bondage, or even *medical* play, and the degree to which the activity becomes less of a *scene* and more of a *lifestyle.* Equipping yourself for a Saturday night *age-play scene* is always going to be a *lot* simpler and cheaper than equipping yourself for a 24-7 *Little's lifestyle.*

BDSM Furniture

BDSM furniture is a truly *fascinating* subject, a subject about which I hope to write an entire book someday. I believe that what makes BDSM furniture so interesting is the fact that each piece is typically a unique, one-of-a-kind work of art, often produced by the owner's own two hands as a labor of love. For that reason, there are few generalizations that can be made about them other than to describe their form and function, but even that can problematic given the boundless creativity that is often used in the production of some of these pieces. In the following pages, we'll take a look at several types of BDSM furnishings in terms of their form, function, variations on the theme, and safety considerations, when applicable. I'll refrain from attempting to make any generalizations about them regarding construction material, workmanship, availability, or pricing, since practically every piece is going to be an exception to the rule.

Crosses

The most common type of BDSM cross is the *St. Andrew's cross,* but it is hardly the *only* type you're likely to see in private or public dungeons. The St Andrew's cross, which is also sometimes referred to as an *X-frame* or *saltire cross,* is patterned after the type of cross upon which the Christian apostle Saint Andrew was purportedly crucified in the 1st century AD. It consists essentially of two cross-beams in the form of a large letter "X", with hardware at the ends of the beams to facilitate the attachment of wrist and ankle restraints. It may or may not be padded, may be completely vertical or canted, and can be constructed from practically any sturdy materials. Sometimes, additional braces, beams, or restraining hardware are added to enable the immobilization of the torso, neck or head. Other interesting modifications may include suspending the cross or placing it upon risers, hinges, or swivels. A raised vertical cross with a centrally positioned swivel can actually allow the cross to be *spun like a pinwheel,* though even just a little of that can quickly become too much of a good thing. Bottoms may be attached facing the cross or facing outward, depending on the type of play being contemplated.

The most common configuration for a cross is to attach it *securely* to a wall; you should always ensure that it is anchored to the wooden studs in the wall, and not just to the plaster dry-wall. Another common practice is to use the cross as a free-standing device with a tripod-base configuration. Never simply lean a cross against a wall or another object. Attaching someone to an *unstable* cross where there is even a tiny risk of it falling over could turn out to be *exceedingly* dangerous.

Other types of crosses that you might encounter include the basic cross (which resembles the familiar Christian symbol), *inverted* basic cross, triangle cross, folding or portable cross, seated cross, cabinet-cross combo, cage-cross combo, or bench-cross combo.

As is the case with *any* form of bondage play, the Top's attention to detail as it pertains to blood circulation, respiration, unintended wounds, and the bottom's mental state or pain tolerance can be the deciding factor that ultimately determines whether or not it is a safe activity.

Benches, Chairs, & Stools

For the sake of simplicity, we will be lumping all BDSM benches, chairs, and stools into the generic umbrella category of *benches.* The near-infinite number of variations in designs and innovations make it increasingly difficult to know where to draw lines of differentiation. In fact, the lines have even become increasingly blurred between *tables* and benches, as well, since many products can serve multiple purposes or are *convertible.*

BDSM benches run a close second to the St. Andrew's cross as one of the most popular types of dungeon furniture. They are typically easy to design and construct, or to adapt from other purposes, which also makes them relatively affordable compared to other types of BDSM furnishings. Unused or discarded weight-benches and exercise contraptions can be particularly well-suited for conversion to kinkier uses, which can make your next trip to the Goodwill store a lot more interesting than it *used to be.* The most popular types of BDSM benches are spanking benches, sex benches, gynecological/medical play, cock & ball torture (CBT), predicament bondage, electrical play, tickle & miscellaneous other forms of torture, and queening stools.

Spanking bench is a generic term which refers to practically any kind of bench used in *impact play.* It need not be limited to spanking alone, as it will probably work just as well for flogging, cropping, whipping, caning, and slapping. There's no single characteristic that makes a bench *definitively* a spanking bench versus any other kind of bench, other than a general tendency to present the bottom's *buttocks* prominently and accessibly.

A *sex bench* is any bench designed primarily to give a Top easy accessibility to a restrained bottom's *genital area and/or mouth.* For that reason, it also tends to be ideal for CBT, gynecological examination play, forced orgasm or orgasm denial play, or any other type of activity that depends upon unfettered access to the restrained bottom's genitalia. Sex benches can come in a variety of forms, including simple short bondage benches, gynecological exam chairs, birthing chairs, leg-spreaders, and modified horizontal crosses.

Any bench that doesn't specifically fall into one of the two categories above can properly and generically be categorized as a *bondage bench* and used in an unlimited number of kinky ways, limited only by your perverse imagination. Two rather unique exceptions would be the *bondage horse,* which typically resembles the sort of *pommel horse* used in gymnastics, and the *queening stool,* which is a specialized stool that allows ready access to a seated person's bare genitals to the person lying on his or her back below. It is used primarily for *forced cunnilingus, or face sitting.* An interesting variation on the queening stool design is the *smotherbox,* which works just like a queening stool, but consists of a box specifically designed to restrain and position the bottom's head in the proper position for forced oral sex.

Suspension Frames & Hoists

Suspension frames and hoists are a handy thing to have around if you want to lift or suspend your bottom, raise specific limbs or body parts, or place your subject into an elevated position for predicament bondage. Most homes are simply not built to support any significant weight from the ceiling and, even when they *are,* not everyone wants to permanently install *bondage gear* there. As a result, some folks find it more convenient to construct or purchase a sturdy frame to which they can attach ropes, chains, or straps for bondage and suspensions that will support the full weight of an adult. Suspension frames can be constructed from wood, iron, construction-grade aluminum, or steel pipe.

One of the advantages of a suspension frame is its relative portability; when you're ready to move into a new home, you should *theoretically* be able to take it with you. Another advantage is the fact that some types of suspension frames can easily be camouflaged as *something else.* A suspension frame in the garage looks an awful lot like an *engine hoist frame*. A suspension frame over your bed might be mistaken for a *canopy support.* Put one on your backyard patio, and it looks like part of an awning or sun shade. Sometimes, the best place to hide something is *in plain sight.*

A *hoist* is any contraption used to raise or lower a weight that is suspended by a rope, cable, strap, or chain. Hoists come in many forms, and can be manually operated, electrically powered, or even pneumatic. A hoist is by no means a *necessity* for suspension bondage, but it *can* definitely make your life easier. Manually operated pulley or ratchet hoists can be purchased quite cheaply from any hardware store, and even electrically operated winches can be surprisingly affordable, if you shop around.

Sex Swings & Bondage Swings

Once you get your suspension frame set up, perhaps you'll want to check out the selection of *swings* that are available in the fetish marketplace. *Sex swings* and *bondage swings* are essentially the same product, differing only in the degree to which one spreads you apart, making your orifices more accessible, while the other binds you up. That, obviously, can make it a tad harder to get to your goodies.

Sex and bondage swings are uniquely susceptible to being marketed as shoddily constructed *novelty items.* I *highly* recommend that you avoid ever purchasing one from your local *sex novelty shop*, as you are virtually *guaranteed* to end up with a *piece of junk* that will not only fail to perform as advertised but may, in fact, be quite *dangerous* to use. Shop, instead, with reputable BDSM retailers. Believe it or not, *right now*, somewhere in the world, there's a marketing executive thinking,

"Hey, you know those crappy leather *thigh cuffs* which have been rotting in our warehouse for the last ten years? Let's connect two of them with a twenty-cent strap, and sell it as a *sex swing!"* Trust me, that sort of thing *really does happen.* How do I know? I know, because *I used to be that guy.*

Stocks & Pillories

Stocks and pillories were popular in medieval times as a form of public humiliation and punishment. Today, they are found only in museums, amusement parks, and BDSM dungeons. The two terms are often used interchangeably, but they are technically two very *different* devices. Both typically consist of hinged or sliding planks of wood with cut-outs used for restraining certain parts of the human body. A *pillory,* however, is generally used to restrain the *hands and neck only,* and is affixed to a pole or set of poles in such a way that the person in it *must stand.*

Stocks, on the other hand, are set *vertically* and used to immobilize only the subject's *arms and legs* while he typically *sits.* There are many other permutations, some of which immobilize *all three* appendages - the neck, arms, *and* legs. For the most part, all stocks, pillories, and similar devices are generically referred to as *stocks.*

There are quite a few online retailers offering stocks and pillories; however, their relatively simple design makes it a do-it-yourself project that is feasible for most people. Some of the fascinating DIY design variations that I've seen have included a *chain-suspended pillory*, a *pillory table* which required the bottom to kneel beneath the table and poke her head and hands through holes in the tabletop, and even a barrel pillory with just a head poking out of the top of a wooden barrel. The possibilities are endless.

Racks

Racks, which are sometimes referred to as *torture* or *stretching racks,* have been used for torture and sometimes even *execution* for over two thousand years. The traditional rack consisted of a wooden frame or table-like device which sat horizontally or at a slight incline, with *ratcheting rollers or cylinders* at each end. Attached to the ratcheting rollers were ropes, chains or cables which were, in turn, attached to wrist or ankle cuffs. A subject would be placed on the rack and restrained by the wrist and ankle cuffs before his torturer would begin ratcheting the rollers tight to put excruciating tension on the arms and legs. Often, the person would be held immobile on the rack by the tension while other forms of torture, such as whipping, burning, or cutting were applied. Eventually, the tension would be increased and the subject's cartilage, ligaments, and bones would begin to pop, tear, and dislocate in a cacophony of gruesome sounds. This form of torture was *so feared,* prisoners would sometimes commit *suicide* rather than be subjected to it.

The modern-day racks used in BDSM play aren't *quite* so draconian, but they *do* apply the same general mechanism to stretch a person out lengthwise by his wrists and ankles, typically to immobilize the subject while *other* things are done to him. Due to the size and complexity of their design, racks tend to be rather pricy if purchased, or a true labor of love if constructed as a do-it-yourself project.

Cages

Cages are *cool.* They just *are.* Even if you haven't got a single kinky bone in your body and have no interest *whatsoever* in the fetish lifestyle, it's still hard to look at a small, elegantly constructed cage made specifically for a human being and *not be completely fascinated by it.*

The cages used by those in the BDSM lifestyle are typically custom-built constructions built as much for their aesthetics as for their functionality.

They can range in size from *coffee-table-sized* to *bedroom-sized*, and their purposes can run the gamut from *comfort space* to *punishment place*, and everything in-between. They don't even necessarily have to be constructed in the traditional box-shaped way, either. Some cages are built to conform to the size and shape of the human body, making any movement within in almost impossible, or tall and narrow, making it impossible to sit or lie down. Others are built specifically to be hoisted into the air, and may even expand or contract in size and shape as they are. There are cages constructed entirely of netting, heavy-gage wire or chain mesh and, though it's technically not a cage, an *entire room* can be transformed into a *virtual* cage by installing a jail-cell-type barred door at the entrance. Some cages are built to punish, others are built as a comfortable refuge and emotional *happy-place.* A cage stokes our emotions and imaginations wonderfully, regardless of whether you are inside looking out, or outside looking in. The possibilities are truly limitless and bound only by your imagination and budget.

The safety issues surrounding cages are typically a bit *subtler* than they are for other types of BDSM play, but *are* critical, nevertheless. Always be sure that cages are secured when not in use and do not become a temptation for children to play in or around. If the cage is *lockable*, be certain to have at least one or more spare keys kept where they can be located in an emergency or in the event a key is misplaced. Avoid leaving someone *unattended* in a cage for long periods of time and *never* leave the premises, even for very short periods of time, while someone is locked in a cage. In the event of fire, smoke, or a medical emergency the cage can become a *deathtrap.*

Ask your bottom about any hint or history of claustrophobia. It may also be possible for an individual with absolutely no history of claustrophobia to suddenly discover a phobia of being enclosed in small spaces, which is why continuous monitoring of your bottom is always a good idea, particularly the first few times. A claustrophobic reaction can put a person into a state of *shock* or *cause an acute stress reaction.* Contrary to popular belief, shock can result in serious emotional *and* physical problems which can persist for days, months, or even years after a triggering event.

BDSM Toys "R" Us

We've covered a lot of ground in this chapter, discussing a wide assortment of kink toys, fetish equipment, and dungeon furnishings, and yet we've barely scratched the surface. We could easily fill *several* books with endlessly fascinating *toy talk*, but that would probably be counter-productive. We can sometimes risk doing much the same sort of thing in our D/s relationships and BDSM activities. There's no doubt that BDSM toys can be *a lot of fun.* Sometimes, they can be so *much* fun that we are tempted to forget that they are supposed to be a means to an end, and not an end in themselves. The toys are there to please your partner and give you both a measure of mutual enjoyment; your partner shouldn't be there just to give you an excuse to use your toys.

There was a time in my life, long ago, when I was all about the toys. Believe me; I totally understand where your head is at if that's where you are right now or if that's where you're headed. I not only had to have all the latest and finest toys, but I eventually built an entire business around fetish toys and equipment. In the final analysis, however, they were just things. Perhaps my perspective is a tad simplistic, but I believe fun is meant to be shared. I have a really nice set of skis, but I don't enjoy skiing alone. I've got an awesome racquetball racket, but hitting the ball against the wall gets old fast. I've travelled all over the world - sometimes with, and sometimes without a partner. I'm sure I don't have to tell you which was more enjoyable. The BDSM lifestyle is no different. It's simply more fun when you can share it with someone special, and that's why I've written this book.

I'm hoping you'll look beyond the toys and focus a little more on your *playmates.*

My Two Cents on BDSM Toys

The year was 1980, and I was a young soldier, stationed at Fort Lewis, Washington as a Forward Observer in the 2/75th Infantry (Ranger) Battalion. I met and became involved with a young lady in town who enjoyed going to storage unit auctions each week and, eventually, I was cajoled into attending a few. To be honest, I was usually far more interested in *people-watching* and sampling the snack bar's nachos and beer than I was in the auction itself. Sometimes, however, the auctioneer would auction off the contents of a *sealed cardboard box* just to make things a little more interesting, and it never failed to stoke my insatiable curiosity.

On this particular night, the auctioneer pointed to a large, unopened cardboard box and told us that it had come from the estate of an elderly doctor. He claimed to have no idea what was inside, and started the bidding at $1. To this day, I have no idea what possessed me to raise my paddle and start bidding on it, but I did. I was the highest bidder at $7, and I left the auction later that night the proud owner of a *medical mystery box.*

When I inventoried the box, I found it full of odds and ends, worthless office supplies, some deteriorating medical texts, a few simple medical instruments, and a curious wooden box with a small metal latch. I opened it and found it full of strange looking *electrical equipment,* oddly-shaped glass tubes and thick black wires. A small metal data-plate attached to a box-within-the-box identified it as a *"Parco Super High Frequency Generator - Violet Ray."*

As you might imagine, I was very much *intrigued* by this intimidating looking contraption, which seriously resembled a prop from an old *Frankenstein movie.* Since I'd never seen anything quite like it before and, considering the fact that this was pre-internet, pre-Google, and *pre-Violet Wand,* I decided to delay *plugging it in* until I'd visited the local library and had a chance to figure out just *what the hell it was.*

What I learned was *fascinating*, to say the least. Violet rays were produced by a dozen or more companies in the 1920s as quack-medical devices marketed to the public as the cure-all for everything from *Aarskog Syndrome to Zygomycosis.* Its high-frequency electrical stimulation and ultra-violet emissions were claimed to be an effective treatment for psychosis, deafness, corns and callouses, "brain fag" *(seriously, look it up!)* and would even increase a woman's *bust size...* all for just $7 plus the cost of a draft beer, two chili dogs, and an order of nachos.

I thought to myself, "Mike, you are the *luckiest son-of-a-bitch* on the planet! And hopefully, when you plug that baby in, it won't explode, electrocute you, or burn your eyebrows off!"

Fortunately, it did *none* of *those* things, *and* I didn't grow bigger breasts, *either.* For an antique piece of equipment that was *sixty years old*, it was in remarkably good shape and it *worked perfectly!* There were two *glass* electrode attachments in the box - one roughly the size and shape of a *bratwurst,* and the other shaped like a *hollow glass garden rake.* When the device was plugged in and turned on, the attachment would light up like a *purple neon light*, buzzing and crackling with electricity, following your touch with an aggressive ticklish sensation, and intimidating the hell out of anyone with a *healthy fear of electrocution* - which, frankly, *ought* to be *everyone.*

My Parco Super High Frequency Generator & Violet Ray was *truly* a beautiful thing to behold, particularly as it crackled and glowed menacingly in in low-light conditions. And what was the very first thing I thought of when I turned it on?

I can't wait to try this thing out on my girlfriend's nipples.

"I refuse to join any club that would have me as a member!"

- - Grouch Marx

CHAPTER 10: BDSM GROUPS & ACTIVITIES

When we first discover that we are *psycho-sexually different* from most of our friends and neighbors, it usually comes as a bit of a shock to our psyches. Whether it occurs in our youth, or much later in life, the first thought that pops into one's head is typically something like, *"What?* Are you telling me *not everyone* likes spankings?" This is inevitably followed by *"What am I, some kind of freak?"* Hence begins our quest to know that we are *not alone* in our unique perspective on sexuality, relationships, and the universe in general; a quest that sometimes brings us to D/s lifestyle or BDSM groups.

Groups and associations that serve the *fetish community* exist in almost every major metropolitan area in the United States. Smaller towns and rural areas can sometimes be problematic when it comes to finding a group, but you may be surprised to learn that they often *do* exist there; they simply try to stay under the radar and are generally a bit harder to find. If you *do* get lucky and find a small-town fetish group, *do* keep in mind that privacy and discretion are *paramount* in such communities, where *everyone* knows *everyone else's* business.

There are many different kinds of fetish groups out there, and not all of them are necessarily D/s or BDSM related. For the purposes of our discussion, we'll focus here only on those that are, with a hat-tip to the fact that some groups cast a very *wide net* that includes pretty much *any* fetish or kink outside of the mainstream. Some groups go out of their way to try to be inclusive of every possible kink, fetish or lifestyle. These groups often include the words *kink* or *fetish* in their names, to draw attention to this *broad* focus. Other groups narrow their focus to specific interests, like *rope bondage, daddy's girls*, or *impact play*. Some groups are formally organized, with strict membership criteria and a rigorous set of rules, while others may consist simply of a loose association of like-minded individuals who get together for an occasional coffee. Finding a group that suits you is often as much about your tastes in *group social dynamics* as it is about your kink and lifestyle.

In addition to learning what BDSM groups are, and what they have to offer, it's just as important to examine *what they are not.* They are *not* swingers clubs, dating services, or brothels. Their gatherings are *not* orgies, hook-up opportunities, photo sessions, or spectator events for the general public. They are simply groups of like-minded individuals who gather to share their experiences and knowledge while making kinky friends and enjoying their company in a welcoming, safe and non-threatening environment.

As wonderful as all of that probably sounds to many of you, there may actually be some good reasons why you may *not* want to seek out your local BDSM lifestyle group. First of all, if you're the sort of person who is exceedingly fearful, prone to anxiety or paralyzed with shyness in group settings, you may find this to be a path to a bridge too far. Even so, many people who are face with these challenges have discovered that becoming involved with their local fetish group was *exactly* what they needed to help them face, and overcome, many of their fears.

Another reason why you might actually want to give some serious thought to whether or not joining a BDSM group is right for you concerns your *temperament* and *social skills*. Are you the sort of person that others might describe as judgmental, abrasive, prone to drama, lacking tact, or even *just plain creepy?* Do your friendships end just as quickly as they begin, as the result of major disagreements, misunderstandings, or arguments? Did your elementary school teachers ever annotate your report cards with, *"Doesn't play well with others?"* Are you are overwhelmed with thoughts of *actual nonconsensual sex and violence*, obsessed with the idea of doing someone serious bodily harm, or fascinated with scenarios involving *death?* If so, you should probably put any notion of joining your local fetish group completely out of your head and proceed, instead, to see a good therapist. Do *not* pass *Go*, do not collect $200.

Even if you consider yourself a *wonderful* person with a temperament of *gold*, and as much as you may think you *want and need* to be a part of what goes on at your local fetish group, you *may* just have to face the remote possibility that they don't quite agree with your self-assessment. Most groups have a screening process that helps to reduce the possibility of a disruptive or dangerous individual showing up at certain types of events. The most common mechanism for doing that is the *public munch*. A munch (sometimes called a *social, coffee, lunch, dinner, meet-up, meeting or get-together*) is typically a vanilla-style gathering which is held in a public venue – usually a restaurant that is willing to set aside table space for a large group. Munches may be held monthly, weekly, or *as-needed*, depending on the level of interest. For the most part, a group munch is indistinguishable from any other large gathering of friends in a restaurant. Attendees are expected to *dress* vanilla, *act* vanilla, and to be respectful of the other patrons of the establishment, which often consist of families with children.

One of the other mechanisms for pre-screening attendees for the group's more sensitive and private activities is the personal interview. Larger, more formerly organized groups are more likely to use this method than the smaller, more casual groups. Often, a group leader or member of a screening committee will be assigned to meet with the prospect for coffee or a drink in hopes of getting some sort of a *vibe – good or bad* – about the person. The interview may or may not include questions about the prospect's preconceptions, intentions, experience, or expectations. Generally speaking, if a trusted existing member of the group can personally vouch for a prospect, such interviews are considered unnecessary.

The customs and protocols that are expected from group members are, for the most part, the same as those expected throughout the BDSM lifestyle, with minor variations tailored to the type of event. The following list of tips may not be applicable to *every* group or event, but it is certainly a *good place to start.*

Customs and Protocols for a Munch

Things You *Should* Do

***Do* give your first name,** and as appropriate, the online username people may know you by. It is generally not a good idea to give the people you meet at these events your *real full name*, even if you have nothing to hide and are not worried about who knows this sort of information about you. The reason is simple. When *you* give your real full name, people may feel as if they're being pressured to give out *their* real full name in return, and *they* may care about who knows that sort of information about *them*. They might also get the idea that you don't understand the *reason* for this unspoken rule, and why it is important to many of the people who have to keep this part of their lives separate from their friends, families and coworkers. The last thing you want at this point is to give your new friends any reason to believe you'd be careless with their personal information. This is, however, a good time to tell them any online usernames by which they may already know you, or by which they may look you up after the munch.

***Do* be yourself.** You may feel as if you're under a lot of pressure to make a good impression, and that can sometimes cause people to say and do strange things. The key to making a good impression with *this* crowd is simple – be *authentic*. Be *yourself*. Nothing raises a red flag in someone's mind faster than the feeling that the person they are talking to isn't being entirely honest about who or what they are. Exaggerating or misrepresenting your experience, orientation, or lifestyle is one of the quickest ways to become a pariah in the fetish community. You should *never* attempt to *bluff* your way through *anything related to this lifestyle*, not even the simplest conversations. *At best*, you'll embarrass yourself. Worse, someone could end up getting seriously hurt, and that someone could be you. Contrary to popular belief, most people in the BDSM community *love to welcome and mentor people who are new to it and eager to learn*.

***Do* try to smile** and be a good conversationalist. Your smile is always your best asset when it comes to making good first impressions! Don't be afraid to start a conversation with those you meet, and try to uphold your end of any discussion that occurs. Giving monosyllabic answers to questions can be a quick way to put a damper on just about any exchange, so try to avoid giving curt *yes or no* responses. Even better, try to work a question of your own into your responses. For example, when someone asks, "Have you been in the lifestyle long?" you could respond with, "No, I am pretty new to it, but I am excited about learning more about it. Are there people in this group who do mentoring?"

***Do* try to find something to like and compliment** about those you meet. This tip works wonderfully in just about any social situation, with any kind of group, not just with fetish groups. One reason it can be very effective in *this* particular kind of setting is because it can help you to appreciate each individual there as more than just a walking collection of his or her kinks and fetishes.

***Do* be observant and listen actively** in order to learn more about the group. Being observant involves watching for the little things that transpire between group members, taking note of subtle customs or traditions, and especially to how people like to be addressed. Pay particular attention to which members are paired-up with others, either as husband and wife, Master and slave, Dominant and sub, or close friends. Being attentive to such things can save you a lot of embarrassment later. Being an active listener means more than just *paying attention*. It means becoming engaged, tactfully asking questions, and getting clarification on the things you don't entirely understand.

***Do* be interested in people.** People usually find *interested* people to be *interesting*. One of the most flattering things that can happen to most of us is to discover that *someone has taken an interest in us*. Show a little curiosity. Admit to being intrigued, amused, or fascinated. Just try not to make it the kind of aggressive, *creepy interest* that causes that person to wonder if she remembered to pack her pepper-spray.

***Do* practice giving a little introduction of yourself** that includes a bit about your interest or experience in the lifestyle. In the business world, this is called an *"elevator pitch,"* and it is designed to deliver essential information about you to another person in a way that might pique his or her interest, and to accomplish it all in *60 seconds or less.* It is fairly common for a group's long-time members to be juggling several responsibilities simultaneously at these kinds of events. They may be acting as hosts and hostesses, welcoming new guests, coordinating things with the restaurant staff, ensuring the right people know when and where the after-party *(if there is one)* will be, and on top of everything else, paying sufficient attention to their spouses, partners, dates or friends. Expecting that person to allot you more than a minute or two for introductions may be just a little unrealistic.

***Do* treat people with respect,** and try to see them as more than just their kink. Proper manners are a *big deal* to these people – possibly more so than to *any other group of people you will ever meet*. Rendering proper respect can include such things as respecting the lifestyle choices of others, the avoidance of stereotypes and judgmental statements, and a quiet acknowledgment of the fact that your standards of beauty, morality or excitement may not be shared by everyone in attendance. If a conversation topic makes you uncomfortable, turn your attention elsewhere. Tactless, inconsiderate or rude behavior can sometimes result in the perpetrator being unceremoniously *"uninvited"* to future events.

***Do* order something off the menu** if the munch is held in a restaurant. This is actually far more important than many people think. After all, you're meeting in a business establishment, the owners of which have a right to expect to get *something in return* for allowing your group to monopolize a large number of tables for what sometimes can turn into an extended period of time. Most restaurant owners and management have a *word* for individuals who sit in their restaurant for hours without ordering at *least* a beverage, and that word is: *unwelcome.* If it happens more than a few times with a certain group, it's usually only a matter of time before the entire group becomes unwelcome in the establishment. If you're flat broke and can't afford to purchase a meal, consider politely asking someone in the group to buy you a beverage.

Things You *Shouldn't* Do

Don't arrive drunk, or plan on getting that way. If you feel the need to have a few shots of "liquid courage" before attending an event like this, don't bother. If you think being *buzzed* makes you more interesting to people, you're probably mistaken. If the restaurant hosting the munch serves alcohol, having a drink or two with the group is usually perfectly acceptable, though you may want to check with a group leader first. If you do drink, don't overdo it. Getting drunk at a *party* can be fun and entertaining. Getting drunk at a *public vanilla gathering of fetishistas* can turn out to be embarrassing for everyone involved and potentially dangerous to people's relationships and careers.

Don't ask for personal details, beyond a first name or online username. This can be a difficult habit to break, since many of us are taught our entire *vanilla* lives to engage in *small talk* that consists mostly of questions like: *What do you do for a living? Where is your office* *located? Are you married? Do you have kids? Where do you hang out after work?* This sort of chit-chat may serve as a social lubricant in other types of gatherings, but at a fetish group munch, it's generally considered *bad manners*. Information is power, and most people in the BDSM lifestyle are simply not willing to hand you – a complete stranger - *that kind of power* over their lives the first time they meet you. If someone *volunteers* that sort of personal information to you without being asked for it, you should always consider it a sincere compliment and a leap of faith concerning your trustworthiness, and never pass that information on to someone else without their express permission to do so.

Don't ask people where they hang out with their vanilla friends. Many people in the BDSM lifestyle live *dual lives*. That means they often maintain two *completely separate* social circles, and as far as they are concerned, *never the 'twain shall meet*. There are usually very good reasons for doing this, since our vanilla friends aren't always able to understand or accept the kinkier aspects of our lives, and even if they could, we may feel that it simply isn't any of their business. Try to respect that, so they won't have to dread the possibility that you'll someday show up at their bible study group with handcuffs and a riding crop.

Don't invite yourself to any activity. Never forget that a munch is more than just a social gathering. A munch also serves as an informal *screening process* which helps to determine whether it is appropriate to invite you to other less public events. You may hear some discussion about an after-party, or other events planned for the near future, but you should resist the temptation to ask for details, or to make it seem as though you are inviting yourself to them. Some groups require you to have attended a minimum number of munches – often as low as one – before you are invited to attend other activities. When the decision has been made by whoever makes those kinds of decisions for the group, you will usually be discreetly informed of it. If a group leader asks you, "Are you coming to the after-party?" you may *then* consider yourself *invited,* and ask for more details.

Don't touch anyone without permission. If it consists of anything other than a handshake, it is considered *touching*. If you don't have permission to *do* it, then it is considered *bad touching*. *Permission* means an expressed verbal authorization to touch that person, delivered personally to *you.* Just because someone has granted that permission to anyone else, or even to *practically everyone* else, does not mean he or she has granted that permission to *you*. The permission must be explicit, not *implied*. You *may not* assume that just because someone *appears* to want a hug from you, that they *actually do* want a hug from you. Usually, it is simply a matter of asking, *"Is it alright if I hug you?"* If a group member is a slave, submissive, pet, or partner in any kind of relationship, then you may be required to ask permission from his or her Dominant, as well. As you might well imagine, if group members are going to get *this* worked up about nonconsensual *hugs*, you probably don't want to test the waters with random gropes or swats.

Don't reveal information about other people. What happens at group events should stay at those group events. The mere mention of someone's attendance or activities at another event may be considered privileged information. For all you know, that new person sitting next to you in the restaurant while you're describing a particularly kinky BDSM scene that occurred last month involving a friend may just happen to be your friend's *boss*. Another good reason for this rule is, in a lifestyle that often involves BDSM play *outside of committed relationships,* it is usually a good thing for someone to hear about the activities of his partner from his partner, and not from some stranger who just happened to be in the audience when it occurred. Granted, it can sometimes be extraordinarily difficult to have animated discussions about group activities without referring to specific individuals by name, but give it your best shot. At the very least, you should avoid passing along gossip and other personal information about anyone at all cost. People love to *hear* gossip, but they will also naturally assume that someday, they'll end up as the subject of your gossip.

Don't assume everyone is there to hook up, get laid, or find someone who shares their kink. The most common reason people have for seeking out a BDSM group is to learn that they are not alone; that there are others out there who are a lot like they are. Yes, there are *plenty* of people who are seeking out others who share their particular kink, but the fact remains, the majority of people who attend a munch are there simply to enjoy socializing with others who understand their world-view. Once you have attended a few events, you'll have a much better understanding of who is or isn't looking to hook up, and you'll have an informed basis for deciding whether or not you're interested.

Don't make your personal fetish the first thing you tell people about yourself. This may come as a *complete surprise* to you, but introducing yourself to complete strangers as *"Bob, the guy who likes to suck semen from another guy's anus"* is probably *not* the best way to make a good first impression. By the way, that's called *felching*, and yes, there *really is a name for it.* A good rule of thumb might be, if it isn't something you'd put in your *Facebook profile*, it probably isn't something you should blurt out in the first two minutes of a conversation with a stranger, either.

Don't take or use a camera at the munch. The reasons for this are the same as for not asking for or revealing too much personal information. People generally don't take photographs unless they plan to *do* something with those photographs, and that thought makes *some* people profoundly uncomfortable. Imagine how the mother of an eight-year-old might react when she looks at someone's Facebook page and sees a photo of a group of people, one of whom happens to be her child's teacher, with the caption, "Here's me, hanging out with my fellow pervs!" It's hard to envision any way that a discovery like that bodes well for anyone concerned.

Don't use it as a place to take advantage of your private knowledge of someone's personal weaknesses, turn-ons, or triggers. As you attend more events, and get to know people better, you'll likely have opportunities to learn intimate details about their likes, dislikes, turn-ons, and triggers. This is an entirely normal part of making new friends in the fetish community. You may even eventually end up in intimate relationships with some of those people, and there's nothing at all wrong with that. But you should take care *never* to use a munch or any other public gathering to reveal someone's private turn-ons or triggers without their express permission to do so.

You may find it very tempting to show off your exclusive knowledge of a person's intimate secrets, but don't do it. *Just don't.* For an example of how this sort of thing can end in disaster, read the story at the end of this chapter.

Customs and Protocols for a Play Party

Once a new person has been vetted and cleared to attend events beyond the regular *munch*, he or she may be invited to attend play parties, demonstrations, and other kinds of fetish gatherings. For the most part, the customs and protocols one should observe at a play party are the same as at a munch, with some additional considerations. Do keep in mind the fact that most play parties and other private events are held in a group member's *home*. That means extra thought must be given to things like children, pets, neighbors, parking, fragile or valuable household furnishings, and privacy. At play party type events, you have as much of a responsibility to look out for the interests of the homeowner hosting the event as you do for the group as a whole.

The major difference between this kind of event and a munch is the high probability of BDSM scenes being played out during a play party. A BDSM *scene* is simply any BDSM activity that is done in front of an *audience*. A scene should be considered a *performance*, and not be interrupted or interfered with in any way. Scenes do not *usually* involve explicitly *sexual* activity, but there are always exceptions, and it is not uncommon for participants to have *sexual reactions* to what might be considered by most to be *non-sexual* activities. Before *participating* in any scene, be sure you are clear on what will be involved, whether or not it will involve sex, and what safety measures will be in effect.

The following is a list of protocols which typically apply to play party types of events. Again, each group generally has rules that are specific to that group, or to the location and homeowner's preferences, but for the most part, these guidelines for BDSM play events are fairly universal.

Don't touch without permission. This rule cannot be stressed enough. Even so, there's a specific reason for revisiting it here, in our discussion of play parties. Resisting the urge to hug a friend at a public munch is one thing; resisting the urge to touch the scantily clad or naked person next to you, particularly if you are both in a highly aroused state, is *another thing entirely*. For *some* people, an event like this is the first time they'll ever witness, with the lights on, anything quite so erotic *that doesn't personally involve them*. It may also be the first time they see, for the first time, their secret fantasies being played out in real life, right in front of their eyes. Needless to say, for certain individuals, this can sometimes have a profound effect, like making them forget that whole no-touching thing. *Don't be that individual.*

Never interrupt a scene. A scene is *called* a scene for a very good reason – it is usually a highly choreographed *performance* being enacted for an appreciative audience. The performance can consist of practically any fetish activity, from the ridiculously mundane to the unbelievably complex or even *dangerous*. It isn't uncommon for scenes to include such things as *open flames, knife-play, electricity, or even asphyxiation*. The very last thing scene participants need, in those kinds of circumstances, is a *distraction*. It should come as no surprise to anyone that the audience will be unappreciative of any individual engaging in running commentary, interruptions, criticisms, or attempts to inject themselves into the scene. If you are so seriously concerned about a *safety issue* that you feel a scene should be *stopped*, you should quietly and politely take one of the group leaders aside in a way that *does not* *cause a distraction to others,* and voice your concerns privately to that person. Chances are you'll discover that your concerns have already been adequately addressed in ways that you are simply unaware of.

If you are planning to be involved in a scene, make no assumptions about sex. This is *particularly* true if you are participating in a scene involving a new group, a new play partner, or a new activity for you. Even if the scene involves something you've done a *hundred times,* with a *hundred other people,* never assume that things will play out the same way *this time*. It is relatively common for people who do a lot of *scening* to develop their own unique and unexpected ways of doing things, so if such a thing is possible, you should expect the unexpected. You should also never presume, just because certain things may be against the group's rules, that your new play partner *knows or cares* about the group's rules. Obviously, and for a multitude of good reasons, the best time to find out about any sex that occurs in a scene is *before* it happens, not *after the fact*.

Don't mess with equipment you are unfamiliar with. For that matter, you shouldn't mess with any equipment that isn't yours, unless the owner of the equipment expressly tells you that it's okay to do so. When it comes to their BDSM toys, some folks can be *very* protective and often downright paranoid about people touching their stuff, and there are plenty of good reasons to feel that way. First of all, as you'll no doubt learn when you start to build your *own* BDSM toy collection, some fetish toys can be *really expensive*. No one wants to see his brand new $400 violet wand being handled like a Wii controller.

Second, despite the fact that items used in BDSM scenes are often called *toys,* they can sometimes be *dangerous* in ways that you may not be able to foresee. It's easy to assume that the *knives* that a certain Dominant uses in his knife-play demonstration are going to be *sharp*, but the dangers associated with other kinds of BDSM toys and equipment may *not* be quite so readily apparent. For example, a *pinwheel* looks like a cute little toy, until you playfully run it across your skin and create a neat little row of puncture marks. The mentholated oils that are used in *cupping* are highly flammable, and could easily turn you into a human torch if spilled and ignited by a cigarette or candle. Larger pieces of equipment or furnishings, such as racks, platforms, suspension harnesses or St. Andrew's crosses can be *especially* dangerous to anyone attempting to place themselves on or in the equipment without the assistance of another person who presumably knows what he is doing. You probably don't want to be forever remembered by the group as that new person who needed to be rescued from the furniture.

Third and finally, there's that awkward issue of *bodily fluids*. Yes, we generally think of bodily fluids as being *on or in people's bodies,* but they also have a curious habit of being on their *sex toys*, as well. In the BDSM community, you'll occasionally hear the term *"fluid bonding,"* which generally refers to relationships between people who have agreed to engage in unprotected sex involving the potential exchange of bodily fluids. A *fluid bond* can also sometimes refer to a BDSM toy or piece of equipment that should be reserved for the sole use of its owner, because it comes into contact with bodily fluids such as semen, secretions, saliva or blood. Even items that you might not often associate with bodily fluids may fit into this category. A simple leather flogger might not *seem* like a logical place for bodily fluids – until you consider things like *pussy floggings*, and other types of floggings that *draw blood* or result in *ejaculation*. Bottom line: Sharing toys for *six-year-olds* is a good thing; for kinksters, maybe *not so much*.

Don't take pictures. This is another rule that cannot be stressed enough, and even though we've already listed it once in the munch protocols, it bears revisiting in the context of play parties. At a munch, the relevant and sensitive issue is generally *who was there.* A play party complicates things *exponentially* for people who must keep their kinky lifestyle and the more vanilla aspects of their lives separate. A photograph of you in a restaurant, having a margarita and *chimichangas* with your pervy friends can usually be explained away pretty easily. Explaining away a picture of you being flogged while hanging upside down and naked in somebody's living room is probably going to be a tough sell.

Don't wander into parts of the house not designated for the event. Try to remember the last time you had a dozen or more people in your house. The thought of that crowd in your living room or family room was probably stressful *enough*, without adding the terrifying notion of them wandering randomly through the *rest of your house.* Respect the privacy of the event hosts and stay in areas that have been set aside for the event. This will usually consist of a main play area *(living room, family room, or rec room)*, a guest bathroom, and perhaps the kitchen/dining area. Stay away from bedrooms, dens or children's rooms, and ask before congregating in outdoor areas like patios, porches, yards or driveways, since voices and noise can carry, and your hosts may have nosy or irritable neighbors.

Protect the furniture. One of the things you can expect to see a lot of at your fetish group's play party is *skin*. Some nudity or partial nudity is fairly common, particularly for those who will be part of a scene or demo. Sometimes, folks who aren't planning to be a part of a scene that evening will still change into *fetishwear* of some sort, just to get into the spirit of things. You shouldn't feel as if you're under any pressure to wear anything kinky or shed any of your clothing, particularly as a new person. But in the event that you do, *remember the furniture*. This may come as a bit of a surprise to you, but most household furniture simply isn't designed to accommodate naked, wet, or sticky people. Not only can it damage the furnishings, but it can be something of a bio-hazard to sit in someone else's couch puddle. Many people bring their own towel to sit on if they're planning on getting naked at an event. Sometimes, the event host will make clean towels available to anyone who needs one. When in doubt, simply ask the host if bare butts are allowed on the furniture.

Your fetish group will likely have a written set of rules governing the behavior of members at their events. Be sure to ask the group leaders where you can find them, and get familiar with them. Every group is different, and their rules may differ significantly from the protocols we've discussed here, but you can be sure that there is almost always a very good reason for any rule that is adopted. Applying a little common sense and consideration for the comfort, health and privacy of others will go a long way towards making you a welcome and valued member or any group.

How to Find a Local BDSM Group

Finding and contacting a local group of like-minded kinksters can have its own peculiar challenges, particularly if you aren't already a part of those social circles. Chances are pretty good that you may already know someone in the D/s lifestyle, but just don't know it yet. As we explained earlier, most of the people in the lifestyle try to stay under the radar, and rarely go around wearing t-shirts that read "Pervy and Proud!" Even so, you probably have a good idea which of your friends and acquaintances is most likely to be connected to, or at least knowledgeable, about the lifestyle. Diplomatically asking them about whether they know of any local fetish groups may just pay off. Who knows, it could even turn into a kinky date for the weekend. The recommendation or invitation of a friend is by far the easiest and most reliable way to find and connect to a local BDSM group.

Another way to learn whether there is a group in your area is through *(duh!)* the internet. While this may seem like the easiest and most obvious method to those who are already in the lifestyle, it can be incredibly confusing and frustrating to someone who doesn't even know where to start. Googling "BDSM" and the name of your town will usually give you about a million results, some nine hundred thousand of which will turn out to be porn sites. Most of the rest will consist of classified personal ads, merchants of kinky toys, and web cam sites. The sad fact is, only a handful of websites out there will turn out to be useful to you in your quest to find a local BDSM group.

One type of web site which you will find extremely useful is the sort that caters specifically to the BDSM fetish *community*. Surprisingly, while there are a lot of web sites that make the attempt, only a few seem to be any good at it, and even that is debatable. Some of the most popular BDSM community web sites include FetLife.com, Bondage.com, Alt.com, and CollarMe.com. Each has its own unique strengths and weaknesses, and boasts a large number of devotees. The utility of any of these sites will depend a great deal upon your preferences and habits, and your ability to separate the wheat from the chaff when it comes to finding useful information and making worthwhile friends. Always remember that there are plenty of people in the BDSM lifestyle who cannot be a part of the online community for a variety of reasons, including career and professional factors, family concerns, or even technical reasons. Conversely, many people are members of multiple web sites and online communities.

You should also keep in mind the fact that *whatever* online forum you use, it is simply a *communications* medium. It is does not necessarily equate to the *real-life group* of people you may encounter. Just because *Joe-Bob* has started a local *FetLife* group related to your home town on the *website* doesn't mean he is the leader of any *actual community group*.

The second internet resource that you may find useful is *social media*. Doing key word searches on social media sites like Facebook, Twitter, or Google + can sometimes give you surprisingly good results. The best way to do it, however, is to know exactly who and what you are looking for. Many BDSM groups have their own social media pages, which are used to keep their members informed about events and other news. Lifestyle-friendly businesses, such as sex toy shops, leather goods merchants, piercing or tattoo parlors, and adult bookstores also are likely to have social media accounts. Following or friending them can often lead you to discover what you're looking for *on their friends list.* You can ask them about their social media sites whenever you visit, or you can make a phone call to the establishment, or you can simply search for the names of the businesses on the web site in question.

Many of the individual BDSM group members will have social media accounts which are specifically used to connect with their kinky friends, and may welcome new friends. Don't be surprised, however, if they expect to have actually met you in real life first. On that same note, if you also plan to use your social media to stay connected with vanilla family, friends and coworkers, it might be a good idea to create a new account specifically for your BDSM lifestyle connections.

Another great place to make progress is with *blogs*. A search of a popular blog portal may lead you to a group right in your own back yard. Since blogs can be a relatively easy way to create a web site, allow for collaborative authorship, and automate the process of registering followers, many lifestyle groups find them to be extremely useful. To see if any of your local BDSM groups have a blog-type website, check out Blogger.com, Wordpress.com, Tumblr.com, LiveJournal.com, Blog.com, Xanga.com, Weebly.com, or Posterous.com. A simple search of the terms "BDSM" and the name of your state or home town should reveal whether or not these blogs will be useful to you.

One online resource that I do *not* recommend, if you're serious about connecting with others in the BDSM lifestyle, is internet chat rooms. Generally speaking, internet chat rooms – while they can certainly be *entertaining* – can be incredibly frustrating and a *huge* waste of your valuable time. A significant number of the people you meet in them will turn out to be clueless, deceitful or both, and even their locations will quite often be deliberately misleading, which makes searching for new friends and groups in your geographical area somewhat problematic. On the other hand, once you connect in real life and make friends with other folks in the BDSM lifestyle, chat rooms can be a great way to *stay* in touch.

Another method that is *not recommended* would be to confuse anything having to do with the *"swinging"* lifestyle with the fetish or BDSM community. Most major metropolitan areas have swingers' clubs, swingers' publications, and swingers' web sites which are, more often than not, completely useless *even to swingers*, much less to those in the

BDSM community. While *vanilla* folk may have a hard time telling a *swinger* from someone in the BDSM lifestyle, the differences can be *quite stark*, and are usually painfully obvious to the individuals in the two lifestyles.

The bottom line is, the best way to locate and connect with a local BDSM group is to use pretty much the same methods you might use to find and join any *other* kind of group. While it's true that you won't be able to just look up "BDSM groups" in the yellow pages, you probably wouldn't find the local model train club there, either. In the end, you will likely get the best results from networking with friends, using social media and blogs, and visiting with the people at lifestyle-friendly businesses.

If done right, being a part of your local BDSM group can be an incredibly rewarding adventure. Not only is it good to know that you are not alone, but some of the friendships you make there will be unlike anything you've ever experienced before. Regardless of your age, experience or expertise in the lifestyle, there will almost always be something fascinating to learn from your fellow *fetishistas.*

# # #

My Two Cents on BDSM Munches

The aroma of sizzling fajitas filled the air as twenty members of our local BDSM group were gathered together, as was our usual custom, at a trendy Mexican restaurant for our monthly social. We chatted amiably over our beverages as we sat clustered around a very long table at the center of the restaurant, and waited for our server to take our dinner orders. To the other patrons of the restaurant, we could easily have been mistaken for members of the local Rotary Club, or a group of co-workers or friends celebrating a promotion or birthday.

As the waitress completed her order-taking, other members of the group would occasionally wander around the table to introduce themselves to first-time visitors, or to give others directions to the after-munch party, which we euphemistically referred to as *"movie night,"* on the off-chance that we were overheard by the other restaurant patrons or staff.

Suddenly, to the surprise of everyone at the table and practically everyone in the restaurant, one of the young women in the group let out a *shrill scream*, burst into uncontrollable sobbing, and ran through the restaurant in a bee-line for the ladies' restroom. One of her friends was quickly dispatched to check on her, while the rest of us were left confused and wondering, *what the hell just happened?*

A worried restaurant manager rushed to our table to inquire about the incident, and we quickly concocted a semi-plausible story about the poor girl and the awful panic attacks that she sometimes suffers in public places. He left, not entirely convinced of the explanation, but thoroughly satisfied that the scream wasn't the result of something important, like a fat, hairy *roach* crawling out of someone's taco salad.

It wasn't until hours later that some of us learned what had upset the young lady. She had recently met, and gotten to know the young man who had escorted her into the restaurant that evening. During the process of getting to know one another, the young woman revealed to him a very private and, for her, somewhat embarrassing kink. She liked to be choked, and when she is, the effect is almost always an immediate and orgasmic experience for her.

She revealed this to her new friend in the expectation that perhaps he might put it to use in the *bedroom*, not in the middle of a crowded restaurant which is, in fact, *exactly* what he did.

In a pathetic attempt to bolster his own inflated ego, and to demonstrate to others that he knew something about this girl that they didn't, this young man had stepped behind her as she sat at the dinner table talking with her friends, and *choked her.* Needless to say, she was not amused.

Don't be that guy.

"The difference between sex and love is that
sex relieves tension and love causes it."

- - *Woody Allen*

CHAPTER 11: SEX, LOVE, D/S, & BDSM

People mistake sex for love (and vice-versa) *all the time*, and that misperception isn't just limited to the *vanilla folk.* This should come as no surprise to *anyone.* Yet, as complicated as *that* can be, try to imagine what happens when you toss *D/s and BDSM* into the mix. It can be enough to make your head spin, even if you've spent your *entire life* navigating those treacherous waters. There are many, many ways that a D/s relationship can be lost on dangerous shoals, but for our purposes, we'll focus here on three of the most common and frustrating: mistaking BDSM for sex, mistaking love for BDSM, and mistaking BDSM for D/s. The following three real-life case studies nicely illustrate not only *what* can go wrong, but *how* it can go wrong. Naturally, names and locales have been changed to protect the privacy of the individuals concerned.

Mistaking BDSM for Sex

Robert D., a twenty-six-year-old restaurant manager in Kansas had always been curious about the BDSM lifestyle, but had never made much of an effort to seek out like-minded individuals or a fetish group in his home town – that is, until *now.* Robert had recently created an account at one of the major online BDSM portals, learned about a local group having a get-together, and decided to attend. The munch was being held at a nearby Pizza Hut, which regularly reserved a semi-private party-room for the large group. Robert was familiar with the place, which helped him to get past his nervousness about going.

Robert arrived at the appointed hour and introduced himself to those who were already in attendance. He enjoyed his pizza and listened to the conversations that seemed to swirl around and across the table. The two-hour social passed quickly and enjoyably, and at the end of it, one of the group leaders approached him discreetly and invited him to the *after-munch play party*. Robert hadn't really been *expecting* that, but was flattered and excited at the prospect. Without hesitation, he agreed to follow his new friend to the home of the member hosting the event. During the ensuing twenty minute drive, visions of decadent, nubile sex-slaves danced in his head. *Alas,* it was not to be.

Robert spent close to three hours at the play party and then returned home feeling deflated and disappointed. Before crawling into bed, Robert took a few moments to journal his reactions to his first-ever BDSM play party, and post them online for his friends to peruse and perhaps comment upon. His personal reflections, which have been redacted here for content and to protect his privacy, reflect what could have been the thoughts of *any* person new to the lifestyle, attending an event like this one for the first time:

> *"I was excited and nervous about attending a BDSM play party for the first time, and wasn't sure what I was going to be expected to know or do, so I decided to just watch and see what would happen... which turned out to be - practically nothing. One of the women there stripped down to a thong as soon as she arrived, but practically everyone else either kept their clothes on, or undressed for specific activities and got dressed again. This was not at all what I expected. I had expected this to be a clothing-free event, and was fully prepared to get naked myself, but I guess I had*

the wrong idea about how they do things. It's probably just as well, since a lot of the people there weren't the sort you want to see naked, anyway."

"Apparently, they do this thing at the start of the play party, where the girls have to identify who is allowed to touch them or play with them, and when none of them designated me as a potential play partner, I felt like a total loser and an outcast. They described their group as friendly, tolerant and inclusive, but this just made me feel excluded and embarrassed. If no one was going to play with me, what was the point of me even being here?"

"People were mostly paired off into couples already, so I felt incredibly uncomfortable talking to anyone, for fear of stepping on someone's toes or intruding. I don't know how a single guy like me is supposed to hook-up with anyone, and even if I did meet someone interesting, I wasn't authorized to touch or play with her, so what's the point?"

"Basically, all I got to do was watch an edge play demo and a couple of scenes. Yeah, I engaged in a few half-hearted, superficial conversations with people who were obviously not very interested in me, but after a couple hours of that, I was ready to go home. I hope not all BSM groups are like this one."

Robert had gone to the event looking for *sex*, but what he found there was – *surprise! - BDSM.* It's unfortunate that one of the most commonly held misconceptions about the BDSM lifestyle is the notion that it is *all about kinky, promiscuous sex.* The lifestyle is *kinky*, without a doubt, almost by definition; but how much *promiscuous* sex *is* there, really? There is *surprisingly little*, actually - typically *far* less than is typically assumed by the general public.

That is not to say that promiscuous sex *doesn't happen* in this lifestyle.

Of course it happens. But, it happens in the BDSM lifestyle pretty much the same way it does in every *other* kind of lifestyle, with the possible exceptions of *the poly lifestyle* and *the swinging lifestyle.* In other words, it happens mostly behind closed doors. The overwhelming majority of people in the D/s and BDSM lifestyles are either *monogamous* or *polyfidelous*. A relatively small minority of those in the BDSM lifestyle consider themselves *swingers*. A good friend of mine likes to explain the difference to his vanilla acquaintances thusly: "We're *beaters*, not *cheaters*."

Robert made more than just the simple mistake of assuming that a BDSM munch group's play party would be a *sex orgy.* He erroneously assumed that these events were all about *nudity* when, in fact, nudity plays a very small role in most group events. He was *judgmental* about the appearance of the others in attendance, even though the BDSM culture is strongly supportive of being *body-positive*. He assumed that mostly *single people* would be attending an event of this type and was *peeved* about all of the couples in attendance, because it reduced his chances of *hooking-up* with someone. He was *extremely superficial* in how he approached and chatted with other attendees, as evidenced by his remark, *"If I'm not authorized to touch... what's the point?"*

Apparently, it never occurred to Robert that if he had actually been *interested* in anyone as *more than just a sex object* perhaps they, in turn, might have been interested in *him* as more than just a creepy stranger who ought to be avoided. Robert ended his narrative with the thought, *"I hope all BDSM groups are not like this one,"* but fails to comprehend that in BDSM groups across the country, there are a whole lot of people hoping that not all of their first time visitors are like *him.*

Mistaking Love for BDSM

People confuse *sex with love* all the time; they also often confuse *BDSM with sex*. *Neither* of those statements should come as much of a surprise to *anyone.* What *might* come as a surprise to many readers is the fact that, *sometimes,* people confuse *love for BDSM,* or confuse *BDSM for D/s.* Let's take a look at a few examples of how those scenarios can occur.

Ian and Natalie were both in their late twenties when they were married, and it was a second marriage for each of them. They each went into *this* marriage determined to avoid the mistakes of their past marriages, and to do whatever it would take to make this one work. Things went swimmingly for the first couple of years. Then, one night, Natalie awoke at 3 A.M. to find Ian's side of the bed empty. Curious, she got up and walked down the hall, where she saw Ian in the den, masturbating to internet BDSM porn. Her immediate emotional reaction was as if she'd caught him cheating with another woman. She felt *betrayed* and inadequate. Physically, it was as if she'd been kicked in the stomach. In that moment, Natalie feared that everything that she believed about her relationship with Ian might be a lie. She was, in a word, *devastated.*

They *fought* until the sun came up. Finally, exhausted and angry and frustrated, they called a truce and pretended to sleep for a few hours in separate rooms. When they spoke again, it was with cooler heads, and Natalie asked Ian the questions that had kept her awake. *"Why* couldn't you just *tell me* that you liked that kind of stuff? *Why* did you have to keep it a *secret?* I am *your wife,* for crying out loud. You're supposed to be able to *tell* me shit like that!"

Ian stared silently into his coffee. Finally, he looked up from his thoughts and said, "Do you remember when we first began dating...? That time we went into that sex shop and checked out all of the kinky toys?"

Natalie nodded. How could she *forget?* They'd had *great fun* poking fun at some of the crazy things they'd seen in there, and drooling over some of the more interesting items and outfits. In fact, she had even gone back to the store a few weeks later, by herself, to purchase a *naughty French maid costume.* She later surprised him with it during their *honeymoon,* since she had always enjoyed role-playing and dressing up in sexy outfits. Suddenly, she realized where he was going with this. While in the store, Ian had taken her to the aisle where the whips, floggers and paddles were displayed, and casually asked her what she thought. In retrospect, her answer must've caught him completely off-guard.

Natalie had been physically and emotionally abused as a child, both by her natural parents and, later, by her foster parents as well. She grew into adulthood equating BDSM with *abuse*, and seeing the leather implements arrayed as they were in the store brought on a flood of unpleasant memories. She told Ian that she simply didn't understand how *anyone* could *willingly* submit themselves to *that kind of abuse,* and characterized the men who were into BDSM as a bunch of *"misogynists and closet wife-beaters."*

Oh god, she thought, *I did this to him. I had no idea he liked that stuff. He was trying to tell me, and I wasn't listening. Instead, I went on a rant, basically calling him a woman-hater and abuser. Jesus, how could I have been so incredibly stupid?*

They kissed and made up. Ian promised that he would no longer sneak off in the middle of the night to masturbate to BDSM porn, and Natalie promised to keep an open mind about BDSM play and to give it a try in the bedroom. Their marriage seemed to be back on the right track again.

There was just one little problem. In Natalie's heart of hearts, the kinky play that Ian loved so much *still felt like abuse,* and never failed to trigger a flood of painful memories from her abusive childhood. Even so, Natalie not only participated in the kinky BDSM play, she *encouraged* it and *pretended to enjoy it* because she loved her husband very much and wanted *desperately* to make him happy. And for a little while, *it very much did.*

Ian had been so thrilled by his wife's decision to try a little BDSM in the bedroom, he probably missed a lot of the little telltale signs of the deception, at first. But as their experimentation became more elaborate and daring, he started noticing the kinds of things that only a husband knows about his wife. He had always *loved* the way Natalie's body reacted *physiologically* when she had an orgasm. Her face, neck and upper chest always flushed crimson red. Her nipples instantly hardened. Her heart pounded. And there was one more thing that Natalie *herself* didn't know about; you could literally *see and feel* her pussy and ass going through a rapid series of tight spasms, repeatedly clenching and releasing, again and again, faster than could ever be accomplished through conscious effort. Once Ian began *paying attention*, he realized that Natalie had been *faking* her orgasms since they *began* experimenting with BDSM. What Ian *didn't* know at the time was that, *now*, it was *Natalie* who was sneaking out of their bed in the middle of the night to masturbate to *vanilla* porn!

When Ian confronted her about the phony orgasms, she admitted everything. She told him that she was just trying to make him happy, and working to keep their marriage strong. She had felt that, *because she loved him so intensely*, she ought to be able to *enjoy BDSM with him* through sheer *force of will*. She had decided to simply *ignore* the fact that the BDSM play actually made her *nauseous*, stirred up awful memories, and gave her nightmares. Ian explained to her that he can usually *tell* when she isn't enjoying herself, and *knowing* that made it next to impossible for *him* to enjoy himself, since he didn't really consider himself a much of a *sadist*. Instead of *pleasing him*, all Natalie had accomplished was ensuring that *neither of them* was having any fun.

Ian and Natalie set aside the impact play and bondage for the time being, and decided to focus instead on some of the kinks that Natalie *did* enjoy. She loved being sexually submissive, enjoyed dressing up in kinky costumes, had developed an interest in *puppy play*, and had always been bi-curious. While doing some research on pet play, she came across an online reference to a local BDSM munch group which had several members who were into pet play, too. She contacted a few of them, and was invited to an upcoming munch. Ian and Natalie soon became members of the group and became friends with some experienced and knowledgeable folks who were able to mentor and guide them in their exploration of the lifestyle. One of those people was a delightfully charming submissive named Gabrielle.

Eventually, Ian and Natalie came to love Gabby and invited her to move in and join them in a D/s poly relationship. Natalie had always considered herself a submissive, but had never realized that it could be possible to explore that facet of her personality *and her relationship* without having to deal with the *"whips and chains"* that she had always associated with submission and *despised.* Gabby shared Ian's love for impact play and bondage, and she *also* shared Natalie's love of *cosplay and pet play.* Having Gabby in their relationship seemed to fill voids in *both* Ian's and Natalie's lives, and Gabby was positively giddy in love with the two of them, as well.

It is unfortunate that Ian and Natalie's experience is not all that uncommon. There are many people in the vanilla world who, like Natalie, are all too eager to equate BDSM with *abuse*. Prior to these events, Natalie was also unable to separate any notion of D/s from BDSM, which prevented her from exploring her submissive side for fear of being exposed to the aspects of BDSM which she found disturbing. She also falsely assumed that, because her *love* for Ian was strong, that she would be able to *power through* her deep distaste for impact play and bondage. Finally, to top off this menagerie of misunderstandings, Natalie had assumed that, because Ian enjoyed impact play as a Top, *he must be a sadist.* She understood that sadists derive their pleasure from the pain and suffering of others, and so her own internal logic told her that *her* lack of enjoyment of their kinky activities *was irrelevant,* as long as she was making *him* happy. But, of course, she *wasn't.* Their tale is a lot like one of those classic *O. Henry* short stories, full of profound misunderstandings and ending with a strangely ironic twist... except *their* story has kinky sex toys and ends with a hot threesome.

Mistaking BDSM for D/s

A wise person once said that *time* exists in our universe in order to keep everything from happening all at once. It's *extremely* rare to find lasting love, great sex, a hot D/s dynamic *and* awesome BDSM all in the same afternoon. *Most* of us would be overjoyed to experience just *one of the four* in any given day, and frankly, that's *usually* the way it happens. Whichever one you *begin* with, you should do your best to avoid assuming that it's going to be a *"buy one, get the other three free"* kind of a day. It's incredibly easy to get caught up in the excitement of the moment and, because we desperately *want it all,* we sometimes can be a little too quick to believe that we *have it all.* Unfortunately, *wishing* doesn't necessarily make it so.

Vicki was a bright, vivacious twenty-one-year-old whose fairly extensive BDSM experience was relatively unusual for someone of her age. She belonged to three different local fetish groups, and attended munches or kink events at *least* a couple of times each week. When she wasn't attending socials or being a rope-bunny at play parties, she was working as a nude vid-cam model, running a blog about boobs, advocating for fetish and LGBT rights, watching bondage porn, or making friends in BDSM chat rooms. She loved practically every aspect of BDSM; there was almost nothing that she wouldn't try as a bottom. She enjoyed spanking, flogging, whipping, paddling, rope play, needle play, breath play, knife play, pet play *and more.* In fact, she was *voraciously* hungry to try new and exciting forms of BDSM play, which is how she met Mark.

Mark was a forty-five-year-old sales executive who had been invited to do a fire-cupping demonstration for one of the local fetish groups, which is where he became acquainted with Vicki. Mark was a Dominant who had just come out of a D/s relationship which had lasted several years. He had just gotten back into the dating scene and was interested in meeting new people, so when Vicki volunteered to be his "cupping bunny" for future demonstrations, Mark readily agreed.

They quickly became very close, and before long, they were practically inseparable. Within a *month,* they were making plans to move in together, and even the normally taboo topic of marriage began to pop up occasionally in their conversations. They were honestly just as surprised by their whirlwind romance as their friends and families, and would often punctuate their discussions with, "This is crazy; *seriously crazy!"* But it all *felt so wonderful,* they decided to just *go with it.* Six weeks to the day after they met, they arranged to be joined in an intimate collaring ceremony which formalized their relationship as Master and submissive. A few weeks after *that,* they began looking for a house. That's when things began to unravel like a dollar-store sweater.

Vicki had always loved being in constant contact with her Master, and often called or texted him throughout her day just to tell him that she missed him, or to ask him for his opinions on various topics or routine decisions she needed to make. Once they found the perfect rental house and began making preparations to move in, she had *even more* reasons to touch base with him. In just one afternoon, she would call or text Mark a *dozen or more times,* asking such questions as: Do you like beige curtains, or blue? What kind of rug should I get for the master bathroom? Should I buy a garden hose, or do you already have one?

At one point, she even felt compelled to ask him *what color panties* she should buy and, frankly, Mark *enjoyed* making those kinds of decisions for her. After all, he was a Dominant, and *that's what Dominants do.* Perhaps that's why, at the end of a long day punctuated by over a dozen calls from Vicki, Mark was surprised to learn that she had failed to mention that she had *gotten her tongue pierced.* Mark was *livid* over the fact that he hadn't been consulted. After a thorough dressing-down, he ordered her to remove the stud immediately. She tried, but was unable to do it. He instructed her to have the stud removed at the piercing salon the following day. She tearfully promised to do so.

The following day came and went, with no discussion or action on the tongue stud. A few days later, Mark asked Vicki about it. She explained that removing the stud so soon would have been *"too painful,"* but promised to have it done on Saturday, which was her day off. The weekend passed, once again with no action being taken on the tongue stud. Mark said nothing at the time, but was beginning to have serious doubts about the sincerity of Vicki's promises and her understanding of *what was at stake.* Those doubts were magnified *exponentially* just a few days later when Vicki cheerfully announced, to Mark's complete surprise, that she had *bought a puppy.* This was something they had discussed earlier; a fact that Mark decided needed to be brought up.

"I thought we agreed that this was *not* a good time to get a puppy," he growled, "Our budget is strained, we're both going to be at work all day long, and we don't even have any *furniture* yet."

If Vicki could sense his irritation, she gave no outward sign of it. She bounced and squealed in her excitement, "I *know,* Master! But just look at him! *Isn't he adorable?* And he was *only $250!"*

Mark *lost it.* For the first time *ever,* he *raised his voice at her.* He railed at her for failing to consult him on the piercing, for breaking two solemn promises to make it right, and for violating their agreement to wait on a pet until they were settled into the new house. His angry tirade was *so* brutal, she shook and sobbed uncontrollably for *hours afterward.* The next day, Mark and Vicki apologized tenderly to each other, and each promised to try harder to understand the emotional needs of the other.

A wary calm settled over their relationship for the remainder of the week, until an innocuous evening discussion reopened their still-tender wounds. Vicki had been experiencing some minor, yet terribly frustrating mechanical issues with her car, and had been hinting that perhaps it was time to trade it in for something a little more dependable. As she paged through the automotive ads, she asked, "What do you know about *auto leasing,* Master?"

Mark gave her the run-down on how leasing worked, the costs involved, and the relative advantages and disadvantages of leasing, as opposed to purchasing. He followed that up with, "My guess is, considering your age, low credit rating, and income level, you probably won't qualify for auto leasing. I'd advise you to *buy."* Vicki looked up from automotive advertisements and said, "When I *want* your advice, *I'll ask for it."*

Mark was *dumbfounded* by what he'd just heard. *"Excuse me?"* he said, "Perhaps you should consider carefully what you're saying, and how you're saying it. I don't think you have *any idea* the path you've just put yourself on."

Vicki was angry and undeterred, however. She continued, "No, maybe *you* need to consider how harsh and uncompromising *you* can be. You think you're always right and, granted, you usually *are.* But I'm sick and tired of having it *rubbed in my face* whenever I screw up. I should be able to make mistakes without you making a *big deal* out of it or saying *I told you so*. You need to be more understanding, you need to show a lot more compassion, and you need to *stop acting like a jerk."*

Mark pondered her words and her emotional state for a moment before replying, and when he did it was with quiet resignation. "I'm sorry, but it is *not your place* to tell me what I should *do*, how I should *feel*, or how I should *act.* If holding you accountable for your *own promises* is harsh, then I guess I *am* harsh. But when you screw up, it's my job to *let you know* that you've screwed up and to apply some corrective action. That's not *rubbing it in your face.* That's called *accountability and discipline."* He continued, "You say I don't understand what you're going through, but you're wrong. Admittedly, it took me a while to figure it out, but I now know *exactly* what you're going through. Part of the reason why this has been so hard for you is you're simply not suited for it. You may be a wonderful *bottom*, but you're a *lousy submissive.* It's just a shame that we've both had to go through so much pain before figuring that out. I'm sorry, but this relationship is going *nowhere I want to go.* You are released."

And with those three simple words, it was over.

Lessons Learned

I hope you are able to glean something from each of these three case studies that will help you to either *avoid* making a similar mistake or, at the very least, *recognize* when you or your partner have started down a similar path. It is easy to believe that this sort of thing can't happen to you, but it *can* and it probably *will* at some point in your life. If you're *very* lucky, *once will be enough.*

So, let's recap. BDSM shouldn't be mistaken for sex. Sure, BDSM is *sexy as hell,* but then so are a nice pair of red stiletto pumps. There are three possible scenarios when it comes to your stilettos and sex: (1) You could wear your stilettos without having sex. (2) You could have sex *without your stilettos on.* And (3) you could have sex with your stilettos on, preferably at my house, and bring a camera. BDSM is a lot like those stilettos. You can have BDSM without sex, sex without BDSM, or you can have both. I recommend option three.

Love shouldn't be mistaken for BDSM. Just because you *love* someone doesn't mean you will enjoy BDSM activities with that person. Love can encourage you to try new things and perhaps even push the boundaries of what you're willing to tolerate. But love isn't going to change how you feel about pain, humiliation, or hard limits on things that *squick you out.*

BDSM isn't D/s. There are many who attempt to weave D/s into even the acronym, but there *is* a difference, and the difference serves a valuable purpose. BDSM is what you *do.* D/s is what is in your *head and heart;* it is what governs your *relationship dynamic.* A Top *may not* be a Dominant. A bottom *may not* be a submissive.

Knowing those simple truths can save you a *lot* of heartache.

# # #

My Two Cents on Sex, Love, and BDSM

I think D/s is sexy.

Perhaps I find it sexy because it is how I *express* my love and how I want someone to express her love for me, in return. Some people express their love with kisses and caresses. I express mine through a D/s relationship dynamic; not that there's anything wrong with kisses and caresses, too. For me, the gift of submission from my partner is the purest expression of love that I can imagine. *Loyalty* runs a very close second.

Conversely and surprisingly to some, I don't particularly find *BDSM* to be *inherently sexy*. Don't get me wrong; with the *right person* and in the *right circumstances,* BDSM play can be *incredibly* sexy. I've probably already beat this analogy to death, but BDSM really is a lot like sex, and let's face it - sometimes, *even sex isn't sexy.*

Just to clarify: I *like* sex. I like it a *lot.*

My thoughts on *love* are a bit more complicated and controversial.

I believe *real love* should be *unconditional*. It simply doesn't have to be as complicated as most people try to make it. Whenever you let *coulda, woulda, shoulda, and ought-to-be get* into the act, you're just mucking up something that, if left alone, is truly beautiful in its simplicity and incredible capacity for creating a lot of joy in your life and in the lives of others.

If you think you love someone, but you're hoping or angling or trying to get something from that person in return, that isn't *real love.* It's just another form of self-gratification. At best, it is *emotional masturbation*; at its worst, it is *emotional blackmail.*

Love is that condition where someone else's happiness matters more to you than your very own.

If you've spent your entire life thinking that love should be all about insecurity, jealousy or drama, chances are your search for happiness is going to be longer and exponentially more difficult. Love shouldn't be about saying *I love you*, therefore, *you should love me back*, or prove to me how much you care, or you must start shaving your back, or settling down to have babies, or riding unicorns into the sunset.

It shouldn't be all about *what's in it for you.*

You either love the person standing in front of you, or you don't. Loving the person that you *wish* he or she could be is a terrible waste of time and emotional energy.

Love the person, not the fantasy.

"The more you love, the more you *can* love - and the more *intensely* you love. Nor is there any limit on how *many* you can love. If a person had time enough, he could love all of that majority who are decent and just."

- *Robert A. Heinlein*

CHAPTER 12: POLYAMORY

Polyamory is the practice of loving, or ability to love, more than one person at a time. The word is derived from the Latin *poly,* meaning *many,* and *amor,* meaning *love.* Polyamory is about *multiple loves*; not necessarily about multiple *sex partners*. Perhaps it would also be best if we establish a working definition of *love* before we go much further on this subject. For our purposes, we'll use Robert A. Heinlein's definition of love, which is, *"that condition in which the happiness of another person is essential to your own."* The elegance of this definition allows us to sidestep the sometimes thorny problem of trying to differentiate between *romantic* love, *familial* love, *sexual* love, or any *other* kind of love that can be imagined.

If you are one of those people who has a difficult time understanding how loving multiple partners can be accomplished without jealousy, instability and strife, consider the love that a mother has for her children. With each new child that comes along, a mother seems to have an infinite reservoir of love to share with each new addition to her family. She doesn't love her first child any *less* just because a second child has come along, nor does she love her *second* child any less when a *third* one is born. Each child is loved for his or her unique and special qualities, and while their mother may love each in a slightly different *way*, it is rare for a mother to love one child significantly more or less than any other. Do siblings often vie for their mother's attention, and sometimes feel shortchanged or jealous? Of *course* they do. Yet, for the most part, these feelings rarely lead to destructive behaviors, nor do they undermine their love for their mother, or for that matter, for *each other*. All things considered, most people believe that a child who grows up with siblings reaps many intangible benefits that an only child does not. So why are we, as a society, programmed to believe that polyamory, which works so elegantly for parents and children, is next to impossible in *other* kinds of loving relationships?

In the D/s lifestyle, polyamory is typically far more prevalent than in the general population for three simple reasons. First, a Dominant usually has far more discretion to do as he pleases than the typical non-Dominant outside of the D/s lifestyle. Second, the D/s lifestyle tends to attract people who are inherently willing to swim against the tide of social conventions. If this were not so, they wouldn't be in the lifestyle in the first place. Third, many of the people in the D/s lifestyle participate in group activities within their local BDSM organizations, and sometimes develop close relationships with the *playmates* they meet there. D/s folk are no more or less likely than anyone else to be sexual *swingers,* however the cultivation of BDSM friendships with common kinks makes polyamory a more likely scenario. Let us not forget, however, that just because polyamory is relatively *common* in the D/s lifestyle doesn't mean that people in the lifestyle are any *better* at it than anyone else. It is a profoundly difficult thing to be successfully polyamorous in *any* relationship, D/s or otherwise.

Any discussion of what polyamory *is* would not be complete without some attention to what it *isn't.* First and foremost, polyamory isn't *promiscuity*. Just because someone loves *more than one person*, does not mean they love *everyone*, nor does it mean they are willing to *have sex* with just anyone. To be clear, promiscuity is defined as having indiscriminate sexual relations with multiple partners on a *casual basis*. A polyamorous person may have multiple sex partners, but he can be just as faithful and loving and attentive to his *two (or three or more)* partners as a monogamous person can be to his *one.* This faithfulness to multiple partners is called *polyfidelity*, and a polyamorous person who practices it is called *polyfidelous*. Promiscuity and similar conditions, such as love or sex addiction, occur about as often in polyamorous individuals as they do in monogamous people.

Another thing that polyamory *isn't*, is a *value judgment*. Polyamory isn't objectively good or bad, right or wrong. It is simply a description of how *some* people think, feel, and love. You are either polyamorous, or you are not. It is virtually impossible to turn a monogamist into a polyamorist, and vice versa. Yes, there *are* things that a person can learn that can make polyamory *easier or more viable* for someone who has polyamorous feelings, but doesn't yet possess the skills and knowledge to make it *work* in their relationship, but you simply cannot turn a monogamous brain into a poly one. Polyamory *isn't for everyone,* and anyone who believes and preaches the notion that polyamory should be universally practiced is just as wrong-headed as those who are moral crusaders for monogamy.

Even for the small minority of people whose brains are *wired* for it, being poly in a predominantly monogamous world *isn't* easy. Since the great majority of people in western cultures equate polyamory with *promiscuity*, *adultery* and *cheating*, the result is a natural tendency to shun or condemn anyone associated with or practicing polyamory. It is rather common, even in these supposedly "enlightened" times, to hear people toeing the politically correct line that "the government shouldn't try to tell us *whom we can and can't love*; people should be able to marry whomever they want." Yet, for many, those very same principles don't apply *when someone wants to marry more than one person*.

Polygamy is illegal in all fifty states of the United States, yet no one has ever made a logically compelling case for why it should be so. Even as more and more states move to make *same-sex marriage* legal on the grounds that the benefits of marriage should be extended to any individuals, regardless of their gender, who wish to get married, the unspoken fine print seems to be, *"as long as they are gay, and there are only two of them."* It's truly ironic that some of society's most enthusiastic advocates for *social justice*, and *tolerance of alternate lifestyles* also happen to be the least likely to support changes in the law that would legalize *polyamorous marriages, or polygamy.*

Group Marriage and Polygamy

Polygamy is simply *polyamory* applied to the institution of *marriage.* There are three types of polygamy: Polygyny, polyandry, and group or plural marriages. *Polygyny* is defined as a man having multiple wives. *Polyandry* describes a woman with multiple husbands. *Group or plural marriages* are umbrella terms used to describe any marriages or relationships resembling marriages that have more than two partners.

Plural marriages have been around, in one form or another, throughout human history. About half of the over 1200 societies listed in the *Ethnographic Atlas Codebook* have a significant incidence of plural marriages occurring in them. In most of those cultures, plural marriages are relatively rare, even when accepted and legal. In modern times, polygamous marriages have been practiced and legally recognized in Tibet, Thailand, Burma, Sri Lanka, and 21 of the 22 countries that are members of the Arab League, with Tunisia being the lone hold-out. In Senegal, 47% of all marriages are polygamous, while in highly-westernized South Africa, it is not only practiced and legal, but President Jacob Zuma has four wives and twenty-nine children.

In the United States, polygamous marriages were practiced by the Church of Jesus Christ of Latter-day Saints (also known as the Mormon Church) from 1832 until 1890, when it was officially renounced by the church's leadership and made an excommunicable offense. Since that time, splinter groups in the latter-day saints movement, most notably the Fundamentalist Church of Jesus Christ of Latter-day Saints, have continued to practice polygamy in isolated communities in the western United States and in Canada.

Another experiment in polyamorous living was founded in 1848 in New York by a group called "Christian Perfectionism" which was led by John Humphrey Noyes. The members of this community, called the Oneida community, practiced a form of group marriage wherein all of the males in the community were married to all of the females, and vice-versa - a doctrine which they called *"complex marriage."* The community thrived for thirty-three years and, at one point, boasted over 300 members before being disbanded in 1881.

In addition to the Mormon and Oneida experiences, there have been other, more modern, institutional attempts at polyamorous living in the United States. One of those experiments was the Kerista Commune, which existed in the San Francisco area from 1971 until 1991. The Kerista Commune pioneered many of the concepts and practices that are now considered doctrinal in the polyamory lifestyle. One of the terms coined there was *polyfidelity,* which we defined earlier in this chapter.

Another concept developed there was the notion of *compersion*. A simple way to define *compersion* would be to describe it as the *opposite of jealousy*. Compersion is a *positive emotional reaction to your partner's involvement from another romantic or sexual relationship*. The Kerista Commune pioneered the practice of modern group marriages; however some of their practices were controversial, even among their members, such as assigning sleeping partners to commune members on a rotating schedule, and discriminating against homosexuals. After twenty years of operation, the Kerista Commune shuttered its doors due to internal strife and legal troubles.

Today, there is still a growing polyamory movement in the United States, and it is nowhere more robust than in the D/s lifestyle. The reasons for this are relatively straightforward. First, the sort of person who is attracted to a *lifestyle* that is outside of the mainstream has a higher probability of having attitudes and beliefs about *loving relationships* that are outside of the mainstream, as well.

Second, the D/s lifestyle is *structured to allow* polyamorous relationships to occur more easily, and with greater frequency. Specifically, Dominants are far more likely *to be allowed* to have multiple partners, and submissives are far less likely to forbid it, than their vanilla counterparts in general society. Third and finally, the BDSM culture encourages experimentation, group activities, and casual fetish play (which may or may not be sexual in nature) that create opportunities for polyamorous relationships to develop.

There are, of course, many *potential* advantages and disadvantages that come with any polyamorous relationship. They can be more or less applicable to any *particular* relationship, depending upon the nature of the relationship, the number of people involved, whether or not children are a part of the relationship, living arrangements, financial arrangements, sexual relations, and other factors.

Potential Advantages of a Poly Relationship

Since this book is ostensibly about D/s and BDSM relationships, we'll focus now on how polyamorous relationships work *(or don't)* in the context of the lifestyle. Not only is the poly dynamic more *common* in the D/s lifestyle, but it generally tends to be more *useful* there, as well. Consider these potential advantages, while staying mindful of the fact that being poly in a D/s context typically means a relationship consisting of a single Dominant and two or more submissives.

Empathy. *Everyone*, in or out of this lifestyle, needs a little *empathy* from time to time, but for a submissive, this need is usually far more *intense*. Yet, when it comes to a D/s relationship, where does a submissive go to find someone who truly understands her situation, and how she feels about it? You're not very likely to approach a vanilla coworker to discuss, over lunch, your relationship with your *Master.* Even if you were to couch everything in purely *vanilla* terms, there would be one crucial part of the equation missing, and that would be the *D/s relationship dynamic.* Any understanding that your vanilla friend would think she had about your situation would be *seriously flawed,* and any advice she gave you would likely be tragically misguided. And while it would certainly be helpful to know and depend upon friends who understand the lifestyle and are also *submissives,* no one knows you, your situation, and/or your Master *the way your sister (or brother) submissive does.* The empathy and understanding that can exist between *co-wives* or *co-husbands* in a poly relationship is unparalleled anywhere else in our culture.

Attention. It's often easy to assume that being part of a poly relationship means having to *share* someone you love with another, and therefore being resigned to getting less of that person's *focused* attention. However, another way of looking at it might be to see the glass as *half full* instead of *half empty,* by realizing that you could also end up on the receiving end of a lot of attention from the *multiple partners* in your relationship, and that group activities have a way of developing their own brand of energy and excitement, if you'll let them.

Complexity. This can be a double-edged sword which cuts both ways, but the very same *complexity* that makes the poly dynamic difficult in the early stages of a relationship can later work in your favor to help keep the relationship from going stale over time. Generally speaking, the sort of person who is willing to swim against the tide of society's expectations and chooses to live an alternative lifestyle is more likely to be attracted to complex relationships than to avoid them. One of the greatest long-term challenges that confronts any relationship - simple or complex, monogamous or poly – is going to be *staying interested.*

Synergy. Synergy is a word that is used frequently in the business world, but less so in discussions about *relationships.* Yet, it is through *relationships* that the true meaning of the word can be demonstrated best. *Synergy* is defined as a process by which we may produce a *whole* that is greater than the sum of its individual parts. In essence, it is how we make *one plus one equal three*. This may seem counter-intuitive to us, until we are reminded that couples do this *all the time*. We call it *making babies*. But synergy in relationships isn't just about procreation, nor should it be. Synergy *should* be all about accomplishing whatever goals you've set for yourselves - whether they are health goals, financial goals, educational goals, or any other dream you may have - and utilizing the full range of the talents, skills, knowledge and *synergy* of the group to *make it happen*.

Teamwork. While it may be closely related to synergy, the teamwork that occurs in a poly relationship has a nuance all its own, and can be an incredible asset and advantage to everyone involved. Problem solving becomes a process that draws on the unique individual strengths and qualities of each individual. Pooled resources, such as property, income, transportation or even *time* can be put to use where it does the most good. Tag-team child care can reduce or even eliminate the need to give up a significant portion of one's income to pay for child care while on the job. Three or more *incomes* can go a long way towards improving the quality of life for everyone in a poly household. Even where separate households are maintained, there will usually be ways that teamwork can make some things easier, cheaper, or more efficient for everyone involved.

Potential Pitfalls of a Poly Relationship

Attractive as some of the advantages may be, polyamorous relationships have their own unique pitfalls and difficulties, not the least of which is the existence of an intense and almost *rabid* anti-poly societal bias. Anyone choosing to become part of a poly relationship must typically be willing to do one of two things: conceal the true nature of your relationship from the great majority of your family, friends, neighbors and co-workers, or *reveal it to all*, and be consigned to endure a lifetime of contention over it. Neither option is particularly appealing to the average person, but then again, no one ever promised you that polyamory was going to be *easy.* Here are a few more of the potential pitfalls associated with polyamorous relationships:

Jealousy. It will likely come as no surprise to anyone that *jealousy* is at the top of the list when it comes to potential pitfalls of a polyamorous relationship. Many people erroneously assume that *being poly* means being *free of jealousy*. Jealousy is, and always will be, a perfectly *normal* human emotion that is fed by fear, rivalry, poor self-esteem, insecurity and envy. It isn't the *emotion* of jealousy that can become problematic in a relationship; it is the way in which that jealousy is *expressed.* A simple parallel, to illustrate this notion, might be to compare it to *anger.* It would be completely *unreasonable* to expect that your mates *will never get angry*, but it is *entirely* reasonable to expect that they will never come after you with a butcher knife *when they do.* Yet some studies *(White & Mullen 1989, Pines 1992)* estimate that 20-35% of all *murders* are motivated by jealousy! Anyone who is considering entering into a poly relationship should do so with the expectation that jealousy *will* occur, and will need to be skillfully *managed* by everyone involved.

So, how does one manage jealousy in a poly relationship? The techniques are essentially the same as those used while managing jealousy in *any* relationship, though your approach may change, depending on whether it is you or your partner(s) who are the jealous parties.

If you are the one who is jealous:

- Learn to identify the emotions you're feeling, and the triggers that prompt them. Sometimes, keeping a journal can help you, in this regard.
- Unlearn the notion that every time you feel a strong emotion, that you are required to *do something about it.* Decisions made in the heat of high emotion will almost always turn out to be *bad decisions.*

- Work on improving your communication skills. One way to do that is to use precise language to avoid coming across as being judgmental or blaming. Instead of saying, *"You ignored me,"* try saying, *"I felt left out."* Discussing your *feelings*, instead of another person's *actions* works far better, because no one can ever deny *how you felt*, yet they could *(and probably will)* argue the issue of what they *did or didn't do*. Avoid *any* language that leads to guilt trips, blaming, martyrdom, tantrums or threats of violence or self-destructive behavior.
- Seek reassurance from your partner(s) on their feelings about you and/or the relationship, their willingness to work with you to resolve the issues, and their understanding of what is actually happening.
- Avoid viewing your jealousy as a problem that can only be solved by a change in someone else's behavior. Yes, it *is* a problem that can be solved, but only by making changes in your *own* thinking and behavior.
- Learn to love yourself, despite all of your flaws and insecurities. Acknowledge that you are loved, and that you have unique gifts, talents and qualities that *no one else has,* and that you have value. This is, and forever will be, true regardless of whether or not your current relationship endures.
- Recognize that your emotional state and any resulting drama also affect *everyone else in the relationship*, and the effect is almost never a good one. This can cause a ripple-effect of unintended consequences, which may become *self-fulfilling prophecies*.
- Consider *desensitizing* yourself to your jealousy triggers by deliberately exposing yourself to them in small, manageable doses with the help of your partner(s). Evaluate how you react to and handle each instance, and look for ways you can improve.
- Be patient, forgiving, creative and strong in your efforts to overcome the negative effects that jealousy can have on your relationship. Ask yourself, at each step of the way, am I making things *better or worse?*

If your partner is the one who is jealous:

- Don't introduce new partners into a relationship that isn't already built on a firm foundation. Polyamory can sometimes make a *good* relationship *better*, but it will almost always be a *deathblow* to a fragile or dysfunctional relationship.
- Avoid dismissing your partner's feelings as *irrational.* Jealousy, almost by *definition*, is irrational – as is emotion in general. Try to acknowledge and validate your partners *feelings*, even if you don't necessarily agree with how they are expressed or the decisions that are made as a result of those feelings.
- Improve your communication skills, and take a hard look at what you may be doing to make matters worse. This may include things like *pushing your partner's hot buttons*, resorting to *low blows* in arguments, unnecessarily stoking your partner's feelings of insecurity, making comparisons, encouraging competitive attitudes and behaviors, and being inconsistent in your standards and priorities.
- Be willing to ask yourself whether you may actually be in the habit of seeking out jealous partners because it strokes your ego or keeps things exciting.
- Keep your cool, and refuse to reciprocate with verbal abuse or emotional outbursts just because your partner does. Refuse to engage in discussions that involve threats of violence or suicide gestures of any kind. Learn to walk away from discussions or arguments that threaten to spiral out of control. You can always pick up where you left off once you've both cooled off.
- If the discussion involves three or more partners, try to avoid any tendency to *gang up* on one individual. That person will typically feel ambushed and overwhelmed, even if you are taking great pains to be scrupulously fair.
- Affirm your feelings and commitment to your partners, and reassure them in ways that tell them that they are appreciated for their unique qualities, and are valued.
- Be trustworthy, consistent and disciplined. If you agree to something, keep your word.

Focus. Another potential disadvantage of poly relationships is the issue of *focus,* which generally falls into two categories: *time* and *attention.* It is always a difficult balancing act to know when to focus these resources upon *one* partner like a laser beam, and when to broaden your focus to include more than one mate and/or others, such as children or friends. One-on-one *quality time*, which is typically comprised of *highly focused attention on one individual,* can often compensate for far larger *quantities* of *unfocused* time and attention. One-on-one quality time usually includes, but shouldn't necessarily be limited to, sex and intimacy. It can just as easily consist of *any* activity that is unique and special to the individual who is the focus of your attention. The key to overcoming this challenge in a poly relationship is to regularly schedule inviolable one-on-one quality time with each of your mates, and stick to your schedule.

Expense and Resources. The *cost and viability* of a polyamorous relationship can be another one of those double-edged swords that we seem to encounter with great frequency in the poly lifestyle. On one hand, a poly relationship can *sometimes* mean multiple incomes flowing into a single household, which *may* equate to a higher standard of living and increased cash flow for everyone involved. On the other hand, it could also consist of a relationship where all of the partners *aren't able to work* and contribute a portion of their income. That could, for example, mean trying to support *three* people with the same income that previously supported *just two* – which rarely works out very well. While there isn't a cookie-cutter solution to these kinds of challenges, it is almost always a good idea to sit down with any potential poly partners to have a frank discussion about personal finances and perhaps even a proposed budget.

Personal Space. Contrary to popular belief, *personal space* can become an issue even in poly relationships where each partner lives in his or her *own home*. Allowing another person to muck about in your kitchen or sock drawer can definitely be a little unsettling for some. Multiply that by two or more people doing it, and it can be more than just unsettling, it can cause some people to become absolutely *unhinged.* Add two cups of living under the same roof and a dash of the common misconception that poly living somehow equates to *communal property,* and *voila!* – you now have a recipe for *epic relationship failure.* If you are considering entering into a poly relationship where your partners will be living in the same household, be sure to hammer out the details of what is or isn't considered your personal space that is off-limits to the other members of the household *before* you move in.

Scorekeeping. One of the most enduring myths concerning polyamorous relationships is the notion that everyone should be treated *equally.* It's even more curious that many of the people who perpetuate that myth just happen to be the very same people who want to be appreciated and recognized for their own unique qualities and contributions to the relationship. How does one recognize an individual's unique qualities, yet still treat everyone exactly the same? Any parent with more than one child knows that *equity* is always an issue that must be dealt with, when it comes to sibling rivalry. The solution typically involves treating everyone *fairly* and *equitably,* even if they are not treated exactly the *same.* Unfortunately, the *adults* in a polyamorous relationship can sometimes behave like children, by engaging in *scorekeeping.* Scorekeeping occurs when you feel *cheated* because another person in the relationship *appears* to be getting more time, sex, gifts, or attention than *you* are. Keeping a tally of the days, hours or even *minutes* one partner spends with another, compulsively tracking expenditures, and attempting to quantify enjoyment are all manifestations of scorekeeping. Imagine a partner who claims, "Yes, I know you spent *all day* with me, and only an *hour* with her, but I still got cheated *because you enjoyed your time with her more.*" Obviously, there can be no effective rational response to an irrational anxiety. Author Erica Jong probably said it best when she wrote, "Jealousy is all the fun *you think they had.*"

Odd-One-Out Syndrome. We live in a predominantly monogamous society and, as a result, our environment tends to be structured in ways that support that paradigm. Think about it. Our cars have one *driver's* seat, one *passenger* seat, and a *back seat*. Free-standing restaurant tables are set up for *two, four, or more chairs*. Booths typically allow two people to sit side-by-side, while the third must sit across the table. You can buy a *double* bed, but not a *triple* bed; larger sizes are called *queen* and *king-sized*, as if only royalty are allowed to have poly sleeping arrangements. Polygamous marriage is still illegal in most western cultures, so only one poly partner gets to be the *"real"* spouse, while others are relegated to being mere *cohabitants*. The list goes on and on, but you get the idea. *Someone* is always forced to be the *odd one out*, and this can often become a sore spot if it is not recognized and dealt with effectively. It may be useful to discourage competition and rivalry for those coveted *number two* seats by implementing a simple system that randomizes or assigns seats fairly for all concerned.

Children. The presence of children in a polyamorous relationship adds a level of complexity and potential for problems that many people would rather not have to think about, but it is a subject that should be given some thought, whether or not the current partners in the relationship *currently* have any children. Typically, when a vanilla person hears, for the first time, that you are in a poly relationship, the very first question they will ask is *"Do any of you have children?"* This question usually arises for one or more of the following three reasons. First, they may be confusing polyamory with sexual *promiscuity* or *swinging*, and are worried that the children will be exposed to orgies in the living room. Second, they worry that having *multiple pervy partners* in a household with kids will increase the potential for child abuse. And third, they worry that the children may grow up believing the *crazy notion* that it's okay to love more than one person at a time. In defense of your vanilla friends, two of the three concerns actually do have some validity, and ought to be considered. Obviously, polyamory is *not swinging*, so that issue can usually be laid to rest with a simple explanation of the differences. But introducing *any new adult* into *any* household *(mono or poly)* with children increases the *potential* for abuse, and this potential can be significantly higher if that person is, for example, a *sadist*. Further complicating the matter is the unfortunate reality that if any allegation of abuse is made, the fact that a person is living an alternative lifestyle will be counted as a strike against the alleged perpetrator in any court of law. Finally, while you *may* believe that polyamory is the perfect lifestyle *for you*, you may want to give some serious consideration to whether you want to pass that mindset and way of life on to your children. For some, the answer may be simple. For others, perhaps *not so much*.

The Final Straw. You may be familiar with the old Arabic proverb that describes how a heavily-laden camel's back is *broken* by a *single straw* that is added to his already heavy load. This *final straw* parable perfectly describes what happens when an already *overburdened* and *barely functional* relationship is transformed almost instantly into a completely *dysfunctional* one by the addition of another partner. When this occurs, it is *not* indicative of any systemic flaw in the concept or practice of polyamory; it is the predictable consequence of introducing unknown variables, new personalities and additional stresses to a *pre-existing bad relationship*. *Stress* is how the mind and body react to perceived changes, threats or challenges that we encounter in our lives. Even positive changes can result in stress; just ask anyone who has ever won the lottery. The introduction of a new partner into a relationship, household or both can be an incredibly stressful event, even under the best circumstances. The closest *mono-vanilla* parallel would be a couple *getting married* and establishing a shared household for the first time; obviously *not* something one should be considering if your current relationship is not a healthy one. Polyamory may have the potential to make a good relationship better, but it also has the potential to be the proverbial straw that breaks the camel's back.

Now that we have discussed the potential advantages and pitfalls which you may encounter in a polyamorous relationship, let's talk about why it may be important to be *familiar* with polyamory, even if you are not poly yourself and never, ever, *not even in a million years* plan on becoming poly. After all, it's highly unlikely that you'll go to bed one night as a monogamist and wake up the following morning with the sudden epiphany that you're now a polyamorist. But there are plenty of *other* scenarios which are far more likely to occur. You could, for example, one day end up the concerned confidant who feels compelled to ask your poly friends, "Do any of you have children?"

Being properly informed about the true nature of poly lifestyles can mean the difference between an expression of *interest* versus an expression of *condemnation*. You probably *already* have poly friends you don't know about who haven't *come out of the closet* simply because they don't expect you to understand or approve of their lifestyle.

You could also end up being a monogamous person who falls in love with a polyamorous person. If this happens to you, *don't panic*. It is entirely possible to not only *survive* the experience, but to *thrive* on it, *if* you can successfully manage your own expectations and behavior. First, you should understand from the beginning that *it isn't going to be easy* being part of what is sometimes referred to as a *mono/poly* relationship. Second, you must be willing to go into it knowing that you have about as much chance of converting your *poly partner* to monogamy as you do of converting a gay partner to *heterosexuality*. In other words, the odds are somewhere between zero and the proverbial *snowball's chance in hell.* Third, don't delude yourself into thinking that just because your poly partner doesn't have multiple partners *now*, that you can somehow prevent them from being added to the relationship *later*. A poly person is *still poly*, even if he or she *currently* only has one partner.

Polyamory is a paradigm; it is a way of *thinking*. It is founded in the notion that the human heart has an *infinite* capacity for love. Perhaps one of the easiest ways to explain the concept of polyamory to a monogamist is to compare it to our attitudes about *friendship*.

When we make a new *friend*, we never ask ourselves whether *this* friend puts us over some imaginary limit on how many friends we should be allowed to have. We don't feel the need to drop one friend in order to make room for another. We instinctively understand that just because someone is our friend, that we don't have the right to control their feelings or behavior, nor should they feel entitled to control ours.

We don't expect each of our friends to meet *all* of our needs and interests, nor are we willing to give up our interests just because our current friends aren't much interested in them. We may enjoy going to the movies with one friend, dancing with another, and enjoying Thai food with a third. Even if it were *possible* for one friend to match every one of our needs and interests, we'd probably *still* want to make new friends. We also *usually* consider any friend who is irrationally jealous of all our other friends to be somewhat *problematic*.

In spite of all of the challenges that must be overcome, a few of our select friends occasionally somehow manage to navigate the tortuous path that takes them from being just *friends* to becoming our *lovers*. And suddenly, *everything changes*.

Perhaps the question we should be asking is, *why does it have to?*

# # #

Poly Glossary

To bring this chapter to a close, here are some useful terms and phrases that are *unique* to polyamory. They are listed *here*, at the end of this chapter, rather than at the back of the book because, for the most part, they are not *inherently* part of the D/s or BDSM lifestyles. While there is often a great deal of *overlap* between the poly and BDSM lifestyles, the majority of the people in the BDSM lifestyle are *not* poly, and most poly folk are *not* BDSM.

The definitions provided here represent my earnest effort to give the best and most useful rendering of the meaning of the listed terms. Please keep in mind that many of the terms listed have been recently coined, may be controversial in their interpretation, or may differ in meaning from one region to the next, or in different organizations or social circles.

Bright-eyed Novice. Typically a derogatory term for a person who has recently discovered polyamory and whose head is full of *theory*, but has little or no actual *experience* with any practical application of a poly lifestyle. Someone who tells everyone how poly *should* be practiced, even though they've never actually done it *themselves*.

Closed Marriage. A marriage that allows for no outside emotional or sexual relationships.

Closed Group Marriage. A *poly* marriage that allows for no outside emotional or sexual relationships.

Cluster Marriage. A poly relationship consisting of two or more married couples living together under one roof and engaging in *cross-couple* romantic and/or sexual relationships.

Cross-couple. Any relationship or activity between a member of one couple and a member of another couple.

Compersion. The joy or satisfaction derived from the knowledge that someone you love is expressing his or her love for another person. *Compersion* is sometimes referred to as the opposite of *jealousy.*

Complex Marriage. A form of group marriage where all of the male members of the group are considered to be married to all of the female members, and all the female members are considered to be married to all of the male members.

Co-husband. Any male in a group marriage who is one of at least two males in the relationship.

Corporate Marriage. A group marriage that is organized as a legal entity (i.e. as a corporation or limited liability partnership) in order to have standing in the courts, and to specify the legal obligations and privileges of the individuals in the relationship.

Cowboy. Slang reference to a monogamous male who becomes involved with a poly female with the intent of separating her from her other poly partners.

Cuddle Party. A term to describe gatherings which encourage the expression of physical affection while at the same time forbidding sexual activity. *(A commercial trademark owned by Reid Mihalko.)*

Cyclic Monogamy. Sometimes referred to as *serial monogamy*. The practice of having multiple monogamous relationships, either serially or concurrently, and often without the knowledge of the multiple partners, who believe their relationships are monogamous.

Democratic Family. A poly relationship where all of the adult partners are considered equal.

Dyad. A couple, or a relationship between two individuals. Poly people in dyads are not considered monogamous simply because there are only two people in the relationship. See also: *Triad, Quad, Group Marriage.*

Emotional Fidelity. A term generally more common to swingers than in polyamory. The practice of reserving strong emotion or love for a particular partner or relationship, even though sex may occur outside the relationship with other people.

Emotional Libertarianism. A doctrine which teaches that each individual is responsible for his or her own emotions; it is a personal choice, since no one else can *make* you feel an emotion. Thinking or saying, *"You made me angry"* runs counter to the teachings of emotional libertariansm.

Exclusion Jealousy. The fear of being neglected or abandoned by one's lover.

Hinge. Typically a person in a poly relationship who is the common denominator, center or crux of a triad or vee, where the other individuals have little or no relationship with each other.

Line Marriage. A poly marriage that periodically adds younger members to replace those who leave or pass away, creating a sort of *immortality* for the relationship that outlives any of its individual members. The term was coined by author Robert A. Heinlein.

O.S.O. An acronym for Other Significant Other.

O.P.P. An acronym for One Penis Policy.

Monogamish. A term used to describe couples who are *generally* monogamous, but allow limited sexual relationships outside of the marriage, as long as they are not viewed as serious or long-term.

M.S.O. Acronym for Most Significant Other. Typically refers to the partner in a poly relationship that has, for whatever reason, greater seniority or standing than the other(s).

Panamory. Refers to the ability to love a person without regard to their sex, gender identity, or sexual orientation. Being capable of loving *anyone* is *not* the same as actually loving *everyone*.

Polyactivist. A person who is actively engaged in advocating for reforms that promote the practice and philosophy of polyamory in the legal, political, social and religious arenas.

Polyandry. Refers to a polyamorous relationship in which a woman has more than one male partner. It is typically used to describe a polygamous or plural *marriage* consisting of a wife with two or more husbands.

Polyfidelous. The practice of being faithful to more than one partner, usually in a polyamorous relationship, is called *polyfidelity*. For example, a polyamorous Dominant with two submissives may choose to be *polyfidelous* to his two partners, not engaging in intimate relations with anyone else.

Poly Friendly. An umbrella term used to describe a person, place, organization, business, or policy that does not discriminate against people who are in polyamorous relationships.

Polyfuckery. A derisive term used to describe those who *call* themselves polyamorous but who are, in fact, just sexually promiscuous.

Polygyny. Refers to a polyamorous relationship in which a man has more than one female partner. It is typically used to describe a polygamous or plural *marriage* consisting of a husband with two or more wives.

Poly/mono or Mono/poly. Any relationship between a monogamous person and a polyamorous one.

Polysaturated. Humorous term used to describe a poly relationship which is *"full."* In other words, adding any more partners would cause problems for the relationship.

Polyunsaturated. The opposite of *polysaturated.* A poly relationship with room for more partners.

Polysexual. Having multiple sexual relationships which do not involve love or intimacy. *(See polyfuckery.)*

Pollywog. A humorous term for a child in a poly household.

Puppy-pile Poly. A term used to describe a poly relationship where *all* of the individuals are romantically and/or sexually involved with one another, without clear lines of relation or hierarchy, reminiscent of the way puppies sleep in a chaotic pile.

Sororal Polygyny. A poly relationship where a man is married to two or more women who are sisters by birth.

Spice. A humorous term that is sometimes used as the plural of *spouse.*

Swolly. A contraction of the words *swinger* and *poly*. A person who has multiple loving relationships, but also has recreational sex that doesn't involve emotional attachments.

Vee. (See Hinge.)

Zee. A poly relationship consisting of 4 individuals forming a "Z", or two *vees* joined by a relationship between the two *hinges*.

My Two Cents on Polyamory

In the unlikely event that you haven't guessed by now, I *just happen* to be polyamorous and *have* been all of my *life*. It hasn't always been easy, and there were plenty of times that I wished I *weren't* poly, but it is what it is, and I am what I am.

Over the years, I've had many opportunities to try and explain what I think it means to be poly to my monogamous friends and potential love interests, with predictably mixed results. Eventually, I came up with something that I like to call my *"Spaghetti Story."* Don't ask me why I chose *spaghetti* to illustrate this little fable; it was a completely random choice, which may or may not have been influenced by an intense craving for Italian food at the time. But, I digress. Here it is:

The Spaghetti Story – A Poly Parable

Imagine that you and I are friends, and that the two of us are sitting alone in my dining room, side-by-side, at a large dinner table. Both of us are hungry, but the table is curiously set. In front of *you*, sits an empty plate. In front of *me*, sits a large bowl of – *you guessed it* - spaghetti. It isn't just your typical large bowl of spaghetti. No. There's more spaghetti here than I could *possibly* eat in one sitting. In fact, this is more spaghetti than I could possibly eat *in a month* of spaghetti dinners. I could *probably* supply one of those Kiwanis Club spaghetti dinner *fundraisers* with all of this spaghetti. We're talking about... *a lot*... of spaghetti, here.

I look over to see you sitting there, behind your empty plate, with your chin in your hands, staring at my colossal bowl of spaghetti. It's fairly obvious that you're *really hungry*. I can almost hear your empty stomach, growling like a dog does when you reach for his favorite bone.

And so, I ask, *"Would you like half of this spaghetti?"*

For a moment, you regard me through suspicious, squinting eyes, as you consider my simple offer. Your suspicion turns to self-righteous indignation, and you respond with a curiously puffed-up air of moral superiority, "No thanks, *I don't like to share."*

# # #

It seriously just *kills* me that I sometimes have to explain the meaning of this little parable to some people. I mean, *come on*. It just *isn't* that complicated. Even so, for the benefit of *those few*, here it is, in a nutshell:

It isn't *your* spaghetti to *share*. *It's mine*.

You may want it *all*, but you end up with a whole lot of *nothing*. In the end, *others* end up reaping the benefits of your pride and greed, but at least you're making *someone* happy, even if it isn't *you*.

I believe that the human heart has an *infinite* capacity for love. And *half* of infinity is still a *hell of a lot of spaghetti.*

With, or *without* breadsticks.

"Of the delights of this world man cares most for sexual intercourse, yet he has left it out of his heaven."

-- *Mark Twain*

CHAPTER 13: D/S, BDSM, & RELIGION

It is often said that the three topics you should never discuss in polite company are sex, religion, and politics. We've already spent much of this tome discussing the *sexual* aspects of the D/s and BDSM lifestyles, and in the *next* chapter, we'll be touching upon some of the legal and socio-political considerations that should be taken into account by anyone contemplating a D/s relationship. In *this* chapter, we'll be exploring the connection between D/s and *religion*, and discussing any significance that the link might have for *you.* According to the American Religious Identification Survey (2008), 76% of Americans identify themselves as Christians, 4% as belonging to other religions, and 15% are atheist, agnostic or have no religious affiliation at all. In other words, religion is important to *80% of Americans*, and yet practically *nothing* has been written about how religion affects the lives of those who are considering or currently in D/s relationships, or living a BDSM lifestyle.

Our objective, in the following pages, will be to attempt to fill that void. Before we go any further, however, I *would* like to make a suggestion: If you happen to be the sort of person for whom *any discussion of religion* causes blood to actually gush from your eye-sockets, this *might* be a good time to *skip ahead* to the next chapter. *Please.* This chapter is for the 80% of Americans who *are* religious, and may have concerns about this lifestyle *from within a religious context.* The other 20% should simply *move along;* nothing to see here, folks.

Questions concerning the compatibility of a D/s or BDSM lifestyle with one's *religious beliefs* are far more common than you might think. All you have to do is browse any random selection of online religious forums or web sites, you'll invariably encounter *a lot* of inquiries similar to this one:

> *"My husband wants to start doing some BDSM stuff in the bedroom, and I have to admit, I am curious and a little excited at the idea. We are both devout church-goers and don't want to do anything that runs counter to the teachings of our religion. The problem is, neither of us is willing to ask our spiritual advisor if it's okay to do the whips and chains thing in the bedroom. We're stuck, and don't know where to go for advice. Help!"*

For every person who gives voice to a question like the one above, there are scores who don't for fear of condemnation or embarrassment. There's a common misconception, both among those with a religious outlook and the non-religious alike, that there must be a fundamental conflict between being devoutly religious and living a D/s or BDSM lifestyle. The reality is that, for most people, nothing could be further from the truth. People are often surprised to learn that we can, indeed, build a very compelling case for both D/s relationships *and* BDSM activities from within a devoutly religious world-view. In the following pages, we're going to take a look at how BDSM and D/s relationships might be viewed through the prism of religion, specifically Judaism, Islam, Buddhism, Hinduism, Paganism, and yes, even *Christianity.*

D/s and Judaism: Could Lead to Mixed Dancing

Judaism is the three-thousand-year-old *Abrahamic* faith which later became the foundation of Christianity. For many, it is simultaneously a religion, a philosophy, *and* a way of life. Interestingly, there are no universally held beliefs or core doctrines that are considered essential to being a Jew. Some historians have criticized Judaism for emphasizing the observance of customs, rituals and observances over any specific dogma or *core religious beliefs*. In fact, there are some who consider themselves Jews while simultaneously considering themselves agnostics or atheists. There is no central authority over Judaism, and doctrine is sourced primarily from the Torah, the Talmud, and Maimonides' *(12th century Torah scholar and Rabbi Mosheh Ben Maimon)* Thirteen Principles of Faith. Even so, there are an infinite number of interpretations of each, which often makes it difficult if not impossible to know what is - *or isn't* - acceptable when it comes to sexual or BDSM practices.

Generally speaking, Judaism teaches that sex within the context of a committed relationship is a *good thing*. The Torah commandment known as *onah* requires a man to have regular sex with his wife. The Talmud even goes even further, specifying how *often* a man should have sex with his wife: Wealthy men should bed their wives *every day*. Common laborers are *cut some slack*, and are only expected to do it twice a week. Donkey-drivers are commanded to have relations with their mates once a week; camel-drivers once every thirty 30 days; and sailors at least once every six months!

When it comes to how the Jewish faith views kinkier activities and fetishes, things can get a little confusing, however. There is an old joke about a Jewish woman who went to her rabbi for advice on whether or not it would be alright if she and her husband tried a little BDSM. She asks, "Would it be alright if my husband tied me to the bed?" The rabbi nods, and says, *"Not a problem, my dear."* The woman then asks, "How about if he puts me over his knee and spanks my bare bottom?" The rabbi replies, *"Nothing wrong with that. That would be fine."*

Somewhat emboldened, the woman asks, "Could we have sex standing up in the middle of the living room?" The rabbi just shakes his head and says, *"I'm sorry, my dear, but that is forbidden. That could lead to mixed dancing."*

In the Judaic tradition, the term *isurei bi'ah* refers to those with whom Jews are forbidden to engage in sex. The list includes:

- Gentiles, meaning *non-Jews*.
- Incestuous relations.
- *Mamzerim*, meaning anyone who is the offspring of a forbidden relationship, such as adultery.
- Any woman during her menstrual period.
- Divorcees

Other acts that are expressly mentioned as being forbidden include extra-marital sex, male homosexual anal intercourse, bestiality, masturbation, ejaculating outside of a woman's vagina, cuckolding, cross dressing by either sex, having sex with the lights on, and males performing oral sex on women.

When it comes to BDSM, however, things can get a bit more complicated. For example, would the restrictions against *incest* and *bestiality* forbid a person from engaging in BDSM *age-play* or animal *role-play?* Cross dressing may be forbidden, but what about *forced feminization?* Activities such as forced masturbation, forced homosexual sex, and queening are just a *few* of the things that may occupy this moral *grey area* in Judaism. When it comes to D/s relationships specifically, *Maimonides* seemed to subscribe to essentially the same *"safe, sane and consensual"* philosophy that many in the BDSM lifestyle follow *today.* He wrote that a married couple should be able to engage in any sexual acts they desire, *as long as both partners consent to them.* He maintained that there should be *no forced sex acts*, and that sexual relations should always be conducted with "dignity and holiness."

D/s and Islam: Keep Your Clothes On

For adherents of the Islamic faith, the Quran, the sayings of Muhammad (called the *hadith*), and the rulings of religious leaders (called *fatwa*) are the ultimate authorities, even when it comes to relationships, sex, and BDSM. Despite the historic tensions between the two religions, Islam and Judaism are both *Abrahamic* religions, and there are a *lot* of similarities in their respective approaches to sexuality. They *both* forbid adultery, incestuous relations, male homosexual anal intercourse, and sex with menstruating women, for example. Some restrictions on sex that are *unique* to Islam include a prohibition on sex with a woman for forty days after childbirth, a prohibition on sex during daylight hours during the month of Ramadan, and a ban on sex while making a religious pilgrimage to Mecca.

One might naturally assume that slavery and the ownership of concubines is accepted in many cultures where Islam is practiced, that the teachings of Islam would be sympathetic to those in the D/s lifestyle. After all, a large number of them consider themselves Masters and slaves, do they not?

Islamic law not only allows for the ownership of slaves *(jariya)* and concubines *(surriyya)*, but even goes so far as to specify a Master's rights to have sex with them, impregnate them, or to sell them. For example, if a concubine has a child by her Master, he must acknowledge his paternity of the child, and no longer has the right to sell or transfer ownership of the mother. A Master may have as many concubines as he wishes, and his wife may have as many slave girls as *she* wishes, as well. However, the Master does *not* have sexual access *to his wife's slave girls*.

For many Muslims, it may be difficult to know which BDSM activities are *halal* (allowed), and which are *haram* (forbidden). For the most part, Islamic law teaches that any form of *consensual* sexual intimacy between man and wife, or man and concubine is *halal*, except anal sex or sex during menstruation. A woman may not, however, be *compelled* by her husband (or in the case of a concubine, her Master) to perform any sex act that may be considered to be physically, emotionally or relationally harmful or demeaning. This, of course, is always open to interpretation. Many Muslim sects have issued *fatwas* regarding the practice of sexual sadism, classifying it as a harmful practice, and essentially forbidding it. Additionally, there are also a large number of authoritative fatwas forbidding any *role play* of an activity that, in reality, would be considered *haram*. This would include BDSM role-play activities like age play, incest play, pet play, rape play, and forced feminization.

Not only do many of the *private BDSM activities* between a man and a woman fall under the auspices of Islamic law *(sharia)*, but participation in various BDSM *social activities* may, *as well.* A large part of the BDSM culture involves social events such as BDSM munches, dungeon play, and play parties. What might Islamic law have to say about *that?* It probably won't come as much of a surprise when we say, *quite a lot.*

The *good* news for Muslims, who are not permitted to consume alcohol, is that alcohol is *rarely* served or consumed at BDSM social events. The *bad news* is, there's a lot of other stuff that happens at BDSM social events that *is* considered *haram* under Islamic law. For example, gender mixing is *a big* no-no, and you won't see many single-sex BDSM events being held in your neighborhood, or *anywhere*, for that matter. Another *haram* practice you'll see quite often at BDSM events is the wear of fetish clothing, which can be quite revealing at times. Not only does sharia forbid exposing any part of the female body to a man who is not her husband, but it *also* forbids exposing a woman's "private parts" *(awrah,* defined as the area between a woman's navel and her knees) to *other women*, as well. So, *exhibitionism* is definitely *off the table*. But as long as you keep *your* clothes on, you should be good to go, *right?* Wrong. According to Dr. Saalih as-Saalih, an authority on such matters, the prophet Mohammed also made it unlawful for a woman to look at the *awrah* of another woman. The bottom line: If you're a Muslim, and you're into BDSM activities, you may just want to conduct your BDSM activities in the *privacy of your own home.*

Sharia may have a lot to say about BDSM *activities*, but there's actually little or nothing in sharia that forbids you from having a fulfilling D/s *relationship*. Whether that relationship is Master/slave, or Dominant/submissive, sharia seems quite accepting of the D/s *relationship dynamic*, as long as it is *heterosexual, consensual,* doesn't harm the participants, and does not *simulate* something that is forbidden.

D/s and Buddhism: Sensual Misconduct

The foundations of Buddhism rest upon what they call the *Three Jewels*: *Buddha*, the *Dharma* (the teachings), and the *Sangha* (the community). The ethical teachings of Buddhism include what are called the *Five Precepts,* which are not *commandments*, per se, but a voluntary training regimen. They consist of the following:

1. Refraining from taking life and practicing non-violence.
2. Refraining from committing theft.
3. Refraining from sensual misconduct.
4. Refraining from lying.
5. Refraining from drugs and alcohol.

Those who wish to further embrace Buddhism learn the Eight Precepts, which adds three more precepts to the original five, and transforms the third into a precept of *celibacy*. The three additional precepts are:

6. Refraining from eating, except from sunrise to noon.
7. Refraining from dancing, playing music, wearing jewelry or cosmetics, or attending performances.
8. Refraining from using high or luxurious seats and beds.

Buddhists also learn about the concepts of *Samsara* and *Karma*. Samsara is the cycle of birth and death, which is affected by our attitudes about pleasure, pain, and suffering. Karma refers to the actions performed by a person, which may bring about a consequence or result, either in this life, or in subsequent lives. While both *positive* and *negative* types of karma exist, they are an impersonal kind of energy which has nothing to do with personal salvation or forgiveness.

Two of the more well-known forms of Buddhism to westerners are Zen Buddhism, and Tantric Buddhism (which has become popularized in America through books and seminars on so-called *"tantric" sex*). Zen Buddhism is focused primarily on the search for direct spiritual breakthroughs to universal truths through meditation, unsolvable riddles called *koans*, and the art of *shikantaza ("just sitting")*.

Tantric Buddhism involves harnessing one's psycho-physical energy through rituals, visualizations, physical exercises, and various forms of meditation. Some practitioners of tantric Buddhism perform *sexual yoga* as part of their training regimen. With the exception of this practice of *sexual yoga*, there is actually very little in Buddhist literature or teachings about sexuality in general.

The Buddhist admonition against "sensual misconduct" can be interpreted in a variety of ways, including the strictest possible interpretation, which would be that *any sensual conduct at all* may be considered misconduct. If that were truly the case, then there would seem to be little point in discussing which *specific* BDSM activities are in harmony with Buddhism. If we assume, however, that sensuality in general is not necessarily a bad thing, then we can attempt to interpret at least a few of the Eight Precepts from within a BDSM context. A case could certainly be made that Precept One, which teaches non-violence, effectively rules out most activities related to sadomasochism, bondage, and impact play. Precept Four, which encourages *truth-telling*, could easily be interpreted as a prohibition on *role playing*. Precept Seven might make it difficult to observe a scene at any BDSM event or gathering, since that would be considered "attending a performance." Precept Eight would likely discourage the use of highly customized BDSM equipment and furniture. It would seem to the casual observer that the basic tenets of Buddhism do *not* mesh well with some of the most commonly practiced *BDSM activities.* But what might Buddhism have to say about the D/s relationship dynamic?

Remember, Domination/submission – *at least as we've defined it in these pages* – refers to the *relationship dynamic* between two or more individuals. It is what is in their *heads and hearts*; it governs how they relate to one another. It is *not* necessarily about *whips and chains.* Given *that* definition of D/s, we can be relatively certain that there would be little in the Eight Precepts of Buddhism that would be inconsistent with being involved in a loving, non-violent D/s relationship.

D/s and Hinduism: You Can't Do It Wrong

Hinduism is the world's third largest religion, after Christianity and Islam, and is sometimes referred to as the world's oldest living religion. It is the predominant religion of India which, in the 13th century, was also known as *Hindustan.* The authoritative texts of the Hindu religion are written in Sanskrit, and are usually divided into two categories of what we might consider scripture: revealed truths *(called sruti)* and remembered truths *(referred to as smitri).* Hinduism shares many precepts with Buddhism, including the notions of *karma* and *dharma,* and a belief in reincarnation. Aside from certain similarities to Buddhism, there are also great differences between the two religious traditions. Hinduism can be exceedingly difficult to pigeonhole as a religion, since the faith has no codified declaration of beliefs that are universally held by all adherents of Hinduism.

As a result of this lack of a codified and unifying belief system, Hinduism allows its followers the absolute freedom to believe and worship as they please. Therefore, *almost by definition,* a member of the Hindu faith *cannot commit heresy or blasphemy.* Even *apostasy* is practically impossible, since there are at least two schools of Hinduism (*Samkhya* and *Mimamsa*) that embrace *atheism!*

Classical Hindu teachings often refer to the four objectives of life as being *dharma* (ethics), *artha* (prosperity), *Kāma* (sensuality), and *Moksha* (freedom). This designation of *sensuality* as one of the *fundamental objectives of life* is a major departure from what we saw in the Buddhist tradition. While some Hindu monks are expected to renounce most forms of sensual pleasure in order to practice celibacy, the great majority of Hindus are free to revel in their sexuality. Ancient Hindu texts dating to 1500 BC discuss issues such as the sexual duties of husbands and wives, the sexual education of young people, polygamy, polyandry, and polygyny. In the second century, the Hindu religion gave the world its first textbook on sexuality and virtuous living, the *Kama Sutra.*

The Kama Sutra, contrary to popular belief in western culture, was far more than just an ancient Hindu *sex manual.* It was, in fact, a compendium of texts that encouraged adherents to live righteously and to enjoy life. Another western misconception about the Kama Sutra is that it teaches the principles of tantric sex. In reality, tantric sexual yoga is a practice of *Buddhism*, not Hinduism, *at all.* The Kama Sutra does, however, devote a great deal of attention to practices that would *today* be considered *typical BDSM activities*. There are, for example, sections of the Kama Sutra devoted to biting and the marking of one's lover with your teeth. Other sections detail various techniques for teasing, slapping, and over 60 other sexual activities and positions.

On the other hand, the Kama Sutra also cautions against ignoring the potential perils of unrestrained sensuality, saying, "Just as a horse in full gallop, blinded by the energy of his own speed, pays no attention to any post or hole or ditch on the path, so two lovers, blinded by passion, in the friction of sexual battle, are caught up in their fierce energy and pay no attention to danger."

Despite the lack of any formally codified belief system that is universal to *all* Hindus (or perhaps, precisely *because* of it) we can confidently say that there are no prohibitions in the Hindu religion against either BDSM practices, or D/s relationships.

D/s and Paganism: Do What Thou Wilt

Paganism is simultaneously one of the world's oldest *and* newest religions. For thousands of years, the term was used *derogatorily* in reference to *any* religion that wasn't one of the "big three" *Abrahamic* religions; Judaism, Christianity or Islam. In more recent times, the name *Pagan* was used *self-referentially* in America for the very first time in 1964, and gained popularity in the 1970s as part of the counter-culture movement which readily embraced this new age, non-institutionalized expression of personal spirituality and communion with nature.

Today, contemporary Pagans comprise just 0.2% of Americans who express a religious preference, or roughly 1 in every 500 people, yet they seem to represent a disproportionately higher percentage of those in the D/s and BDSM lifestyles. That linkage may well be rooted in the counter-culture character of contemporary Paganism which flaunts social conventions and celebrates, rather than represses, the natural carnality of man.

Modern Paganism is an *umbrella term* that covers a wide range of religious beliefs and practices drawn from many cultures and traditions, spanning several millennia. There is no single organization, doctrine or sacred text that is recognized by *all* Pagans as being authoritative or binding. Paganism includes a host of diverse belief systems, to include Wicca, Witchcraft, Druidism, Shamanism, Animism, Nature Worship, and the Goddess Movement.

Pagans rarely engage in theology, and generally prefer a holistic, nature-based *personal spiritualism* that is often expressed *singularly*, rather than in doctrine or as part of a congregation. What might appear to *outsiders* as a hodge-podge of diverse religious beliefs and practices when viewed in the *aggregate*, superbly serves *each individual Pagan* as a unique and practical expression of his or her own personal spirituality. Even so, there are some common themes that can be found in most expressions of Paganism which typically include reverence for the sanctity of nature, rejection of traditional values and institutional religion, celebration of diversity, and the philosophy of *"doing what thou wilt, but harming no one."*

Perhaps it is this *"do what thou wilt"* ethic that serves as the subtle connection between the Pagan belief system and the D/s and BDSM lifestyles. Their practice of *personal spirituality* and focusing upon the sanctity of *nature* and the way things *are*, as opposed to moralizing on how they *should be*, allows for a freer expression of the D/s dynamic and fetish-related sexuality. It would be reasonable to expect to find a higher incidence of *Primals* among Pagans in the lifestyle as a consequence of their reverence for *nature and instinct.* On the other hand, one should *not* expect many followers of the Pagan *goddess movement* to be lining up to become *Gorean kajirae.* But then again, *who knows?* A Pagan *doeth what he wilt.*

D/s and Christianity: Similitudes of Submission

The Christian religion is based on the life and teachings of Jesus of Nazareth, who lived two thousand years ago in Israel, and who later became known to his followers as the *Christ*, which means *the Messiah*. Christians believe that Jesus was conceived the Son of God and born of a virgin for the primary purpose of atoning for the sins of the world. At the end of his mortal ministry, Jesus was crucified by the Romans and his body placed in a tomb, where Christians believe he was resurrected and appeared again to his followers before ascending to Heaven to reign with God the Father.

Worldwide, there are 2.2 billion Christians, with the three largest sects being comprised of Roman Catholics, Eastern Orthodox, and Protestants. In the United States, those who self-identify as Christians account for 76% of the population. *Self-identification,* for the purposes of this book, shall be the standard by which we categorize a person or sect as *Christian.*

This is an *important distinction* which must be acknowledged before embarking on any discussion which involves the contentious topics of sex and religion. If we *do not* do so, we run the risk of allowing those with an agenda to tailor their definition of Christians and Christianity to fit their own preconceptions and biases. You may not realize it, but that is *exactly* what is occurring when someone says, *"You can't be a Christian if you're into BDSM."* A Christian's response to that, and to similarly wrong-headed statements, should be, *"You* don't get to define who is, or isn't a Christian, *especially* in *my* case. If *I say* I'm a Christian, then *by-golly*, I'm a Christian."

The five largest Christian denominations in the United States are:

- The Catholic Church, with 68.2 million members
- The Southern Baptist Convention, with 16.2 million members
- The United Methodist Church, with 7.7 million members
- The Church of Jesus Christ of Latter-day Saints, with 6.2 million members
- The Church of God in Christ, with 5.5 million members

Among these and the many other Christian denominations and sects in the United States, one can find a wide variety of doctrines and creeds, some of which are distinctive enough to seriously push the boundaries of what it is to be a Christian. The doctrinal commonalities, however, usually far outweigh the differences. While we could probably write an entire *book* on this subject *(and perhaps will, someday),* we're going to focus *now* on three pillars of Christian doctrine, as they may pertain to D/s relationships and the BDSM lifestyle: the Ten Commandments, the Bible, and the words of Jesus Christ, himself.

The Ten Commandments

The Ten Commandments, sometimes referred to as the *Decalog*, actually appear *twice* in both the Hebrew and Christian Bibles, making their debut first in *Exodus*, and then being restated in *Deuteronomy*. On the *off-chance* that it's been a while since you brushed-up on your Ten

Commandments and don't have a Bible readily available, here they are:

1. *I am the* L*ORD your God, who brought you out of the land of Egypt, out of the house of slavery. You shall have no other gods before me.*
2. *You shall not make for yourself a carved image, or any likeness of anything that is in heaven above, or that is in the earth beneath, or that is in the water under the earth. You shall not bow down to them or serve them, for I the Lord your God am a jealous God, visiting the iniquity of the fathers on the children to the third and the fourth generation of those who hate me, but showing steadfast love to thousands of those who love me and keep my commandments.*
3. *You shall not take the name of the Lord your God in vain, for the Lord will not hold him guiltless who takes his name in vain.*
4. *Remember the Sabbath day, to keep it holy. Six days you shall labor, and do all your work, but the seventh day is a Sabbath to the Lord your God. On it you shall not do any work, you, or your son, or your daughter, your male servant, or your female servant, or your livestock, or the sojourner who is within your gates. For in six days the Lord made heaven and earth, the sea, and all that is in them, and rested on the seventh day. Therefore the Lord blessed the Sabbath day and made it holy.*
5. *Honor your father and your mother, that your days may be long in the land that the Lord your God is giving you.*
6. *You shall not murder.*
7. *You shall not commit adultery.*
8. *You shall not steal.*
9. *You shall not bear false witness against your neighbor.*
10. *You shall not covert your neighbor's house, or his wife, or his male servant, or his female servant, or his ox, or his donkey, or anything that is your neighbors.*

At first blush, it's hard to see *anything* in the Ten Commandments that could be interpreted as forbidding a D/s relationship or BDSM lifestyle. Even if there were, the Commandments are unclear on such things as the penalties for breaking them. Some might be tempted to conclude from the first commandment that God isn't too keen on the institution of *slavery*, but then again, Egypt's enslavement of the Jews in the time of Moses was *hardly safe, sane, or consensual.*

The admonition to "have no other gods before me" *could* conceivably be problematic for any submissive in a D/s relationship with a *Lesser God* or *Pharoanic Lord* as her Dominant. Luckily, she does have a convenient *loophole*. All she has to do is appraise her *Dom* as being slightly lower in stature than the God of Abraham and Isaac. Of course, getting her Dominant to *agree* with that appraisal is another matter, *entirely*.

The second and third commandments, which forbid the worship of graven images and taking the Lord's name in vain, are more or less irrelevant to the D/s and BDSM lifestyles. The fourth commandment, however, could become an issue if you're in the habit of engaging in BDSM activities on the Sabbath day. Interestingly, not all Christians observe the Sabbath on *Sunday*, so perhaps you have a little wiggle-room to work with, here. That is, assuming that *wiggling* is allowed on the Sabbath.

Honoring Mom and Dad shouldn't have to be antithetical to living a BDSM lifestyle. If your parents don't agree with your lifestyle choices, perhaps the best way you can honor them is by not rubbing their faces in it. That way, you're *also* helping *them* avoid breaking the sixth commandment by *killing you*.

The seventh commandment, which forbids adultery, is often cited by opponents of the BDSM lifestyle as being relevant to the discussion. The *problem* with that argument, however, is that it is based entirely on the commonly held misconception that BDSM equates to promiscuous sex that occurs outside of committed relationships. Not only is it entirely *possible* to engage in BDSM *without sex*, it's *relatively common.* In fact, *many* BDSM events and facilities do not allow sex on the premises *at all.*

I do realize this is a difficult thing for some people to wrap their heads around, and I hope you are able to grasp what it is that I'm trying to say here. BDSM and sex really do *go great together.* All *I'm* saying is, *they don't have to.* Think: sex and television. You can have sex without television, and you can certainly watch television without sex. Sometimes, you can even do *both (gasp!) at the same time.* So, is watching television during sex inherently a good thing or a bad thing? It probably depends on who you're doing it with, what you're watching, and *why.* Watching a little *porn* to spice things up during sex *could* turn out to be *great* for your relationship. Watching *SpongeBob Squarepants reruns,* perhaps less so. Regardless, if turns out to be a *bad* thing, it is hardly the *television's* fault. The bottom line, as far as the seventh commandment is concerned, is simply this: If you're predisposed to commit *adultery*, the presence *(or absence)* of BDSM in your life probably *isn't* going to change that.

The last three commandments are easy. Don't lie, cheat or covet. Frankly, if you are having problems with any of *those*, you have bigger problems than the challenges of living a BDSM lifestyle, and should probably be reading a completely *different* kind of book – perhaps something like, *"How Not to Be a Complete Jerk."*

Were you at all surprised to learn just how *lifestyle-friendly* the Ten Commandments could be? Believe it not, we've somehow managed to wade through the entire Ten Commandments without encountering a *single* potential deal-breaker for someone who might be considering the BDSM lifestyle! I don't know about *you*, but I really do think that's kind of *cool.*

What the Bible Says About D/s

As we stated earlier, many of the harmful misconceptions about the lifestyle commonly held by those outside the BDSM culture can be traced to equating BDSM with sex. Unfortunately, the scriptures are usually about as *clear as mud* on the subject of *sex,* and much *less* so on any activities which might be associated with BDSM. This is primarily a consequence of the many ways the world and the meanings of key words and phrases have evolved in the course of two thousand years. Take, for example, how the following biblical terms and doctrines have changed over time:

- Early Christians interpreted *fornication* to mean *adultery, incest, and bestiality.* Today, it is generally understood to mean *any* sex outside of marriage, to include premarital sex.
- The New Testament (Matt 5:32) taught that anyone who married a divorced woman was committing *adultery.* Today, adultery is interpreted to mean *sex outside of marriage.*
- Sex *before* marriage was widely tolerated, if not accepted, throughout much of Christianity until the Anglican Church made it taboo in 1753.
- Most of the biblical passages that are today interpreted as references to *masturbation* are actually references to *coitus interuptus,* or the practice of pulling out of a woman's vagina before ejaculation.

Given these and other examples of linguistic and doctrinal evolution, it's easy to see how the various Christian sects and denominations would be forced to develop their *own* ideas on what is and isn't acceptable, as far as *sexuality* is concerned. A casual student of the Bible who might be looking for specific guidance on how to apply biblical principles to twenty-first century sexuality would have a daunting task ahead, indeed. The good news is, the focus of our examination isn't so much *sexuality* as it is about viewing *Domination/submission* through the prism of *Christianity,* and that - *surprisingly* - isn't as difficult as you might think.

The Bible is literally *chock-full* of advice on things like how to submit to God or to your husband, how to treat your slave or wife, and how to respect and obey those who have rule over you. In fact, viewing the scriptures as a collection of *similitudes and parables* which can serve as templates for healthy D/s relationships can prove to be very useful indeed! For example, consider the advice that the apostle Paul gave in his letter of instruction to the members of the church in Ephesus, when he wrote:

> *Giving thanks always for all things unto God and the Father in the name of our Lord Jesus Christ; Submitting yourselves one to another in the fear of God. Wives, submit yourselves unto your own husbands, as unto the Lord. For the husband is the head of the wife, even as Christ is the head of the church: and he is the saviour of the body. Therefore as the church is subject unto Christ, so let the wives be to their own husbands in every thing. Husbands, love your wives, even as Christ also loved the church, and gave himself for it.*
> *(Ephesians 5: 20-25)*

It is fascinating to me that Paul admonishes the saints in Ephesus to "submit yourselves one to another," and goes on to encourage wives to submit to their husbands as they would to the Lord. He even plainly states that the church should be viewed as a similitude for the relationship dynamic between a husband and wife. He ends this passage by reminding us that the gift of submission should always be reciprocated with love and sacrifice.

We should reiterate something here, which may or may not be obvious to the casual reader, and that is simply that in this era, husbands were expected to be Dominants, and wives were expected to be submissives. It was not then, nor is it now, a *value judgment of any sort.* It was simply a *fact of life.*

In his letter to the Hebrews, Paul expounds upon the subject of obedience:

> *Obey them that have the rule over you, and submit yourselves: for they watch for your souls, as they that must give account, that they may do it with joy, and not with grief: for that is unprofitable for you.*
> *(Hebrews 13:17)*

Not only does Paul again encourage us to *submit,* but he goes into some detail on *why* we should do so in a fashion that facilitates "those who have rule" over us. First, they are held accountable for what we do and second, if we make it a miserable experience for *them*, it always ends up hurting *us* in the long run. In his epistle to the Colossians, Paul expounds on the subject even further:

> *Wives, submit yourselves unto your own husbands, as it is fit in the Lord. Husbands, love your wives, and be not bitter against them. Children, obey your parents in all things: for this is well pleasing unto the Lord. Fathers, provoke not your children to anger, lest they be discouraged. Servants, obey in all things your masters according to the flesh; not with eyeservice, as menpleasers; but in singleness of heart, fearing God: And whatsoever ye do, do it heartily, as to the Lord, and not unto men.* (Colossians 3:18-23)

Finally, Paul admonishes the Masters, or heads of households with servants, of Colossae to deal fairly with those who are under their charge, and leaves them with a friendly reminder:

> *Masters, give unto your servants that which is just and equal; knowing that ye also have a Master in heaven. (Colossians 4:1)*

Obviously, there is *no* shortage of passages from the Old and New Testaments to support a religious foundation for a D/s lifestyle. The Bible *clearly* teaches that *submission to one another* teaches us how to be submissive to God, and therefore should be considered *a good thing.* It also teaches that husbands and masters are expected to be just and fair, to honor those over whom they have charge, and that they will be held accountable for their welfare. That advice is just as valuable today as it was two-thousand years ago.

D/s Advice From the Master

The third authoritative resource that we should consider in our examination of Christian doctrines as they pertain to a D/s lifestyle should be the teachings and life of the *Master* himself, *Jesus of Nazareth*. Jesus was considered something of a *radical* in his time for teaching doctrines that were considered heretical by the established religious authorities. A prime example would be the way Jesus took existing religious doctrines, precepts as simple as *"Love thy neighbor as thyself"* (Leviticus 19:18), and turned them on their heads to confound the religious establishment. Jesus taught, instead:

> *Ye have heard that it hath been said, Thou shalt love thy neighbour, and hate thine enemy. But I say unto you, Love your enemies, bless them that curse you, do good to them that hate you, and pray for them which despitefully use you, and persecute you. (Matthew 5: 43-44)*

Jesus understood the power of *love* in teaching, guiding, and overcoming obstacles to submission, such as pride or arrogance. British author Mary Cowden Clarke once wrote, "Fear may induce the show of submission; but love only can truly subjugate a haughty spirit." Among those whom Jesus taught were the twelve disciples, some of whom were initially skeptical and headstrong. Our modern usage of the term *"doubting Thomas"* is a biblical reference to the Apostle Thomas, to whom the divinity of Jesus had to be *proven* before he would believe it. Even so, Jesus won them over with *love* and so, too, will any D/s relationship depend upon liberal helpings of it.

Another of Jesus' unconventional doctrines concerned his confrontational approach to the religious hypocrisy of the established order, and resisting the temptation to share liberally with them the details of a philosophy and lifestyle that they would never be able to understand. Though his *intent* was clearly focused upon the sharing of the *gospel* with those who are incapable of appreciating it, his advice is probably just as applicable *today* to those in the D/s culture who may be tempted to share just a little too much of their lifestyle with their vanilla friends:

> *Give not that which is holy unto the dogs, neither cast ye your pearls before swine, lest they trample them under their feet, and turn again and rend you. (Matthew 7:6)*

Just as the Christian faith *isn't for everyone*, neither is the D/s lifestyle. There will always be those who are simply *not suited for it*, regardless of their religious affiliations or beliefs, or even their professed devotion to the principles and tenets of a D/s philosophy. Not everyone who embarks upon a voyage of self-discovery into the worlds of domination/submission or BDSM will find fulfillment or meaning there. Not everyone you encounter in the lifestyle will be as equally committed to the same underlying philosophy or ethical constraints that you may be. In this lifestyle, as in *any* lifestyle, there will always be pretenders and predators in seek of prey. Even so, the *Master* explains how you can easily spot them:

> *Enter ye in at the strait gate: for wide is the gate, and broad is the way, that leadeth to destruction, and many there be which go in there at: Because strait is the gate, and narrow is the way, which leadeth unto life, and few there be that find it. Beware of false prophets, which come to you in sheep's clothing, but inwardly they are ravening wolves. Ye shall know them by their fruits. Do men gather grapes of thorns, or figs of thistles? Even so, every good tree bringeth forth good fruit; but a corrupt tree bringeth forth evil fruit. (Matthew 7:13-17)*

I shall leave it to your imagination and, of course, to your particular life-circumstances to determine what those "fruits" - *be they good or evil* - might *be.* It should suffice to say that there are usually some very good reasons why certain individuals are *shunned or ignored* by others in the lifestyle. When evaluating someone as a potential D/s relationship partner, you would be well served to take note of the fruits of their labors and the outcomes of their previous relationships.

Skepticism and reason should certainly be your companions on any voyage of discovery towards a life of Domination/submission, but one should never underestimate the critical role of *faith* in this journey. By faith, I am not referring to *religious faith,* despite the fact that it happens to be the subject of this chapter. No, in this instance, I mean *faith in the process, faith in your partner, and faith in yourself.* Jesus proved the critical importance of faith to his disciples when he demonstrated to them that *he wasn't the only one who could perform miracles:*

> *But the ship was now in the midst of the sea, tossed with waves: for the wind was contrary. And in the fourth watch of the night Jesus went unto them, walking on the sea. And when the disciples saw him walking on the sea, they were troubled, saying, It is a spirit; and they cried out for fear. But straightway Jesus spake unto them, saying, Be of good cheer; it is I; be not afraid. And Peter answered him and said, Lord, if it be thou, bid me come unto thee on the water. And he said, Come. And when Peter was come down out of the ship, he walked on the water, to go to Jesus. But when he saw the wind boisterous, he was afraid; and beginning to sink, he cried, saying, Lord, save me. And immediately Jesus stretched forth his hand, and caught him, and said unto him, O thou of little faith, wherefore didst thou doubt?*
> *(Matthew 14:24-31)*

Many Christians are inexplicably *unaware* that Jesus' disciples were able to perform miracles in much the same fashion as their Master. This retelling of how Peter walked on water is just one of *many* examples chronicled in the scriptures.

Because of his faith, not *just* in Jesus, *but also his faith in himself,* Peter was able to walk upon the surface of the sea just like Jesus. When he became distracted and frightened by the wind and the waves, his faith waned, *and he sank like a stone.* What miracles might *you* be able to accomplish through *your* faith as you explore a relationship in this lifestyle?

Filling a Void

I wrote this chapter hoping to fill a *void* for those of you who may have been concerned about potential conflicts between your deeply held religious beliefs and your interest in a D/s or BDSM lifestyle. I chose the six most prevalent religions in America, and gave you an admittedly *cursory* glimpse at their theologies in general before attempting to *extrapolate* from that their perspectives on D/s and BDSM in particular.

I fully understand that writing on such matters is an undertaking that is virtually guaranteed to satisfy *no one* and, in fact, may even upset or *enrage* some readers. If you happen to be one who has been offended or outraged by my characterization of your religious beliefs or by my conclusions, I would like to sincerely *apologize.* I am, after all, *not a theologian,* and no one can ever *truly* know your religious beliefs and convictions like *you* do. I can only hope that what I have written on this particular topic has helped someone who may have been praying for answers to some difficult questions. At the very least, I hope it will encourage others to ponder this lifestyle from a novel perspective.

I leave it to *you* to judge whether I have succeeded in either endeavor.

"There is no happiness where there is no wisdom; No wisdom but in submission to the gods. Big words are always punished, and proud men in old age learn to be wise."

- - Sophocles (497 BC - 406 BC)

My Two Cents on D/s and Religion

I have never felt that there was, nor should there be, any conflict between a person's D/s lifestyle and his or her deeply held religious beliefs and, for me, there never *has* been. I've always just assumed that this was probably because I've always been really *bad* at anything having to do with *guilt*, and have always been pretty *good* at compartmentalizing things in my own head, even if they happen to be competing or contradictory notions.

I subscribe to the idea that simultaneously entertaining completely contradictory beliefs is a great way to give your brain a good *workout*. Blaise Pascal once said, "Contradiction is not a sign of falsity, nor the lack of contradiction a sign of truth," and I agree.

On the *other* hand, I have recently had an epiphany which leads me to think that there may be *another* reason why I've never been cognizant of any real divide that separates D/s and religion. The more I think about it, the more credible and profound the notion becomes, at least in my own head. Or, it could just be the *tequila*.

Wherever it came from, *this* was my epiphany: Maybe, just *maybe*... D/s ***is*** my religion.

If that boggles *your* mind, just try being in *my* head sometime. *Boggled* is pretty much my normal state. Just once, I'd like to know what it's like to be *unboggled*. *That* would be *cool*.

If God exists, he's *got* to be a Dom.

If he *wasn't*, he probably wouldn't even have been considered for the position. The help-wanted ad probably read something like: "Seeking self-motivated self-starter with unparalleled project management skills and who can work well without supervision. Must be willing to provide guidance and supervision to billions of subordinates. Limited opportunities for advancement, but plenty of perks and recognition. *Subbies need not apply."*

That last part *stings*, I know, and probably violates all kinds of cosmic equal opportunity laws. I'm guessing the universe has a really *crappy* H.R. Director, but *hey*, that's *not my circus; not my monkey.*

I think religion in general has unfairly gotten a pretty bad rap. Many people, when they see the word *religion*, think *church.* And let's face it: There are a lot of crazy-ass churches out there. But the existence of stupid churches doesn't make *religion* wrong any more than the existence of stupid algebra students makes *mathematics* wrong.

Let's stop blaming God for *our own* stupidity.

When we think of religion, we should think of the unique *relationship* between us and God, and also between us and our fellow human beings. If God is a Dom, that makes him a teacher, guide, and example. Perhaps we are simply meant to *emulate* him, explore that relationship that exists between us and him, and then try to *apply* those principles in our relationships with our fellow human beings.

Monkey *see*, monkey *do.* And, yes, I realize that's three *monkey* mentions in the last five minutes. I blame the *tequila*.

Perhaps D/s really is my religion. It has but one commandment, which is a slightly modified version of the Golden Rule:

Dom unto others as you would have God Dom unto you.

"This is a pleasant surprise, Archie. I would not have believed it. That of course is the advantage of being a pessimist; a pessimist gets nothing but pleasant surprises, an optimist nothing but unpleasant."

- - *Rex Stout*

CHAPTER 14: WHAT COULD *POSSIBLY* GO WRONG?

I am utterly convinced that there are just three kinds of people in the world: optimists, pessimists, and realists. The optimist sees the glass as *half full.* The pessimist sees the glass as *half empty*. A realist sees the glass as *twice as large as it needs to be*. Which are *you?*

If you're seriously considering entering into a D/s relationship or adopting a BDSM lifestyle, it would be wise to *realistically* contemplate *all* of the potential issues, and *not* just consider the *rainbows and unicorns* perspective. It can be incredibly *easy* to leap headlong into a new relationship or scenario without having a full appreciation of the potential pitfalls which might lie ahead. I *know.* I've *done* it. I've done it more times than I care to admit. In those instances, would I have been receptive to an offer of some friendly advice on the potential for problems ahead? *Probably not.* So then, what makes me think you'll take anything I say in this chapter any more seriously than *I* would have, when I was in your shoes?

Only this: *I'm hoping that you're a lot smarter than I was.*

There are a *lot* of things that can go wrong in *any* relationship. You don't need *me* to tell you that. You most likely have a collection of relationship horror stories of your *own* that would *curl my toes,* and most of them probably have nothing to do with D/s-related issues. Relationships, *in general*, can be complicated, messy things. Adding *any* new variable to the mix tends to make it even *more* so. When those variables just happen to exist on the fringes of acceptable societal norms, as do D/s, BDSM and polyamory, it gets *infinitely* more complicated.

Honestly, not everyone *wants* to ponder all the things that could possibly go wrong in a complex relationship. Humorist Dave Barry noted that one of the major differences between men and women is their affinity for understanding complicated relationships, saying, "Your basic guy is into a straight-ahead, bottom-line kind of thought process that does not work nearly as well with the infinitely subtle complexities of human relationships as it does with calculating how much gravel is needed to cover a given driveway." Even so, *neither* sex likes to contemplate a relationship that is complicated to the extreme of being *unworkable*. Some might say that to do so makes one a *pessimist* in outlook. I would beg to differ.

Considering the pitfalls is not quite the same thing as *expecting* them. One *educates* himself and *prepares* for a possibility *not* because he *expects* it to happen or *hopes for it*, but to be better able to *recognize* it as it approaches, and perhaps even prevent it from having a disastrous impact. A person living in Florida learns something about hurricanes, *not* because he is a *pessimist*, but because it is a *perfectly rational thing to do* for anyone choosing to live on a penis-shaped peninsula which is bounded by sadistic seas and regularly flogged by killer storms.

Make no mistake, the topics we're about to discuss in the following pages are *possibilities*, not necessarily *probabilities*. My goal is *not* to sway you from your natural world-view and disposition, whether you are habitually an optimist *or* pessimist. My goal is to assist you in *reducing the chances* of a negative outcome by educating yourself, recognizing the tell-tale signs of an impending train wreck, and knowing how to respond to some of the challenges you *could* encounter. *Hoping and expecting* things to always work out for the best is fine, but when it comes to relationships, we should always be cognizant of our ability to *influence the outcome*. *Hope* is not a viable *strategy*.

A final note, before we dive headlong into this tumultuous sea of negativity. You're going to find plenty of generalizations and anecdotal examples based on my observations and experiences from 35 years in the lifestyle and in a variety of D/s relationships. Before anyone becomes incensed and offended, let me just say that I *know* that not all Dominants and submissives are *typical*. I understand that *my* perspective on what is typical may differ from *your* idea of what is typical. I'm aware that many of *my* experiences may have been an anomaly. I *get* it. I really *do*.

Every day, *someone* asks me, *"What makes you an expert on BDSM relationships?"* I usually respond thusly: "Frankly, I *don't* consider myself an expert on this subject, any more than someone who has been married for thirty-five years is an expert on *marriage*. I do, however, think I may have some insights for those who may be seeking answers to some tough questions about the kinds of relationships that I've spent my entire adult life in." That's my *diplomatic* response. A somewhat harsher alternative might be:

Possible insights ahead. *Use 'em*, or *lose 'em*. It matters not to me. I get paid *either way*.

Unclear on the Concept

The first possible pitfall we're going to talk about is probably the most *prevalent*, both in and outside the D/s lifestyle. It is not, *by any means*, a problem that is unique to the chronically clueless. It often occurs when and where you *least expect it,* and with people that you'd never, ever in a million years, suspect as sufferers. It is what we will call *"being unclear on the concept."*

Take, for example, the commonly confused terms, D/s and BDSM. D/s, or Domination/submission, is *not* synonymous with BDSM, despite what many would have you believe. D/s is an expression of *how people relate* to one another as Dominants and submissives. It is about *who they are, and how they love.* It has very little to do with whether or not they *act* upon those feelings. It is, in many ways, analogous to *gender identity* or *sexual attraction.* We are not defined as much by our reproductive organs, as we are by *how we feel about them.* We aren't classified as gay, straight or bisexual by whom we've had sex with, but by *how we feel about it.*

D/s is what happens *between our ears,* at least inasmuch as it is an expression of our innate dominant or submissive character traits *as they pertain to the relationship dynamic.* But there's also an awful lot that can happen between our ears that *isn't* necessarily D/s-related, even if it *is* thoroughly infused with bondage, discipline, sadism and masochism, the components of BDSM. The attraction, pleasure and satisfaction that a person derives from his or her BDSM activities *certainly* occurs as much in our brains as it does in our bodies, but that doesn't *necessarily* have much to do with a *relationship dynamic.* In other words, if you're heavily into BDSM *impact-play,* then *any* competently delivered spanking from a trusted play partner is probably going to be considered a *good one, whether or not your play partner loves you.* That's because it isn't about the *relationship,* it's all about the *activity* and the sensations.

There are, of course, those who are lucky enough to have *both* - a BDSM play partner *and* a loving D/s *relationship* - all neatly wrapped up in a single person. Wouldn't it be great if *everyone* could have that? Shouldn't this *"perfect balance"* of D/s and BDSM be the goal of just about everyone in the lifestyle? The answer, in a word, is *no.* There are plenty of people who want the *relationship* without the whips and chains. There are still others who are all about the whips and chains, but have no real interest in the trappings of a D/s relationship dynamic. And yes, there are those who not only want *both,* but they honestly *cannot conceive of one without the other.*

It should come as no great surprise to *anyone* that it is exceedingly difficult for a member of *one* of these groups to understand and empathize with someone from one of the others. It's almost as if someone who cares only about *love*, to the exclusion of sex, were trying to understand what motivates a friend who cares only about *sex*, and not a bit about *love.* As difficult as that would be, imagine further what might be the result if suddenly, those two individuals *found themselves in a relationship with each other?* You might be tempted to laugh off the possibility, since it's hard to imagine how someone who *doesn't want love* would seek out a *relationship*, right? Frankly, it happens *all the time* in this lifestyle.

Every day, thousands of submissives and slaves who are *not* emotionally involved in any significant way with them are *collared* by their Dominants. Often, Dominants will offer and submissives accept these collars without any thought whatsoever to what their new partner hopes or expects to gain from the arrangement, or whether they share any commonalities *at all.* One may be seeking D/s, while the other simply wants BDSM. One may want *love*, the other, *sex. Both* may be accustomed to calling the shots in a relationship, even if one of them *thinks* he or she is a submissive. In short, they are *unclear on the concepts of D/s and BDSM.*

There are sometimes those even in the BDSM lifestyle who confuse being a *"top"* with being a Dominant, or being a *"bottom"* with being a submissive. These terms are *not* interchangeable. Acting in the *role* of a top doesn't make you a *Dominant* any more than standing in the kitchen makes you a *cook.* Similarly, the fact that you enjoy being on the receiving end of a lot of BDSM play doesn't necessarily make you a submissive, either. *Topping and bottoming are activities,* not core character traits. Anyone who thinks, *"I like to be spanked, therefore I must be a submissive,"* is unclear on the concept.

Incredibly, there never seems to be a shortage of people who are unclear on the concepts of sadism and masochism. I have seen countless examples of dysfunctional D/s relationships that failed for the simple reason that, apparently, *someone didn't understand what it means to be a sadist.* For the record, a *sadist* is a person who *enjoys inflicting pain and suffering upon you.* For the most part, the more you protest, *the more he's going to like it*. Complaining about how mean or insensitive your sadistic Dominant is being towards you is a little like complaining that *sugar is sweet*, or that *fire is hot*. If pain and suffering *isn't* what you want, if you're *not* a masochist *yourself,* here's a novel idea: *Don't get involved with a sadist.* You'd be *amazed* at the number of people I have known who claimed that they *"didn't like pain"*, yet were collared to *hard-core sadists.* There's really only one way imaginable that such a thing could possibly be a good idea, and that would be *in the mind of someone who was unclear on the concept.*

Masochists are similarly misunderstood, more often than you might think and occasionally, in unexpected ways. Perhaps it would be a good idea to restate now, for the sake of clarity, exactly what it means to be a masochist. A masochist is someone who *enjoys being beaten, sexually humiliated, bound, tortured, or otherwise made to suffer.* Most masochists do not enjoy pain outside of a BDSM context, but there are some who *do.* If there *were* such a thing as the *Prime Directive of Masochism*, it would have to be, "If you don't like being beaten, humiliated, bound, tortured or made to suffer, then please *don't claim to be a masochist."* To *most* of us, this would seem like *common sense*. Apparently, common sense *isn't* quite as common as it used to be. For whatever reason, it has become *popular* among many teens and young adults to *claim* to be masochists, when they are obviously *unclear on the concept.*

True masochists are quite often misunderstood by their own partners, who may not be able to wrap their heads around what a masochist *wants and needs* out of a relationship. If you're someone who is intimately involved with a true masochist, and yet can't bring yourself to *actually hurt that person*, you're like the guy wearing a red uniform on a Star Trek away-mission: *expendable.*

Other frustrating and sad examples of being *unclear on the concept* include those who seek out D/s relationships because it's the *trendy or popular* thing to do, Dominants who seek submissives because they can't get laid *any other way*, submissives who want a Dominant who will *"fix"* them in some way, and of course, the determinedly self-destructive or even *suicidal* person who just needs a helping hand from an all-too-cooperative but clueless sadistic Dominant. Sooner or later, you're bound to meet some of these people. Will you recognize them, when you do?

Trust Issues

Trust is hard; *not* just for you, *not* just for me, it's hard for *everyone*. Even those who claim to trust often and easily will usually *tell you so* in a manner that suggests that they consider this to be something of a curse. For some, trusting is something that is difficult to do, for others it's easy to *do*, but difficult to live with the consequences. Either way, *trust can be hard,* and that is why *trust issues* account for a significant slice of the underlying issues that can plague D/s relationships.

When we think of *trust* as it pertains to relationships, we typically contemplate notions of *fidelity*, and questions about whether or not one partner may be *cheating* on the other in some way. This is truly unfortunate, since *trust* can mean *so much more*, particularly in the context of a D/s relationship dynamic. In the early stages of a D/s relationship, a Dominant may ask his submissive-to-be the *seemingly* simple question, *"Do you trust me?"* The novice sub may respond, *"Yes, I do trust you,"* by which, she almost certainly means something like, *"I trust you not to betray me or break my heart."*

Unfortunately, that's *probably not* what was going through the

Dominant's head when he asked the question which is, in fact, *deceptively complex* and difficult to answer. What the Dominant may *really* be asking is, *do you trust me to be competent as your Master? Do you trust me to do the right thing, and to know what I am talking about? Do you trust me to put your needs before my own, and to always act in your best interests? Do you trust me to have a plan for us, to execute that plan, and to accomplish what I say I will?* The submissive simply responds, *"Yes, I do trust you,"* and thus, the *first* major misstep of a budding D/s relationship goes *completely unnoticed by either.*

In later stages of the relationship, the submissive may engage in activities which *she* considers to be well-intentioned acts of *relationship maintenance* - asking questions, getting feedback, trying to better understand her Dom's motives and plans - without realizing that her Dominant *may* interpret this as a *loss of trust* and a *violation of her earlier promise*. A relationship *death-spiral* begins to swirl around the couple as the submissive becomes more agitated and confused, and the Dominant becomes increasingly angry. Not only does she *not understand what she's done wrong* in the eyes of her Dominant, *he* can't understand why *she can't seem to see it.*

To be sure, not every Dominant is going to be *worthy* of a submissive's trust. Obviously, in those cases, a submissive should not accept his collar in the first place, or if his unworthiness is only made apparent at a later stage of the relationship, she should ask to be released. It isn't *trustworthiness* itself that we're talking about here, however. The issue *here* is, *are these two people even speaking the same language* when they say they *"trust"* one another?

A Dominant needs to be able to trust his submissive too, and once again, that trust needs to be more than the simple assurance that he won't be betrayed. He trusts that she will be earnest in her efforts to learn what she must about the lifestyle, her role in the relationship, and about *him.* He trusts that she understands the concepts of loyalty, devotion, service, and respect. He trusts her to reveal to him her thoughts, feelings, and activities of her day. He trusts her to represent him in all ways, in everything that she does. He trusts her to take him seriously, and that she will follow his guidance, instruction or advice. When these things do *not* happen, or they *stop* happening at some point in the relationship, the dynamic changes *radically*, and in most cases, it's *not for the better.*

Hidden Agendas

When it comes to hidden agendas, D/s relationships can provide fertile ground for what is, even in *vanilla* relationships, *always* going to be a complex issue. A *hidden agenda* exists when a person is focused upon and is actively working to achieve a goal that differs significantly from his or her *stated goals.* The most common examples are the Dominant who *says* he wants a D/s *relationship*, when all he *really* wants is a *sex slave,* and the submissive who *says* she wants a *Master*, when all she *really* wants is a *collar.*

Another great illustration of a hidden agenda is what happens when a *monogamist* becomes involved with a *polyamorist* and *at least one* of the partners secretly harbors an unstated plan to convert the other to his or her own way of loving.

The unfortunate thing about hidden agendas is the fact that they are rarely discovered until *after* you've made a significant investment into the relationship of time, effort, emotional energy and financial resources towards a destination or goal that *isn't* necessarily the same place your *partner* wants to go to. There's really only one way to avoid hidden agendas or mitigate the damage that can be done by them, and that is to be observant for *inconsistencies.* Any apparent *disconnect* between what a person *says* they hope to accomplish in the relationship, versus their *actual behavior* should probably be considered a yellow flag.

Incompetence

I recently learned that, in the jungles of Central and South America, *sloths - which live their entire lives in trees* - are sometimes so inept, *so incompetent*, that they will frequently grab their *own arms and legs,* thinking they are *tree limbs*, and fall to their deaths. In some ways, I suppose, it is regrettable that natural selection doesn't work *quite* so efficiently in the D/s lifestyle.

Incompetence, unfortunately, is no stranger to D/s relationships or to the fetish culture in general. People in this lifestyle are typically *tolerant in the extreme* of other people's kinks, even when it *looks* like they may be *completely clueless*. After all, *who are we to judge?* What gives us the right to tell them that they're *doing it wrong?* Unless and until we see something that involves *breaking the law, non-consent* or doing *permanent damage* to someone, we *generally* avoid trying to tell other people how to get their jollies. I honestly *do* believe this almost-universal atmosphere of tolerance is a *good thing*, even though I also believe it can sometimes have unintended consequences.

D/s, in its purest form, may be a *mindset or an attitude*, but relationships and BDSM activities often require *skills* of one sort or another. They may be as simple as *communication skills*, or as complex as *kinkabu suspension* skills. And where do we *go* for that kind of training? If we're *lucky*, we are *mentored* and guided by someone who is not only *competent*, but capable and compassionate. A less fortunate group, consisting of those who aren't blessed with competent mentors, will *at least* be diligent enough to do a little *homework* so they can learn whatever possible from books, articles, online forums, and other available resources. The third and final group consists of *everyone else.* These are the people who are simply *making it up as they go.* In a nutshell, their trial-and-error-based strategy is to *"fake it, 'til they make it."*

If we were talking about *any other kind of lifestyle*, this strategy probably wouldn't be much of a problem. For example, if I wanted to adopt a *surfing lifestyle*, I could easily adopt a trial-and-error strategy to learn how to surf, what kinds of surfboards I should buy, where to go to catch the best waves, and *so on*. And while *some* of those lessons might turn out to be embarrassing, expensive, time consuming or even *painful* to me *personally*, there is going to be very little chance that I can *destroy someone else's life* in the process. A Dominant can, *and often does*, assume that risk when he accepts full responsibility for practically *every aspect* of another person's life. Similarly, a submissive holds her Dominant's fate in her hands in ways that the average person cannot even *begin* to comprehend. What happens, for example, if a *"slave"* decides *long after* a turbulent Master/slave relationship has *ended*, that there *never* really was any *consent* involved? What do *you* think your chances would be of convincing a judge and jury that someone actually *wanted* to be treated like a slave?

The bottom line: incompetence can be encountered *anywhere* in this lifestyle and it can have far-reaching, sometimes *unimaginable* consequences. Keep it at *arm's length*, whenever possible.

Abuse

Let's start this section off by stating what *should* be fairly obvious to just about anyone capable of *reading*. Abuse, in *any* form, should never be tolerated by *anyone* in, or out, of this lifestyle. That includes *physical* abuse, *sexual* abuse, *financial* abuse, and even *emotional* abuse. There are *many* misinformed and, frankly, *bigoted* individuals who equate the D/s and BDSM lifestyles with an inherently abusive relationship dynamic. They often claim without any evidence *whatsoever* to support their allegations that these lifestyles promote violence and the objectification of women, as well as a host of other societal ills which apparently *must* be blamed on *someone,* before they can be *"eradicated."* My perspective on this is if you believe that either of these problems will ever be *eradicated*, then I have some *prime Everglades real estate* deals I'd like to discuss with you.

Abuse *does* exist in the D/s and BDSM lifestyles, just as it occurs in *every* lifestyle. The *false impression* that it occurs with greater frequency in *our* lifestyle than elsewhere can likely be attributable to the increasingly popular and insidious notion that people are *stupid* and can't be trusted to make their own life choices; therefore they *must be rescued from themselves.* In this *nanny-state* worldview, a masochist woman who is happily married to a sadistic man *hasn't* made a valid lifestyle choice *at all.* She is a *brainwashed* and perhaps even *mentally ill victim* of a sadistic *misogynist* who married her *not* because he loves her or because they have mutually complementary interests, but because *he hates women*. This twisted sort of logic is applied just as frequently to people involved in plural marriages, age play, humiliation play, pet play, and a host of other activities that offend the sensitivities of the *nanny-state* elitists who think they know what's best for you.

One of the rather unfortunate consequences of the political exploitation of the D/s lifestyle to serve political ends has been that *real abuse* may sometimes be overlooked. When *everything* related to the lifestyle is mischaracterized by *outsiders* as abuse, people *within* the lifestyle tend to circle their wagons and adopt a mutually defensive stance. This can *sometimes* result in a community-wide spirited defense of someone who, frankly, *might not deserve it.*

I believe the answer, for both the community *and* for its individual members, is to examine any allegation of abuse independently and fairly, and to avoid the natural tendency to assume that *any* accusation of abuse is the result of misinformation and bigotry. In the final analysis, we must be able to presume that consenting adults are going to be fully capable of knowing when and whether they are being abused, without any help from you, me *or* the *nanny-state busybodies*. The discerning criterion should be, *are they happy?* If *so*, then *butt out.*

For anyone who cares to look beyond the superficial, it's usually pretty easy to discern the differences between a consenting, trusting and mutually pleasurable activity and abuse. The differences are stark, and obvious. D/s is about *loving*; abuse is about *hurting*. A healthy D/s relationship is built on *trust and real consent;* abuse is almost always a *breach of trust* and a matter of *coercion.* A healthy D/s relationship requires and builds mutual *respect;* abuse is demonstration of a profound *lack of respect.* A healthy D/s relationship *builds* self-esteem; abuse *destroys it.* Healthy D/s and BDSM activities involve the *planned, controlled* application of pain, restraint or humiliation; abuse is typically *spontaneous and out of control.* In any consensual BDSM activity, a Bottom can stop the scene at any time *with just a word;* in an abusive situation, a victim *wishes* such a thing were possible, *but it is not.*

Dom/sub Type Mismatch

In the first few chapters of this book, we described different types of Dominants and submissives, and even went into some detail on which types of partners might be more suited to each. What we *didn't* do was describe in any real detail the kinds of *unholy messes* that can result from a Dom/sub *mismatch*. One might reasonably assume that such things do not happen often, and in truth, *most people* have a pretty good idea of what it is they are seeking in a mate, even if they are brand-spanking-new to the lifestyle. And, then again, there's always that slender minority of people who don't.

Most likely to find themselves in a D/s mismatch are the lifestyle novices, who have not yet accumulated enough experience to differentiate between the various types of Dominants and submissives, or to discern the nuanced ranges of intensity even within those categories. A lifestyle novice is likely to assume, for example, that the only real difference between a *Daddy Dom* and a *Sadistic Dom* is what they *like.* As a result, a novice *may* attempt to tailor her *presentation,* behavior or appearance to appeal to the Dominant in question, without giving much thought *at all* to the fact that these two types of Dominants *think and behave very differently.* The novice may also fall into the dangerous trap of believing that *because she is compromising to please her Dominant*, that he will do *likewise* and behave *less* like the Daddy or

Sadist *that he is.* Chances are, he *won't.* These characteristics are, for the most part, *non-negotiable.*

What follows are some of what I consider to be the most common D/s relationship mismatch types, accompanied by some pithy commentary on how it happens and the typical outcomes:

- The Sadistic Dominant and *anyone* who isn't *truly* a masochist. I *do* realize I am probably beginning to sound like a broken record here, but this point simply *cannot* be stressed enough. Anyone who gets involved with a *sadist* should expect to get *hurt.* After all, that's the *whole idea.* That's *why* people get involved with sadists. It won't be an unfortunate turn of events when he inflicts pain and suffering upon you; *it's the plan.* I *do wish* there was a way to say it even *plainer* for the benefit of those who may still be unclear on this concept.
- The *evolving* Dominant and *hardwired* submissive, or vice versa. These relationships somehow actually manage to get off on the right foot *from the start*, but then meander down a dangerous path when *one* of the partners begins to explore *other* roles. Typically, this evolving partner is *completely unaware* of the gut reaction of his *hardwired* partner, who is unwilling or incapable of switching roles to accommodate him. This really only becomes an issue if one partner in the relationship is *flexible*, while the other *is not.* Role evolution can be a wonderful thing, *as long as both partners have signed up for it.*
- The polyamorous Dominant and monogamous submissive, or vice versa. It *happens* all the time, and *sometimes*, it even *works out,* but the odds are overwhelmingly stacked against it coming to a good end. To be fair, *most* people go into these things with the best of intentions, earnestly believing that they can be *taught* the secrets of polyamory or monogamy when, in fact, it is actually quite *rare* for someone to be able to change his or her outlook in this way. Certainly, there are *techniques and strategies* which can make the adoption or practice of a new way of loving *easier* for someone who is *predisposed to it, but merely unskilled.* But there are no silver bullets that will transform a monogamous person into a poly one, or

vice versa. I *do not* recommend entering into a committed D/s relationship with the unrealistic hope of *converting* your partner to *your way of loving*.

- The pure BDSM Dominant and pure D/s submissive, or vice versa. As I've said in previous chapters, *most* of the people in the fetish community like to *integrate* their D/s and BDSM, just as *most* people generally prefer their *sex and love* conveniently wrapped up in one person. But there are many who *don't,* and to further complicate things, it isn't always easy to figure out who those people are. There's nothing *wrong* with simply wanting to participate in BDSM activities, without seeking a relationship. There's also nothing wrong with simply wanting a D/s relationship dynamic, without the whips and chains. The important thing is that both partners are getting what they want and need out of the relationship.

It is certainly easy to assume that certain types of Dominants and submissives will never be happy together in a relationship. Of course, that's a little like assuming that cats and dogs will never be able to tolerate each other, a generalization that isn't always supported by the facts. Can a babygirl submissive be happy with a sadistic Dominant? Would a Lesser God Dominant be able to tolerate a brat submissive? Should a non-Gorean Dominant ever consider a kajirae for a collar? Your first impulse might be to doubt the long-term viability of mismatched relationships such as these. Pure *probability* in such cases certainly *favors* a train wreck in the not-too-distant future. Sometimes, however, *people can surprise you*. They *change.* They *grow.* They learn and adapt and, occasionally, they succeed in a relationship which completely defies explanation. This, however, is generally the *exception*, rather than the rule.

Poor Communication

Make no mistake about it; communication is a *skill*, and a *critical* one at that. D/s relationships are no more prone to communication breakdowns than vanilla ones, but their complexity and potential consequences can be *mind-boggling.* At the end of this chapter, I share a simple example of how two people having two completely different notions of the definition of the word *"extreme"* can change *everything.* Just because you and your partner both speak *English* doesn't necessarily mean you *speak the same language.*

Words can have *drastically* different connotations and meanings to people, but when you are part of a *fetish culture* that habitually frames things in double entendre and euphemism, it becomes even more complicated. For example, when is *"whips and chains"* just another way to say *BDSM*, and when does it *literally* mean *whips and chains?* It's not unusual *at all* to hear someone in the lifestyle who claims to be into *"whips and chains"* to go pale when an actual *bullwhip* is brought out, saying *"Oh no,* I didn't mean an *actual* whip! *Got any nice, thuddy floggers?"*

When we hear a term like *"age play,"* we generally assume that it involves a mature individual acting in a *child-like role*. In reality, *age play* is any activity where one person assumes the role of someone *any age* that significantly differs from his true age, while another person interacts with him age-appropriately. The most *common* expression of age play is found in the *Daddy Dom - babygirl* relationship dynamic, but there are *plenty* of other possible permutations, including role play *gerontophilia*, which is a sexual attraction to the *elderly*.

Examples like these can be humorous or even ironic at times, but when a relationship goes off the tracks because of a basic misunderstanding, it can be heartbreaking. Some of the most common communication breakdowns occur as the result of a *lack of clarity* on such things as the differences between a slave and a submissive, or what a *collar* represents to each of the parties involved. A simple word like *respect* can mean *completely* different things to different people, and a slave contract specifying that *"each party shall respect the other"* is virtually *worthless* unless the term can be adequately defined.

The *disagreement* is another communication minefield which must be navigated *cautiously* in any D/s relationship. Learning how to disagree without becoming *disagreeable* can be a challenge that simply overwhelms many couples. Other couples may find it difficult to stay engaged and communicating constructively when the first impulse of many submissives is to *withdraw* in order to avoid conflict with his or her Dominant. Ideally, couples should look for a solution that exists somewhere between all-out war and silent sulking.

Each relationship is different, but you should be able to work together to identify *"hot buttons"* to be avoided, tell-tale signs that a discussion has gone off-track, and *"lines in the sand"* which must not be crossed under any circumstances. Couples must also learn to *read between the lines* to divine the true meaning of what is, *or isn't*, being said.

Years ago, I was chatting online with one of my submissives when, *seemingly out of the blue,* she said, "You're angry with me." And frankly, I was. But I was also very *surprised* that she had picked up on it, because I *thought* I'd done a pretty good job of concealing my annoyance at some silly thing she'd said. I may be *easily annoyed*, but over the years I've learned that if I can just resist for ten minutes the urge to *say or do something about it*, it usually passes quickly, and everyone is happier for it.

So I asked her, "How did you *know* I was angry?"

She hesitated. She really didn't *want* to reveal the *source* of her superpower, but now she was trapped and had no choice but to come clean. She reluctantly said, "It's your *punctuation*, Master."

I was completely baffled. "My... *punctuation?"*

She explained, "Yes, your *punctuation.* You never use *periods* when chatting online. *Ever.* That is, unless you're *angry* about something. Then, suddenly, *periods* start appearing at the ends of your sentences. And even though you might be *saying nice things*, I know what the periods *really* mean. They mean, *I am so done with this conversation."*

I scrolled back to see if what she was saying could *possibly be true*, and sure enough, *there they were.* All this time, I thought I was being clever, yet I'd been betrayed by the little dots at the ends of my sentences. I definitely learned something about how my subconscious mind worked that day. More importantly, I also learned that an *observant and motivated partner* can find helpful lines of communication in even the *tiniest* details.

Unstated Relationship Rules

If you don't know what the rules are that govern your relationship, there's a pretty high probability that you won't be *following* them. D/s relationships are often *all about the rules.* Generally speaking, Dominants love to *make them*, and submissives love to be *subject to them*. When one or the other fails to fulfill his or her responsibility in this regard, or steps outside the boundaries of what is expected by the other partner, it usually doesn't end well.

The most difficult rules to follow in any relationship are the *ones that no one told you about.* Being held *accountable* for something that you're unaware of is manifestly *unfair.* Unfortunately, there will always be things left unsaid because it is simply *assumed* that we *know* certain things, and understand the implications of what we're doing.

One of the things typically assumed by practically everyone in the D/s lifestyle is the notion that Dominants, *almost by definition,* make the rules. If you consider yourself a Dominant, yet are subject to a rule-set not of your own making, *I have bad news for you*. Similarly, if you consider yourself a submissive, yet are telling your Dominant what he should or shouldn't be *doing, thinking or feeling*, then *I have bad news for you, too.* Here it is, the awful, unvarnished truth: *You're probably far more vanilla than you care to admit.* The *good* news is, I'm told the survival rate for people with this condition is quite good.

Role Drift, Role Abandonment, & Role Reversal

When an individual is *hard-wired* for dominance or submission, he is likely to remain so for as long as he lives. It is extremely rare for anyone to be able to change these core personality traits in any meaningful or significant way. This is *not* the case, however, for anyone who may be *consciously or unconsciously acting out a role* of Dominance or submission. In those cases, a D/s relationship which is based on the assumption of a Dominant or submissive *role* by one or both partners runs a high risk of falling victim to *role drift, role abandonment, or role reversal.*

Role drift is what happens when a partner's assumed role incrementally changes over time. It should come as no surprise to anyone that this sort of thing happens in *all* kinds of relationships, *not* just in D/s related ones. The impact of this phenomenon is relatively more severe in D/s relationships for the simple reason that most D/s relationships *exist primarily for the sake of the Dominance/submission dynamic.*

Role drift can occur at either end of the D/s spectrum, and for a wide variety of reasons. Quite often, it is a natural consequence of a person's maturation or the simple broadening of his horizons. It is fairly common and almost reasonable for people to assume, for example, that just because they *want* to be Dominants, or because they happen to be particularly *good at performing in a Dominant role*, then *that's what they are.* Unfortunately, *it ain't necessarily so.* These folks would more accurately be described as *Tops.*

A *Top* is a person who *situationally or temporarily* assumes a Dominant role as appropriate for BDSM scenes, specific relationship or sexual partners, or simply as the mood strikes him. A Top may, in fact, be *very, very good* at what he does, which is *assuming a Dominant role.* But that doesn't *necessarily* mean that he finds lasting joy or fulfillment in it. Perhaps he assumes the role of a Top to please his partner. Perhaps he continues doing it simply because he is very *good at it*, and it's really *nice to be good at something.* Or, perhaps he does it in an earnest effort to *discover his inner Dominant.* Whatever the reason, it ultimately comes down to this: It is *something he does,* and not necessarily *who he is.* It is a *role,* and eventually, *all roles become tedious.* Once fulfilling his role starts *feeling like work,* it's only a matter of time and opportunity before the inevitable process of role drift begins.

Bottoms are equally as susceptible to role drift, and for essentially the same reasons, with one notable exception. Subs and bottoms *both* depend on their Dominants and Tops to *act like Dominants.* That means they are expected to make important decision, handle problems, and generally provide for the wants and needs of their subs. When they *fail* to fulfill these obligations, it isn't as if those needs *just go away*. Obviously, *someone has to do it,* and that usually means the submissive must take up the slack. Over the course of many months, or perhaps even *years*, the submissive's cherished role is whittled away bit by bit until one day, she suddenly wakes up to the realization that she somehow ended up in a place where she never wanted to be. She's *in charge.*

A folk tale that is often used to illustrate this principle of *gradual, almost imperceptible change over time* involves what happens when you toss a *live frog* into a pot of boiling water. According to the earthy folks who love to tell this tale, your frog will immediately *leap right back out of the pot.* Apparently, this is a *bad thing,* because (this is the part that strains credulity) I am *supposedly really hungry for a boiled frog.* When I was first told this story, I was more than just a little *skeptical.* But then again, my only real experience at tossing live critters into boiling water involved *lobsters,* and they're not exactly known for being *big leapers.* They do, however, make a *creepy sound;* but I digress. There's apparently *more* to this *how-to-boil-a-frog* story, and we're just getting to the good part: If you were to put your frog, instead, into a pot of *cool water* and raise the temperature *incrementally,* he will simply *sit there* like a dope and *tolerate* the increasingly hot water until he is fully cooked, through and through. This is great little story, for everyone but the frog. The moral of it, obviously, is *don't be that frog*. Or, perhaps, *don't marry that frog*. Or, just *don't eat frog.*

Role abandonment occurs when a partner in a relationship suddenly just *discards* his or her previous role. It happens in many different ways, and for a variety of reasons, but it is almost always a *surprise* to almost everyone concerned. The most common scenarios leading to role abandonment include such things as the termination of a relationship, unforeseen difficulties in assuming the role, catastrophic failure in fulfilling his responsibilities, or the sudden realization that while *he* is role playing, *his partner is not.*

It is, in a nutshell, the so-called-adult version of *"I don't want to play anymore... I quit."*

Giselle was a petite, ambitious twenty-six-year-old lifestyle submissive when she met Carl. Carl was a few years older, ruggedly handsome, and relatively successful in his chosen career as a real estate agent. There was just one little problem with Carl. He was as *vanilla* as they come, and Giselle had vowed after her recent divorce that she would *never again* be involved in another *vanilla relationship*. And so, over the course of the next few months, Giselle introduced her new beau to the D/s and BDSM lifestyles. To his credit, Carl was a good pupil who found everything about this new culture fascinating and, as a result, he caught on quickly. Giselle reveled in this once-in-a-lifetime opportunity to *"create the perfect Dom"* by mentoring and teaching him how to be *decisive*, yet collaborative. He would be *strong*, yet compassionate. He would be *aggressive and confident*, yet gentle and humble. And when it came to *BDSM* skills and knowledge? Carl was going to be *legendary.*

Giselle's mentorship of Carl continued apace with the growing intensity of their relationship and five months later, to absolutely no one's surprise, they were married in a simple traditional wedding for the benefit of their families. Later that evening, a private *collaring* ceremony was conducted for the couple and their friends in the lifestyle. Giselle was *living her dream*, and couldn't have been happier.

Carl, on the other hand, was secretly beginning to feel a little *overwhelmed.* He certainly *appreciated* the faith that Giselle had placed in him, he enjoyed the kinky BDSM play, and he loved his new friends in the lifestyle. But he never expected this stuff to *take over his life. Everything* now seemed to revolve around their kinky *activities*, their kinky *toys*, or their kinky *friends*. Even the *collaring ceremony*, in his view, had been way over the top, but he had gone along with it because he wanted to make Giselle *happy.* She was always seeking *new skills, new thrills*, and *new play partners* for increasingly challenging scenes and it was becoming increasingly difficult for Carl to deal with it all.

Then, the economy took a turn for the worse. The real estate market tanked, and Carl was laid off. Giselle began having health problems that seemingly defied treatment and mystified her doctors. Their savings were gone, their retirement accounts devastated, medical bills were mounting, and there were no jobs to be had. Throughout it *all,* Giselle continued to have faith in Carl, telling him daily, *"I know you'll be able to turn things around."*

One sunny Saturday morning, Carl woke up to the sure knowledge that he *just didn't want to be a Dom any more.* He told Giselle, "I'm sorry, but it's just *too hard.* I want to go back to being just a *regular guy*, with *regular problems.* You know, *like before we started doing all this BDSM stuff.* I feel like I'm being expected to manage *your* life, *when I can't even handle my own.* It's just too much. I'm *done."*

A year later, Carl and Giselle were divorced. Today, Giselle is still active in the lifestyle, and is still seeking her *perfect Dominant.* Carl has put the D/s lifestyle behind him, and prefers now to immerse himself deeply in the *cosplay and furry cultures*. The two of them have managed to remain dear but distant friends.

Role reversal is characterized by a polar shift from Dominant to submissive, or vice versa. It occurs for many of the same reasons as *role shift* and *role abandonment*, but the starkly contrasting consequences of such a complete reversal of roles can be jarring or even *traumatic* to the other partner in a D/s relationship. The depth of the emotional impact that this kind of sudden metamorphosis can have on one's partners may be difficult to comprehend for anyone who is not, himself, defined primarily by D/s roles and traits. In some ways, it could be compared to how a typical person might react if he came home from work one day to discover that his spouse had undergone a *sex-change* operation, or had switched her sexual orientation. Yes, it's *that big of a deal.*

Like any other lifestyle, the D/s lifestyle is *defined* by what we think is *important*. Unsurprisingly, we believe that *Domination and submission* are central to our way of life, our way of relating to one another, and our sense of purpose and self-worth. Assuming either character trait as a part of one's *role play* activity may be a perfectly *legitimate and entertaining* thing for many people to *do*, but it makes a terrible foundation upon which to build a lasting and meaningful D/s relationship.

Religion

Here we go again, talking about that thing *no one likes to talk about* - religion. In the previous chapter, we discussed how religion, *for the most part*, should *not* be an obstacle to a healthy D/s relationship or for *most* BDSM activities. In *this* section, we're going to explore some of the ways it *can be.* In the *vanilla* world, religion typically becomes a stumbling block to relationships in one of two ways. The first occurs when one partner in a relationship is religious and the other is *not.* The other occurs when *both* partners are religious, but their religious views are *incompatible*. As unpleasant and complicated as those two scenarios can be, they can't hold a candle to the absurdity and magnitude of the potential mess that can *sometimes* result from mixing kink and religion.

You probably don't need to be told that couples in D/s relationships are just as prone, if not more so, as *anyone* to the two scenarios we just mentioned. Having different religious beliefs can be hard on *any* relationship, but this is a problem that has been around for as long as religions and relationships have existed. Exercising a little tolerance and the ability to moderate your natural desire to share your beliefs can go a long way to reducing any potential for religious friction in this regard. It starts to get just a little more complicated, however, when the major point of contention between these two religious viewpoints becomes D/s or BDSM *itself.* Fortunately, this isn't terribly common, but it *does* happen.

A devout Buddhist, for example, may be profoundly uncomfortable with the thought of even *simulating* an activity that, in reality, would be considered to be harmful to others or might cause them pain. Examples *might* include spanking, paddling, bondage, torture, and a host of other traditional BDSM activities. The Buddhist practice of avoiding *performances* could make BDSM scenes, *even as a spectator*, taboo. If the Buddhist distaste for being *elevated* above others applies even to *chairs and beds*, it's a pretty safe bet that *aspiring to become a Dominatrix* would probably be *frowned upon*. Many people are perfectly willing to ignore or overlook what their *religion* thinks of their BDSM activities, but it certainly becomes a lot harder to do that when it's your *relationship partner who is doing all the frowning*.

If the only potential religious problems for D/s couples simply involved religious differences that could arise *within* the relationship, life would be pretty simple. Unfortunately, life in a D/s relationship is *never quite so simple.* Let's consider, for example, what happens in a hypothetically scenario where a D/s relationship develops into a personality cult with a Lesser God Dominant at the helm and an assortment of acolyte submissives worshipping at his feet. In essence, a private, insular religion has been formed, with its own unique beliefs, doctrines, and practices. You or I might view this scenario with some bemusement or even fascination but, even so, our *first* instinct as members of this lifestyle is typically to tolerate and respect the informed consensual choices of others. But what if you were *not* a member of the D/s lifestyle? What if you were, *instead*, an influential member of the community who was profoundly vanilla and devoutly religious, and your *eighteen-year-old daughter* just became one of those acolytes? It's hard to see a hypothetical scenario like this one developing into anything other than a *train wreck* for everyone concerned.

The point of this story is to illustrate the fact that, once you adopt an alternative lifestyle or become part of a non-traditional relationship, you run the very real risk of having *religion used as a club* against you by people outside the relationship who may, for whatever reason, believe they have a stake in the outcome. Those people are *typically* going to be family members, or concerned friends and associates. But there may even be times when your neighbors, your church, the community at large, or even the heavy-hand of government is arrayed against you. Consider the April 2008 raid of an FLDS *polygamist compound* in Eldorado, Texas, where state troopers and Child Protective Services agents swooped in with *armored vehicles* and placed over 400 children in "protective custody" on the basis of a *prank telephone call.*

Think something like that couldn't ever happen to you? *Think again.*

Legal Issues

It's *easy* to have faith in the courts and in our judicial system, until you actually find yourself suddenly at its mercy. When you consider the fifty U.S. states, five major U.S. territories, the District of Columbia, and the Uniform Code of Military Justice, there are close to *sixty different sets of laws* governing what is or isn't legal to do *in the privacy of your own bedroom.* As if *that* weren't bad enough, each legal jurisdiction gets to arbitrarily decide which laws they want to enforce and/or prosecute in the courts. That discretionary latitude is *not* reserved solely for the states themselves; it is often exercised by cities, counties and townships. As late as 2012, twenty-three U.S. states still had laws against *adultery* on the books, but when was the last time you heard of someone being *arrested* for that particular crime? In Massachusetts,

Idaho, Michigan, Oklahoma and Wisconsin, *adultery is a felony*. In the other eighteen states that consider it a crime, it is a *misdemeanor.*

Did you know that, as of 2013, mere *cohabitation* with a person of the opposite sex who is not your spouse is still illegal in three U.S. states? Those states would be *Mississippi, Florida and Michigan,* by the way. This is *despite* the fact that, according to the Census Bureau's 2009 American Community Survey, 58% of all women aged 19-44 have, at some point, lived with a man who was not their legal spouse. In fact, these arcane laws are still on the books despite the landmark ruling in *Lawrence vs. Texas (2003),* in which the U.S. Supreme Court ruled that *laws against cohabitation were unconstitutional.* And yet, there they are.

You *probably* think you know what the word *sodomy* means, and if so, you're probably *wrong*. U.S. courts have historically interpreted *sodomy* to mean *"any sexual act deemed to be unnatural or immoral."* Traditionally, the courts have defined that further to mean *oral sex, anal sex and bestiality;* but the implications of the broader definition for someone in the fetish lifestyle are *seriously scary.* What it means is if the authorities *don't like what you're doing*, and even if there aren't any specific *laws* against it, *they can always charge you with sodomy. Consent* is not an acceptable defense.

In fact, the entire notion of *lawful consent* is riddled with so many traps, pitfalls and legal loopholes, the mere thought of attempting to build a trial defense based upon it should be enough to strike fear into the heart of any competent trial attorney. We like to think that whatever happens between *two consenting adults* should be no one's business but their own, but that's *not* necessarily how the *law* sees things.

Let's take, for example, the crime generally known to most people as *battery.* The basic definition of *battery* is: *the unlawful application of force upon the person of another which results in bodily injury or offensive touching.* The first thing we should take note of here is the glaring lack of any mention of the word *"consent."* In *most* states, the law is pretty clear on this. *Battery is battery, regardless* of whether or not the alleged victim *consented to* or *enjoyed* the activity. Obviously, if the victim is the only available witness to the alleged battery, and isn't inclined to cooperate with the prosecutor's case, then there really isn't much of a case for the prosecutor to work with. But there *have* been plenty of cases prosecuted in the courts where an alleged victim has declined to cooperate with the state, yet the case was prosecuted *based solely on the testimony of police officers, other witnesses, or medical personnel.* Many people erroneously believe that if an alleged victim *"refuses to press charges"* against his or her *"attacker,"* then that person cannot be charged with *battery.* It's a *myth.*

While the notion of legal consent may be considered *irrelevant* to the crime of *battery*, it can be a critical factor to prove *other crimes*, and in some types of cases, it is essentially the *only* relevant factor. Without *consent*, sex becomes *rape*, heavy petting becomes *sexual battery*, bondage becomes *unlawful imprisonment or kidnapping*, impact-play becomes *aggravated battery* or *assault with a deadly weapon*, and even pillow talk turns into *sexual harassment.*

You may be thinking, *"Not a problem.* I *always* get my partner's consent before engaging in any sexual or BDSM activity." If that is *so,* then that is a truly commendable strategy *indeed.* There's just one little problem with it. Could you prove it in a court of law? Could you do it *ten years, or even twenty years from now?* Some states have recently acted to extend or *eliminate entirely* the statute of limitations for the crimes of rape and sodomy. In those states, you could *theoretically* be charged with one of those crimes *at any time while you are still alive.* The odds of such a thing happening are, of course, *infinitesimally* small, but it is a sobering thing to contemplate.

Family Issues

Among the many other things that could possibly go wrong with a D/s relationship, we shouldn't neglect the very real possibility that your *families* may not be entirely thrilled with your involvement in this lifestyle. Much of this negativity will be rooted in misconceptions and false stereotypes, but that doesn't make the *effects* any less stressful, and the potential consequences can run the gamut from *comical* to *catastrophic.*

I always enjoy telling the story of what happened a few days *after* I presented Jade, my former submissive, with her beautiful new collar. She was still riding high on a wave of euphoria when she called me to tell me those three little words which can have such a profound impact on the psyche of just about any Dominant: "I told Mom."

I'm rarely rendered speechless, but *this* was one of those times. I stammered, "You. Told. Your. Mom. *What, exactly, did you tell her?"*

She nonchalantly replied, as if she were discussing her last load of laundry, "I told her I was *collared*; that I now have a *Master*, and that my heart, body and soul belong to *You.* And I told her that I was deliriously *happy* about it.*"*

"I see..." said I, struggling manfully to stay calm, "and how*, pray tell,* did she *react* to this news?"

A long pause followed, no doubt fueled by an internal struggle over how to best phrase her response. She finally decided on, *"Not so good."*

"Not so good?" I asked. "Please define *not so good."*

"Well..." she replied, "She wants your full name and address, and she said she'll use the *police or private investigators*, if necessary, to track you down and rescue me from whatever crazy kind of cult you've gotten me into. So, *yeah... Not so good."*

I like to think I took the news *calmly*, with a stoic resolve to weather whatever storm would be coming our way. Jade, however, remembers it in a *slightly different* way. Today, she describes it thusly: "You totally freaked out." *Whatever.* Eventually, her mother *(and I)* calmed down, and life returned to *abnormal.* But this amusing little anecdote is illustrative of how *family* can sometimes become a critical factor in your D/s relationship in unpredictable or unexpected ways.

Take for example, what typically happens whenever you tell someone outside the lifestyle that you are in a committed D/s or BDSM relationship. *Almost without fail*, the very first question they will ask is: *"Do either of you have children?"* The unspoken assumption, of course, is a suspicion or belief that you may be *putting your children at risk*, or raising them in an amoral or immoral environment. Those misconceptions can be relatively easy for you to discount or ignore *until those busybodies act on them*. The fact that they can do so *anonymously* in most cases just makes it all the more dangerous. It is unfortunate that our legal system grants almost *unlimited powers* to agents of state child protective services when they have any reason to suspect that children are being endangered, even when those reasons may be entirely *bogus.*

Family-related D/s relationship issues don't *always* have to be quite so potentially disastrous. Sometimes, they can be simply annoying, frustrating or even *amusing*. I once made the mistake of telling my eighty-three-year-old father about my D/s lifestyle during a long and monotonous road trip we took across the states of Texas and Louisiana. To this day, I still can't fathom what might have caused me to think that it would be a good idea to have that particular conversation with him. All I know is, we each have very different tastes in music, and after hours of driving in silence, I was about ready to *crack.* So I gave him some background about the BDSM lifestyle in *general*, talked a little about the D/s and poly *mindset and philosophy*, and even tried to put it all in the proper *context* by explaining how the poly D/s relationship I was in at the time worked. I *thought* I had done a pretty good job of it all, until I realized that, in the course of the last thirty minutes, he'd really just focused on *two little words*.

"Sex slaves?" he asked. "You're telling me you have *sex slaves?"*

"No, Dad." I replied, "Technically, they're not *slaves*, they're *submissives.* There's a difference. And besides, that's what I've been *trying to explain* to you. It's *not* all about *sex."*

"Right," he nodded, and pondered the point for a moment before continuing, "But, they're basically *sex slaves, right?* You can tell them to do *anything*, and they *have to do it*, no matter what?"

I silently cursed myself for starting this conversation, but knew I had no choice now but to continue with it. I explained, "Dad, *it's not like that.* It's not like that at *all.* These are loving relationships. My girls do what they do out of love and devotion, and an intense desire to serve and please their Master. They don't do it because they *have to."*

"But... you're their *Master*," he countered. "That pretty much makes them your *sex slaves*, right?"

Desperately wanting this line of discussion to end, I simply replied, *"Yes,* Dad. I guess you could say they are *sex slaves."* I suddenly understood what it was like to be one of those poor bastards who confesses to a crime he didn't commit because he just wants the world to start making sense again; *he just wants to wake up and have it be over.* At that point, I probably would have told him that my girls were *sex slaves from the planet Gor* if that's what he wanted to hear, *especially* if it would drive a stake through this discussion's heart and *finish it.* Unfortunately, Dad was nowhere *near* done.

"What about that little blonde girl you introduced me to a couple of years ago, when I came for a visit. Was *she* a sex slave?" *Yes*, Dad. "And that tall brunette you brought with you to my wedding? Was *she* a sex slave?" *Yes,* Dad. "And what about that hot *Eurasian* girl, the one with the epic tits? Was *she..."* *Yes,* Dad, *all of them!* They were all *sex slaves, every last one of them!* Can we just talk about *sports, or something, now?*

But, no such luck. My father spent the next half hour naming or describing *every woman I have ever known* since I was a teen, asking,

"Was she a sex slave?" I started looking for spots along the highway where I might be able to slow down just long enough push him out of the car into a *hedge* or culvert. I sought solace in the fact that he would eventually run out of names to ask me about, but then he did something just plain *weird.* He began listing practically every woman that *he'd* ever been involved with, *and asking me if I had ever dated their daughters.* Perhaps it was just his *oh-so-subtle* way of saying, *"Hey, I've had my share of experiences, too!"* but all it *really* did was make me want to run up to the nearest Louisiana State Trooper and lunge for his gun in the desperate hope that he might *shoot me* and put me out of my misery.

The rest of the trip passed without any discussion of my lifestyle or my relationships and for that, I was *exceedingly* grateful. A few days went by, and I began to think that perhaps I'd been a bit *hard on him;* that maybe my perceptions had been *tainted* by my tendency to become easily annoyed. In fact, I'd forgotten all about it when I took him by my office to introduce him to my boss and to a few of my co-workers. Dad was spry for an eighty-three-year-old, but his *hearing* had gotten progressively worse over the years. This sometimes resulted in the volume of his *own voice* being inappropriate to the circumstances, and unfortunately, *this* turned out to be one of those circumstances.

At the office, we chatted with my boss for a few minutes and then I took Dad down the hall to meet a colleague and friend, who just happened to be a *stunningly beautiful,* shapely brunette. Dad slipped effortlessly into the role of a charming and witty *raconteur*, telling funny stories and flirting shamelessly with her and the other women who worked in that department.

As we said our goodbyes and turned to leave, Dad leaned in close to me to deliver a stage whisper which was, in fact, *loud enough for everyone within fifty feet to hear.* He said, "Please tell me she is one of those *sex slaves* you've been telling me about."

Health Issues

When you have your health, you are truly blessed. Conversely, when age, illness or injuries prevent you from doing the things you enjoy most, *life sucks.* It's a sobering thing to contemplate the fact that *we will each* someday have to come to terms with age or circumstances that make certain types of BDSM play impractical, painful, or dangerous. It's at times like these that it is important to remember that we are more than the *sum total of our kinks*, and that we should never allow ourselves to be defined solely by our *dungeon activities.*

Who you are trumps *what you do.*

I once had a friend tell me, "I could *never* be a submissive." Frankly, I hear this *all the time*, and I'm rarely surprised by the reasoning or misconceptions behind such statements, but this woman was the exception to the rule. I asked her *why* she believed she could never be a submissive. She replied, "I could never be a submissive *because I have bad knees."*

In *her* mind, a submissive was *someone who kneels. Bad knees* meant *no kneeling*, and therefore, she concluded that she could never be a submissive. I told her that *kneeling doesn't make you a submissive;* any more than standing in my garage makes you a *car.* Since then, she has enjoyed many happy years as a submissive in the lifestyle.

Other health issues which could significantly complicate your D/s relationship include BDSM play-related injuries, mental health issues, and sexually transmitted diseases. The wisest strategy to employ in each of these cases is to take preventative precautions, seek immediate medical treatment as appropriate, and don't let these setbacks make you bitter. As long as you are able to find some measure of joy within yourself and in your partner, *there's hope.*

The D/s Break-up

Break-ups *happen,* but they should never be allowed to break your spirit, or to convince you that there aren't *good people* out there who are definitely worth the effort of loving them. It can sometimes be all too easy to fall into the trap of thinking: *there were problems in this D/s relationship, therefore D/s relationships must be the problem.* D/s relationships fail for many of the same reasons other kinds of relationships fail, many of which we've already covered in this chapter. One way to cope with the disappointment and sadness associated with the end of a relationship is to think of the experience *not as a failure,* but as a process of *discovering one more way not to do it in the future.* You may end up *kissing a lot of frogs* before finding your *Prince (or Princess) Charming.*

Once you and your partner have reached a point where you have made every possible and reasonable effort to save your relationship without success, then it's time to do the right thing and put an end to the mutual misery. The challenge, of course, is to do so without recriminations or by causing unnecessary pain for your partner. Just because your relationship has become dysfunctional or you can see no clear path to where you had hoped to be going *doesn't mean you've stopped caring* about your partner. Be sure to let your partner know that your *feelings* probably haven't changed; the only thing that *has* changed is your ability to make the relationship *work.*

When a break-up occurs, I think it's critically important that we do whatever we possibly can to avoid lashing out at or hurting our former partners. I like to think that there are really just *two* kinds of break-ups. The first is the *"I'm a cat person; you're a dog person, and I love you but this is never going to work out, so let's stop hurting each other"* kind of break-up. And then, there's the *"I'm a cat person; you're a dog person, and I thought I loved you, until you put my cat in the microwave oven"* kind of break-up. I probably don't need to tell you which type we should be striving for.

Regardless, a D/s break-up is *never* an easy thing, nor should it *ever be.* The saddest and most painful experiences of my life have been those instances where I had to say goodbye to someone I loved deeply. Sometimes, love simply isn't enough to sustain a broken relationship. Sometimes, mistakes are made that *can't be undone*, or things are said that *can't be unsaid.* Frankly, it pains me greatly to even *think* about some of those agonizing, gut-wrenching decisions and experiences, much less *tell* you about one. But I think it's important, *and so I will.* Her name was Joanne, and I loved her very much.

Joanne sat on the edge of the bed, wringing her hands and looking deeply troubled. She'd been anxiously waiting all day to speak to me, and now that I was there, she wasn't quite sure where to begin. She knew that bringing a grievance to me always required a certain amount of tact, and to be sure, she was usually quite adept at it. But today she just didn't know if she would be able to keep her volatile emotions in check long enough to say what needed to be said.

"Master, this rift between Jade and me doesn't seem to be getting any better. I know you said that I should be patient, and give her a little time; that I should try to see things from her point of view, but..." she sighed, struggling to contain her emotions. Joanne had moved here from Colorado a year ago to form a polyamorous family with Jade and me, and while the two women were certainly close, they weren't as close as Joanne had initially hoped they would be.

Over the course of the past twelve months, it had become increasingly apparent that Jade was essentially a monogamous heterosexual submissive who envisioned herself in a poly *vee* relationship, with me as the hinge. Joanne, on the other hand, was a poly bisexual submissive who had envisioned herself in a full triad relationship, where all three partners are equally loved and sexually attracted to one another. Obviously, this was a source of some frustration for the two women, and frankly, I wasn't exactly crazy about how things had developed, either. But this was not a perfect world, and on the whole, the three of us were generally happy.

"I love her like a sister. I really do, Master. You know that." She continued, "I would do anything for her. But she has this wall that she has built around herself that I just can't seem to break through."

I nodded, looking into her lovely blue eyes, and wiped away the tears that were beginning to well up there. "Maybe that's the problem, baby." I said, "Maybe you're trying just a little too hard. The more you try to break through her defenses, the more she will fortify them. You can't break into a person's heart and expect to be welcomed with open arms. You need to wait for her to open a door and invite you in."

She pondered this for a moment, and replied, "But Master, she isn't going to invite me in. She is perfectly happy with the way things are. And what makes this even more frustrating to me is the fact that you're not doing anything to fix this!"

I was surprised and somewhat perplexed by this charge since I had, indeed, been working quite diligently both in the open and behind the scenes to keep the peace between my two wonderful submissives, and to subtly nudge each toward compromises that they could both live with. I said, "Believe me - I've been working very hard on this. You're just going to have to trust me to work this out."

That's when Joanne blurted out the sentence that changed everything in an instant. I'll probably never know if she really meant what she said. All I know is that some things, once said, can never be unsaid, nor forgotten. What she said was, "That's the problem, Master. I don't *believe* you, or *trust* you."

I replied, "If that is true, then we obviously have nothing more to say to each other. You may consider yourself released. Goodbye, Joanne."

I stood up and walked out of the front door and out of her life forever.

Avoiding the Train Wreck

It may seem as though we've just been through an *exhaustive* list of things that could possibly go wrong in a D/s relationship, but the sad truth is *we've barely scratched the surface.* My goal is *not* to sour you on the idea of pursuing your D/s lifestyle dreams, if that's what you're considering. But I *do* want you to be aware of what *could* possibly go wrong, so you *can see it coming and, perhaps, even avoid it.*

We began this chapter with a wonderfully illuminating quote by Rex Stout: "A pessimist gets nothing but pleasant surprises, an optimist nothing but unpleasant." Perhaps you've noticed how trouble always seems to follow certain *so-called optimists* the way fat kids go for cake. *Happy thoughts* don't keep potential problems at bay. The truth is trouble doesn't really *care* whether you're *happy or unhappy*. Trouble only takes notice when you are *prepared*.

Relationship train wrecks *don't just happen*. *Something* sets that train in motion. *Someone* has their hand on the throttle, as the engine accelerates ever faster to its cataclysmic demise. *No one* expects it to happen, so precautions may seem just a tad *silly.* Yet, after the fact, everyone will say they *saw it coming.*

For the ill-fated passengers on board, the discussion is entirely *moot.*

# # #

My Two Cents on What Can Go Wrong

As much as I hate to admit this, I didn't learn what I know about these kinds of D/s blunders and catastrophes *second hand.* Many of these mistakes, I've made *myself.* Sometimes, I made the same mistakes *again and again* before coming to my senses. Sure, it's easy to look back *now,* years or even decades later and think *"Could I have been any stupider?"* Unfortunately, the answer is, *yes, I probably could have.*

There will always be limits to what we can know, but *our potential for stupidity is infinite.*

Earlier in this book, I promised to end each chapter with a brief, yet intimate peek into my head as my way of giving you the only truly unique thing that I have to offer. For the most part, it's been an enjoyable exercise. This installment, however, is personally painful to me.

It's often been said that a Dominant is never wrong. This, of course, is a *myth*. We're wrong *all the time*; we just hate *admitting* that we are wrong. Mark this day on your calendar, because I am about to admit that I was once absolutely *unclear on the concept* of extreme masochism.

Her name was *Faithie* and she was a chat room friend who seemed like the *ideal submissive*. She was an engaging, intelligent, spirited and beautiful woman who loved many of the same kinds of BDSM play that I did, so we seemed perfectly matched to one another. *Sure*, she'd mentioned that she was an *extreme* masochist, but the word *extreme* means different things to different people. I was swimming in a sea of *new relationship energy,* so I didn't pay a whole lot of attention to that particular fin in the water.

Eventually, our relationship progressed to the point where we believed we were deeply in love, and that she should be *collared.* To that end, we arranged to spend three days together at a posh resort in Santa Fe,

New Mexico. We met for the first time in the hotel lobby and retired to our suite, where we spent the next 48 hours in *fetish heaven*. There was spanking, whipping, paddling, rope-play, and *oodles of kinky sex.* I was one happy Dom. But apparently, Faithie *needed more.* On the afternoon of the third day, she reached into her suitcase and pulled out a small block of wood, a hammer, and some ten-penny nails. *Would you please drive these nails through my nipples? That would be lovely, Master. Thank you so much!*

I thought about it. *I really did*. And I politely declined. I realized in that moment that I'd just learned about a limit that, up to that point, I never even suspected that I had. Faithie, however, was undeterred. She put away her hammer and nails, and returned with a small pouch containing the biggest damn *safety pins* I'd ever seen. *Master, would you be willing to use these safety pins to close up my pussy? Pretty please? Just this once?* This time, I didn't have to ponder it long *at all.* My answer was a polite but firm *no.*

I will not pin your pussy once.
I will not pin your pussy twice!
Not with a needle. Not *even* with ice!
Won't close it with a safety, or other sharp pin
Won't close it at *all!* Might want to get in!
I don't want to nail your pretty pink nipple.
Not *one* of them, *both* of them, or even a *triple!*
I will not do it on the table.
And not on the floor. I'm just unable!
Masochists, I *do* understand.
I'll give them spankings with my hand.
I'll paddle, and whip and *chain* their asses.
I'll even dip them in *molasses!*
But I never have, nor shall I start,
Punch bloody holes in body parts.
The closest I'll get, is *I'll cut you loose...*
and send my regrets to *Dr. Seuss.*

"Many have a wrong idea of what constitutes true happiness.
It is not attained through self-gratification,
but through fidelity to a worthy purpose."

- - Helen Keller

CHAPTER 15: RAINBOWS & UNICORNS

This final chapter is about *happiness. Your* happiness. We've spent a great deal of time discussing the almost infinite number of ways that a Domination/submission relationship can go off the rails. To leave you in a state of apprehension, viewing this lifestyle from a cynical perspective would be unfair, both to you *and* to the lifestyle. While this life and these kinds of relationships *aren't for everyone*, there is a *lot to like* about the lifestyle for those who are well-suited for it. Actually, that is an understatement. There's a lot to *love* about it.

My greatest concern, while writing this book, has been that by describing some of the pitfalls to be avoided, that I might inadvertently convince you to avoid the lifestyle *entirely*. I have worried that I spent too much time *describing* the BDSM culture and not enough time explaining how to be a *part* of it, or even why you might *want* to. I have been vexed by the thought that I may have spent too much time describing different kinds of D/s relationships, and not enough time telling you *how to have a good one.* I really do wish I could let you peek into my heart and see the wonderful relationships and the lifetime of joy that this lifestyle has provided me.

This lifestyle ought to be fun and fulfilling. If it is *neither* of those things for you, then perhaps you're *doing it wrong.* I wish there was a one-size-fits-all recommendation that I could give you that would ensure that your future D/s relationships and BDSM lifestyle will always and forever be fun and fulfilling. The key to finding that kind of happiness is going to be different for each individual, but it will always come from the same place. It will come from somewhere deep within *yourself.* If you're seeking it elsewhere, you're looking in the wrong place.

I like to tell the tale of a man who was out one night for his usual evening stroll, when he happened upon a neighbor, crawling around on all fours in the street under a streetlight:

> "Hi there, Ralph!" he greeted his neighbor, cheerily. "What are you *doing?"*
>
> Ralph looked up from his studious examination of sticks, leaves, and other gutter debris and said, "Oh, hey there, Bob. I'm looking for my cellphone. I think it may have fallen out of my pocket when I got out of the car."
>
> Bob furrowed his brow and asked, "What makes you think it would be here? Is this where you parked your car earlier?"
>
> Ralph shook his head, and pointed to a spot about a hundred yards further down the street. "No. Actually, I'm parked over there, *under that tree."*
>
> Bob peered down the street to where the car was parked in the dark shadow of a large elm tree. He turned back to his friend and, just a little confused, asked, "So, why are you looking for your phone over *here,* Ralph?"
>
> Ralph looked up from his gutter-rummaging, pointed to the streetlamp above, and replied, "Well, *duh!* The light's better *over here!"*

How many of us have expended precious time, resources, energy, and emotion seeking happiness in all the wrong places, in all the wrong ways? How often have we chosen the easy *wrong path* over the hard *right one?* Are we hoping that our partners will *fix us,* rather than working to heal our own injuries and scars? Are we trying too hard to know and love someone else, before really knowing and being capable of loving ourselves?

Only *you* know the answers to these questions. Are you willing to be honest with yourself?

Frankly, if anyone *could* help us to find those keys to happiness within ourselves, it would be the people in this lifestyle. They are quite simply the *best.* I have always loved the fact that kinksters are typically very open to exploration, and not just exploration of the lifestyle, but of *themselves.* They are generally far more willing than the average vanilla person to push the boundaries of what they know, what they think, how they feel, and even *what they like.*

As a general rule of thumb, there's also far less *self-censorship* in the fetish lifestyle. Kinksters tend to say what they mean, mean what they say, and care not about what others might think about that. This, of course, can be a double-edged sword. The good news is, for the most part, *what you see is what you get.* The bad news is you're not going to *like* a lot of what you see. But at least you'll be making *informed choices* and know that *compared to all of that*, you're not as much of a pervert as you might have thought!

This is a culture that is *incredibly* diverse and places a very high value on *tolerance.* Just because *my* kink is not *your* kink doesn't necessarily make *me* right and *you* wrong. You may view another person's fetish with disdain or even revulsion, but you should never forget that the world is full of people who might look upon your kinks with equal repugnance. It is this community's respect and reverence for diversity and rejection of judgmental posturing that makes it very special. That does *not*, however, mean that we should tolerate absolutely *anything.*

I won't pretend to be able to tell you how you should set your own moral compass. Just know that when you come into this lifestyle, you shouldn't leave your ethics at the door.

D/s relationships can be among the happiest and most intense, loving, passionate, and fulfilling kinds of relationships you may *ever experience*. A very small percentage of people will be lucky enough to find the right D/s partner at the right time under the right circumstances, and literally *live happily ever after*. Another small slice of those in the lifestyle may get just a brief taste of *what could have been*, and spend a lifetime hoping once again to *recreate* that magical spark. Still others may *never* get a chance *at all* to experience the thrill of hearing or saying, *"I am yours,"* and knowing it is *not just a figure of speech.*

The rest of us - *the great majority of us* - will do what we have *always* done, *in or outside* of the lifestyle.

We will find those special people who make us smile so much that our cheeks hurt, who spark our imaginations, who make us unafraid to show our secret selves, who *want* the very best for us and prove it every single day, the ones who make us *ache* for them, day and night. When we *find* those people, we hold them close and live, love, lust, and laugh with them for as long as we possibly can.

Rinse. Repeat.

You *can* find joy and fulfillment in a loving, healthy D/s relationship.

There are no guarantees, no sure things, and no secret formulas for success. It could last a *day*, or it could last a *lifetime.* Regardless of how long it lasts, if you keep your focus on bringing joy to your partner, and savoring the personal fulfillment that springs from that, you'll be on the right path.

# # #

My Two Cents on Happiness

Guess what? We're at the end of the book. I don't know about *you*, but that makes me a little sad. When a trusted colleague tentatively suggested that I include some personal experiences, anecdotes, and observations in this book, I wasn't particularly *thrilled* by the notion. Yet in the course of the writing, I've come to see not only the profound wisdom of her advice, but I have warmed to it immensely and now think of them as a series of intimate letters to a treasured friend who knows all of my flaws, and *likes me anyway*.

Now, with this - my final *Two Cents* - it comes to an end, and I will miss our little talks. I will miss *you.*

My consolation prize is the knowledge that I may have helped someone. *That* makes me *happy.* At the beginning of the book, I described myself as a *White Knight Dominant.* In short, I *live* to slay dragons, rescue those who are in distress, and solve problems. *You,* of course, will be the ultimate judge of whether I have been of service to you in any way. If so, please do me a favor and *let me know*. It would *seriously* make my day.

I'm usually a pretty happy guy. I once had a psychologist tell me that I was like *a bi-polar person who didn't have a down-side.* The old label for people like me used to be *"manic"* but that term went out of style when *"manic-depressive"* did. Now, the politically correct, technical term for people like me is *"too-damn-happy"* or, sometimes, *"consistently, nauseatingly cheerful."* I *do* realize that I drive most of my friends *bonkers*, but I *yam what I yam.*

When I'm *not* happy, I seek out the people, places, and things that bring me joy. For me, that usually means visiting a cherished friend, treating myself to a root beer float, working on my koi pond, or digging my toes into the sand at the beach and watching the sun dip into the sea. In general, I have found that I am happiest when I am engaged in a meaningful project, faced with an interesting challenge, or performing *service* for someone in need.

I *highly* recommend performing service. Seek out someone who may be experiencing some misfortune, someone with critical needs, and *do something nice for them.* It doesn't have to be a *big deal.* Pay them a compliment. Drop off a hot meal. Mow their lawn. Sing them a song.

Trust me. You'll feel like a *million bucks.*

My point is simply this: *You* are responsible for *your own* happiness. If you're sitting around waiting for something or someone else to *make you happy,* it could turn out to be a very long wait. Frankly, most people are so wrapped up in their *own* emotions that *your* happiness isn't even on their radar.

You want to know the *real* secret to achieving true and lasting happiness? Here it is: Get off your ass, and *do something.*

May your days be happy ones.

Mike Makai

"When I use a word," Humpty Dumpty said in rather a scornful tone, "it means just what I choose it to mean - neither more nor less."

- - *Lewis Carroll*

Appendix A:

Glossary

This glossary is provided for quick reference to certain words, terms or phrases one might encounter in the D/s or BDSM lifestyles. It is not intended to be an all-inclusive laundry-list of every possible kink-related term or toy. In some instances, the terms *play, role play, or fantasy* may be interchangeable, however, generally speaking, *play* refers to an activity, *role play* refers to a scene or scenario, and *fantasy* refers to something that is primarily a mindset, even if that may lead to related activities and role play.

In instances where a word or phrase may have multiple meanings, particularly in differing contexts, this glossary will always favor the BDSM context and usage. The mere inclusion here of any term describing a BDSM activity *should not* be considered an *endorsement* of it as something that you should try. Many of the activities described in this book can be *incredibly* dangerous, and should only be attempted after proper precautions are taken, and after being trained by a qualified person.

Just because something is *listed* here, doesn't necessarily mean you should *run out and try it*. By the same token, if something that you think is important is *not* listed here, it is more likely an oversight than a commentary on its significance in the lifestyle.

AB/DL. Acronym for Adult Baby / Diaper Lover. Adult babies and diaper lovers enjoy activities that involve at least one of the partners in a scene or relationship assuming the role of a baby or toddler still in diapers. *(See also: Age play, Bathroom use restrictions, Diaper play, Forced bed wetting, Littles, Role play, Urine play)*

Abandonment Fantasy. This refers to a fantasy or role play involving leaving a person, typically a submissive being disciplined, in a remote or isolated area such as in the middle of the desert, or on an open and empty stretch of highway. Abandonment fantasies are most often used as a way to induce fear, particularly in individuals with abandonment anxiety, and are often used in role play scenarios involving coercion, humiliation or punishment. *(See also: Abduction play, Interrogation play)*

Abduction Play. *(See: Abandonment fantasy, Interrogation play, Kidnapping fantasy, Role play)*

Abrasion Play. Stimulating, over-stimulating, or causing the skin to become hyper-sensitized through the application of abrasive materials such as sandpaper, brushes, the edges of coins, or special instruments designed specifically for this activity. Often, this stimulation of the skin also involves certain salves, ointments or chemicals which add to or enhance the sensations, either during or after the abrasion activity. The most commonly used enhancer is mentholated oil, such as the kind found in muscle rubs and ointments. *(See also: Sensation play)*

Acupuncture. *(See: Needle play)*

Adelphogamy. *Adelphogamy* refers to a specific form of polyandry, which consists of a two or more brothers in a committed relationship *(usually, but not limited to marriage)* with the same woman. It is sometimes referred to as fraternal or leviratic polyandry. *(See also: Polyamory, Polyandry)*

Aftercare. *Aftercare* refers to special attention and consideration which should be given to *all* scene participants immediately following any

BDSM scene, and should *not* be limited *solely to bottoms.* Even though it is primarily the responsibility of the Top to provide aftercare for his or her bottom, it is not uncommon for *both Top and bottom* to require some transition time after a scene to allow their focus, physiology, and mental states to return to a normal state. Immediately following a scene, participants may appear disoriented, flushed, exhausted, weak, confused, or inwardly focused. Even if there are no outward signs, they may require time to refocus their thoughts and emotions. The time required to recover will vary from individual to individual, which is why it is important to monitor their condition. It is usually a good idea to refrain from attempting to engage someone in conversation or activity until they show signs of recovering and begin initiating interaction themselves. *(See also: Scene, Subspace, Topspace)*

Age Play. *Age play* is BDSM *role play* activity or behavior that involves the interaction of at least two people, with at least one of them assuming the role of a person whose age differs significantly from his or her real age. While age play is most often used as a euphemism for *Daddy Dom – babygirl* role play, it can also refer to portrayals of any age, from newborn to the elderly. Age play can involve behaviors that are overtly sexual, mildly sexual, or completely asexual, and may or may not incorporate incest-related role play scenarios. Age play is not related to, nor considered pedophilia, since it does not involve an actual attraction to biologically underage children, but rather to the emotional state associated with playing the role, or interacting with a person exhibiting child-like behaviors. *(See also: AB/DL, Daddy Dom, Diaper play, Littles, Role play)*

Anal Play. *Anal Play* consists of activities involving the rimming or penetration of the anus with the fingers, fist, penis, vibrators, dildos, plugs, beads or other miscellaneous items. For many, stimulation of the anus with the tongue, fingers or sex toys can stimulate the nerves surrounding the anal sphincter and create a more intense orgasm than normal. For males, stimulation of the prostate gland, which can be reached by finger through the anus, can often hasten or intensify an orgasm. *(See also: Pegging, Strap-on)*

Ankle Cuffs. *(See: Restraints)*

Arm/Leg Sleeves. Arm and leg sleeves are typically items placed on the arms and legs of a person to immobilize or restrict the movement or use of those limbs as part of bondage play. They differ from *wrist and ankle cuffs* by being elongated tubes or sleeves which often are longer than the limbs themselves, in much the same way that strait-jacket sleeves are used to immobilize the arms of the wearer. *(See also: Bondage, Cuffs, Restraints)*

Asphyxiation. *(See: Breath Play.)*

Ass Worship. *Ass worship* is a form of *body worship* that focuses primarily on the buttocks. This erotic obsession usually involves a submissive kissing or licking a Dominant's ass, and it is often combined with *facesitting, smothering, spanking, humiliation or enemas.* The person whose ass is the object of the submissive's devotion typically remains aloof throughout. *(See Body Worship, Facesitting, Queening, Queening stool, Smotherbox)*

Auctions. In many BDSM lifestyle circles, auctions are held to raise funds for charity or to fund the group's activities or facilities. Often called *slave auctions*, the events essentially ask volunteers to auction themselves, or at least their complete *obedience* for a set period of time, off to the highest bidder. Since the "purchased" slave is sometimes expected to engage in BDSM or sexual activity, the law typically takes a dim view of slave auctions, and considers them a thinly veiled form of prostitution. *(See also: Role play, Slave)*

Autoerotic Asphyxiation. *Autoerotic asphyxiation* refers to masturbation while cutting off your own oxygen through the use of nooses, straps, plastic bags or other devices. This is an extremely dangerous practice which was blamed for the death of film actor David Carradine in a hotel room in Thailand on June 4, 2009. The fact that it is an activity that is typically engaged in while *alone* makes it potentially even deadlier. *(See also: Asphyxiation, Breath play, Edge play)*

BDSM. Acronym for Bondage, Discipline, Sadism, Masochism. Some people attribute the D or DS portion of the acronym to *Domination/submission,* but this is the result of a fairly recent effort by activists to rewrite the definition of BDSM to be "more inclusive" of the D/s lifestyle. For the purposes of this book, BDSM refers primarily to kink and fetish *activities*, while D/s refers primarily to a *relationship dynamic* or mindset. While there is often a great deal of overlap, this does not make them the same thing. *(See also: Bondage, D/s, Discipline, Masochism, Sadism)*

Babygirl. *(See: Little.)*

Ball Busting. *Ball busting* is a form of cock and ball torture (CBT) that involves striking, kicking, kneeing or squeezing a person's testicles to produce intense pain and humiliation. This practice can be extremely dangerous, as it can cause serious and permanent scrotal damage. *(See: CBT, Torture)*

Ball Crusher. *(See: Ball Busting, CBT, Torture)*

Ball Stretching. *Ball stretching* is a form of cock and ball torture (CBT*)* that involves applying devices or weights to a male's scrotum that elongate or stretch the testicles. Ball stretching devices can be constructed of steel, leather, rope, string, or any other materials designed to be attached to the scrotum and pull them away from the body. Ball stretching can be extremely dangerous, as it can sometimes result in a blockage of blood flow to the testicles, or a testicular hernia. *(See: Ball Busting, CBT, Parachute, Torture)*

Barebacking. *Barebacking* refers to having *unprotected sex,* which can potentially result in pregnancy or the transmission of sexually transmitted diseases (STDs). *(See also: Fluid bonding)*

Bathroom Use Restrictions. *Bathroom use restrictions* refer to the practice of a Dominant limiting, deferring or denying altogether the use of a toilet to his or her submissive. This is typically done to produce discomfort, pain, or humiliation – particularly if the denial of toilet privileges leads to the submissive soiling or wetting herself. *(See also: Diaper play, Humiliation, Torture, Urine play)*

Beating. *Beating* typically refers to any form of *impact play,* to include spanking, slapping, whipping, flogging, clubbing, caning, paddling, cropping, and punching. *(See also: Impact play)*

Being Serviced. A common euphemism for a Dominant or Top receiving oral sex from a submissive or bottom in a somewhat aloof fashion.

Bipoly. A person who is *bipoly* is both *bisexual and polyamorous. (See also: Polyamory)*

Blindfold. *Noun:* Any strip of cloth, accessory or device designed to be worn over the eyes to prevent a person from seeing. *Verb:* To cover the eyes of a person. Blindfolding is typically a form of sensory deprivation used in BDSM play used to heighten the wearer's fear or unease, and sometimes, to simulate anonymous sexual activity. *(See also: Bondage, Sensation play)*

Body Worship. *Body worship* is an obsession with another person's body, typically the form, musculature, genitals, or buttocks. This obsession is typically demonstrated through reverence, prostration, kissing, licking, sucking, and other types of oral sex. *(See also: Ass worship, Cock worship, Pussy Worship)*

Bondage. *Bondage* is the practice of binding, tying, strapping, boxing, caging, suspending, or otherwise restraining a person for sexual, psychological, artistic, or decorative purposes. Bondage is often combined with other forms of BDSM play such as humiliation, torture, impact play, or acting out rape fantasies. *(See also: Restraints, Self Bondage.)*

Boot Worship. A fetish that involves the obsessive adoration of a Dominant's boots. *Boot worship* often involves prostration, kissing, licking, or masturbation involving the Dominant's boots. It is commonly a part of the dynamic between a sadistic Dominant and a submissive that enjoys humiliation and forced behaviors. *(See also: FemDom, Foot fetish, Humiliation)*

Bottom. A term used in both the BDSM and gay lifestyles to refer to a person in a submissive, passive, receiving or obedient role. The term is usually applied to describe a person's *actions and behaviors* demonstrated at any given moment in time, rather than his or her deep-seated *character and thought-processes*. In a nutshell, one's actions may make him a *bottom*, while one's character may make him a submissive. There is often some overlap and it is entirely possible to be a *submissive* who is, for whatever reason, *not* in the role of a *bottom* at any given time or circumstance. *(See also: Dominant, Role play, Scene, Submissive, Top)*

Branding. *Branding* is a form of body modification, similar to tattooing, that is far more common in the BDSM lifestyle than in the general population. It typically involves the use of hot metal implements to produce burns and scar tissue on a person's skin for a variety of reasons, to include sadomasochistic pleasure, aesthetic or artistic reasons, to demonstrate ownership of a slave or submissive, or as a badge of honor. Branding is almost exclusively practiced by hard-core masochists or those with an extreme body modification fetish. *(See also: Edge play, Fire play, Scarification)*

Brat. Typically a submissive who is *generally* well-behaved, but has made misbehavior, teasing, and limited kinds of defiance or disobedience an *integral* part of her Dominant-submissive dynamic. Preferably, this occurs with the full awareness and approval of her Dom. When such is *not* the case, problems will invariably arise. *(See also: S.A.M./Sammy, Submissive, Topping from the bottom)*

Breast Bondage. *Breast bondage* involves binding the breasts with rope, straps, tape, cloth, leather, chain, or any other material to create a sensation of pressure or pain. This is often done as much for the aesthetics as it is the intense sensations produced, and is considered by some to be an art form. *(See also: Breast whipping, Kinbaku, Restraints, Rope play, Shibari)*

Breast Whipping. *Breast whipping* usually refers to the practice of striking the breasts with a flogger, crop, whip, or slapper. This is often combined with other types of breast torture, such as binding or nipple clamps.

Breath Play. Often referred to as *choking*, breath play generally consists of being sexually aroused either by choking your partner or by being choked, either as foreplay or during sex. It can involve a wide range of activities ranging from simulated or actual choking from hands around the neck, to *autoerotic asphyxiation. (See also: Asphyxiation, Autoerotic asphyxiation, Edge play)*

Brown Showers. *Also sometimes referred to as scat play.* A *brown shower* refers to any activity which involves the act of defecating on another person, or having it done to you. It is sometimes combined with *enemas* to create a more fluid experience.

Bruising. *Bruising* generally refers to the black and blue or purplish marks on the skin as the consequence of tiny capillaries in the skin being damaged or broken as the result of either impact play such as *spanking, caning, slapping, flogging, whipping or paddling*, or aggressive handling during bondage, choking, or rough sex. Bruises are quite often worn as a badge of honor by masochists and bottoms.

Caging. The practice of using a cage, crate, pen, or barred cell to restrain a person for sexual, psychological or aesthetic reasons. Caging can be used for just about any reason, to include punishment, reward, foreplay, humiliation, or even to produce a sense of security for the submissive being caged. Some submissives enjoy sleeping in cages, or staying in cages when their Dominants are away. Others use the cage as a refuge, or as a place to be sent when they feel that they have done something wrong, and must do pennance. Caging is also a favorite activity of many people in the D/s lifestyle who are into pet play. *(See also: Abduction play, Cow/Pig Submissive, Pet Play, Prison Fantasy.)*

Caning. *Caning* is a form of corporal punishment that typically consists of striking the buttocks with a thin, rattan cane. It is often erroneously assumed by those outside the BDSM culture that caning refers to the use of a heavy, stiff implement that resembles a *walking cane*, but such is *not* the case. The *cane* used in *BDSM* canings is a lightweight switch that is generally used to deliver strikes to the buttocks, but sometimes to other parts of the body, hands, or feet. Strikes are referred to as *cuts* or *strokes*, and can sometimes be severe enough to break the skin. *(See also: Cropping, Flogging, Impact play, Whipping)*

Castration Play. Though it may seem somewhat oxymoronic for most to see the words *castration* and *play* used in the same phrase, the role play aspects of this activity have a great deal of appeal to those who enjoy the use of *fear, anxiety, medical play,* and/or *knife play* as part of their BDSM activities. Typically, *castration play* consists of causing another person to fear being castrated *(having one's testicles surgically removed).* Far less common is the sort of castration play that involves a participant who actually has a *castration fantasy*, i.e. is aroused by the thought of being castrated. *(See also: CBT, Medical play, Torture)*

Catheterization. *Catheterization* typically refers to the insertion of a thin, highly flexible, surgical grade plastic tube into a person's urethra. This is usually done by medical professionals to drain urine from the bladder when a patient cannot use toilet facilities. In a BDSM context, catheterization may be done for a wide variety of reasons. The simplest might be that a person has developed a catheter fetish and simply derives pleasure from it. Other reasons for catheterization my include *humiliation, torture, prolonged bondage, caging, bathroom restrictions, or medical play*. *(See also: Bathroom Restrictions, Bondage, Caging, Humiliation, Medical Play, Torture.)*

Cattle Prod. An electrical device typically used by cattle ranchers to deliver a high-voltage, low-current electrical shock to cows to get them to move in the direction desired. When used on human beings, cattle prods produce significant pain and sometimes the loss of muscle control, and may cause burning or scarring if continuously applied to the same area. With the advent and growing popularity of *tasers and stun guns*, cattle prods have become less common in the BDSM community. *(See also: Electricity play, Torture)*

CBT. Cock and Ball Torture. This usually involves binding, caging, and/or applying pressure or other forces on the penis and testicles as to cause pain, restrict erection, or create the expectation of such. *(See also: Ball busting, Ball stretching, Parachute, Torture)*

Chamber Pot. This generally refers to a bowl, pot, pail or other receptacle used as a makeshift toilet. Traditionally, chamber pots were used by people who either did not have indoor plumbing, or could not conveniently get to a toilet in the middle of the night. Victorian era chamber pots often had a lid, and were kept under the bed. In a BDSM context, chamber pots are used in a wide variety of activities. (See also: *Bathroom Restrictions, Brown Showers, Caging, Closeting, Golden showers, Humiliation, Scat Play.)*

Chastity Belt. This refers to a device worn, and usually locked, around the pelvis and crotch of the wearer to prevent sexual intercourse and, sometimes, masturbation. It is generally believed that chastity belts were used during the Middle Ages, to ensure the chastity of wives left behind by crusaders to the Holy Land. However, there is little evidence to support this notion, as the earliest known chastity belts appeared much later, during the Renaissance. In a BDSM context, chastity belts are used on both males and females, and can be designed to prevent intercourse, masturbation, and in some cases for males, erections. *(See also: Bondage, Restraints, CBT, Humiliation, Orgasm Denial.)*

Chauffeuring. *Chauffeuring* refers to the duties of a *service submissive* that consist primarily of driving, delivering, picking up and running errands for a Dominant and possibly for other members of his or her household. Chauffeuring may or may not involve sex, wearing a uniform, and/or performing these duties in public. *(See also: Domestic, Service Submissive.)*

Choking. *(See Breath Play.)*

Closeting. Typically refers to the practice of punishing a misbehaving submissive by locking him or her in a closet or similar enclosed space. *(See also: Caging.)*

Clothespins. *Clothespins* have become a bit of an anachronism for many people who have never had to hang their just-washed laundry out to dry on a clothes line, but they *do still exist*. In the BDSM lifestyle, they are often used to apply pain and pressure to sensitive body parts, such as the lips, tongue, nipples, labia, penis, or scrotum.

Cock Worship. Cock worship describes any sexual or pseudo-sexual activity where the primary focus involves demonstrated love, adoration and reverence of a man's penis. The practice often involves kneeling, prostration, or assuming other submissive poses to emphasize the Dominant-submissive dynamic. While there is sometimes an element of humiliation or even discipline (i.e. spanking, caning, or bondage) involved, it is far more common for the Dominant to assume a somewhat aloof role while the submissive "worships at the altar." *(See also: Body worship)*

Collar. Collars are viewed by those in the D/s lifestyle in much the same way that *rings* are considered by those outside of the lifestyle. Just as a ring can symbolize anything from friendship to marriage, or have no symbolism whatsoever, so too can a collar. A collar can be comprised of just about anything, to include a ribbon around the neck, an actual pet collar, custom designed fetish-wear, or even a traditional necklace that only you know the significance of. A collar is simply *what the people involved agree that it is,* nothing more, nothing less. When a Dominant no longer feels his submissive is worthy of the collar, the submissive may be "released," meaning the collar is revoked. Alternately, a submissive may ask to be released from her collar, though generally speaking, this is a mere formality that is done out of respect. *(See also: Collar of consideration, Collar of protection, Day collar, Play collar)*

Collar of Consideration. A *provisional* collar that is offered by a Dominant to a submissive that he is considering as a potential submissive who'll presumably become eligible for a collar of greater significance at the end of the probationary period. It is typically used to give some recognition to the process of getting to know each other by formalizing a *tentative* commitment by a submissive to discontinue shopping for a Dominant while being considered by this one, and by the Dominant to treat her as his for the duration of the agreement. The terms of this tentative agreement should be negotiated *prior* to the collaring, and are typically set to expire after a relatively short period of time. *(See also: Collar)*

Collar of Protection. A collar of protection is similar in many ways to a collar of consideration, and in fact, there are often areas of overlapping functionality. Most collars of consideration are *also* collars of protection; however, *not all* collars of protection are collars of consideration. A Dominant will sometimes extend his *protection* to a submissive out of friendship or charity, even though *neither person* has any intention whatsoever of establishing a more serious relationship with the other as a consequence. The *protection* offered to the submissive in these circumstances often includes advice and guidance, approving play partners and events, and interviewing and/or approving prospective Dominants who may wish to consider the submissive. *(See also: Collar)*

Consent. *Consent,* for BDSM purposes, refers to the *informed agreement to engage in an activity,* scene or relationship, assuming that all parties have a mutual understanding of what is meant by the agreement. Evidence or proof of a partner's prior consent *may* be difficult to prove *after the fact,* which can be *problematic* considering the fact that it is typically the critical factor when it comes to criminal charges such as assault, sodomy, and rape. Even so, *documenting* consent is a relatively rare thing in the BDSM lifestyle. *(See also:*

Consensual non-consent, R.A.C.K., and S.S.C.)

Consensual Non-consent. *Consensual non-consent* is the term for a somewhat controversial practice of ostensibly *giving up the right to say no in advance* of an activity, scene, or relationship. The reason it is controversial is the simple fact that such an agreement has no legal standing whatsoever in any court of law. (So-called *slave contracts* are similarly illegal and unenforceable.) This makes the practice of consensual non-consent not only illegal, but dangerous for the Top, who could find himself - *perhaps even years later* - unexpectedly faced with criminal charges. Even *documentation* of the agreement is futile, since the agreement itself is technically *illegal.* Despite these risks, consensual non-consent is widely practiced and enjoyed by many in the lifestyle. *(See also: Consent, R.A.C.K., Slave contract, S.S.C.)*

Corset/Corsetting. A *corset* is a garment that reshapes the torso, making it appear more slender or shapely through non-elastic materials, lacing and ribs, stays or *boning*. A corset differs from a girdle, which is typically elastic and contains no lacing or ribs. Corsets may be worn by Dominants to give them a more commanding appearance, or by submissives for aesthetic, restrictive, or body-modification purposes.

Crops. *Crops,* which are sometimes referred to as riding crops or horse whips, typically consist of a long, slender and flexible shaft which is thicker and reinforced at one end to form a handle and has, at the other end, a tongue of leather, neoprene or cord called the *keeper.* The traditional shape of the keeper can be a square, rectangle, circle, half-circle, fiddle, or half-fiddle. Keepers can also come in a variety of novelty shapes, as well. The flexible shaft adds leverage and speed to the strike, while the keeper is designed to come into contact with the target. *(See also: Caning, Floggers, Impact play, Whips)*

Cuffs. *(See: Restraints)*

Cutting. *Cutting* is the practice of cutting the skin with a blade or other sharp instruments to produce pain, fear, excitement or decorative scars.

(See also: Abrasion, Branding, Castration Fantasy, Knife Play, Scarification)

Daddy Dom. A *Daddy Dom* is typically a Dominant whose primary attraction to the D/s lifestyle is a unique form of *paternalism*. The relationship dynamic may involve sexual or nonsexual *age play*, incest role-play, erotic or nonsexual spankings, and other expressions of an imagined parent-child relationship. Daddy Doms are *not* attracted to *children*, they are attracted to *adults* who exhibit childlike behaviors. *(See also: Age play, Little)*

Day Collar. A *day collar* refers to anything that is worn throughout a person's day-to-day *vanilla life*, to include at work, school, and family or social gatherings, to symbolize the collared relationship between a Dominant and submissive. A day collar may consist of just about *anything*, and need not necessarily be worn about the neck like a traditional collar. The most common varieties of day collars are necklaces, chokers, ribbons, bracelets, anklets, and rings. *(See also: Collar, Collar of consideration, Collar of protection, Everyday collar, Play collar.)*

Deferred/Delayed Gratification. *(See: Orgasm denial/control, Masturbation restrictions, Mitts)*

Diaper Play. A form of age-play involving the wear of traditional or adult-diapers while assuming the role of an infant. Sometimes used in play involving the control (or lack of control) of the bodily functions. *(See also: AB/DL, Age Play, Infantilism, Littles.)*

Dilation. *Dilation* refers to an activity which involves the use of a medical speculum to open a woman's cervix as part of a medical scene. This procedure can be dangerous if done by an untrained person.

Discipline. Traditionally the "D" in BDSM. Generally speaking, it refers to various forms of corporal punishment, such as spanking, caning, beating, flogging, whipping, or slapping. In a more subtle sense, discipline can also refer to the mental discipline required to be a good

Dominant or submissive, which sometimes requires a disciplined mindset that allows a person to resist his or her natural impulses. *(See also: Caning, Crops, Flogger, Impact play, Paddles, Spanking, Whips)*

D.M. Acronym for Dungeon Monitor. Typically someone in authority whose role is to monitor the activities of a particular establishment to ensure that none of the house rules are being broken.

Domestic. The Domestic, sometimes referred to as a *service submissive,* is a submissive who is expected to perform domestic duties in the Dominant's household, such as cooking, cleaning, childcare, and yard work. More often than not, the Domestic is also expected to be available sexually to the Dominant, his other submissives, or guests. It is entirely possible, but relatively rare, for a Domestic sub to be in a nonsexual D/s relationship. *(See also: Service submissive, Submissive)*

Dominant. One who acts in a domineering or authoritative role in life, and especially in relationships. A Dominant may be a "true Dominant" in the sense that this trait is firmly hard-wired into his psyche and he simply doesn't know any other way to be, or he may be acting out a role, whether consciously or unconsciously. A Dominant is defined primarily by his need to control his environment and personal interactions and his skill at being able to do so.

Domme. A female Dominant, sometimes referred to as a Dominatrix or Mistress. Generally speaking, a Domme may refer to *any* female Dominant, however, outside of the D/s lifestyle, the stereotype typically fits the FemDom Mistress. The correct pronunciation of *domme* is identical to *dom. (See also: Dominant, FemDom)*

Dungeon. - A place designed and furnished for BDSM play. Some dungeons are private homes or communal playspaces managed by local BDSM groups, while others are commercial establishments. Dungeons may host events such as workshops, demos, classes or parties. Dungeons typically have an area set apart from the playspace for conversation and/or refreshments. *(See also: Munch, Scene)*

Edge Play. *Edge play* refers to BDSM play that is generally considered to have a *higher-than-usual* risk of serious harm or death (i.e. breath play, knife play, or gun play), or may be of a particularly sensitive nature (i.e. age play, rape play or scat play). The definition of edge play is highly subjective, and ever-evolving. What might have been considered edge play a few years ago may be considered relatively mundane today, and *vice-versa*. Before the advent of HIV/AIDS, a scene involving *wet play* (blood) would not have been considered particularly risky; today bodily fluids are a *big deal.*

Electricity Play. *Electricity play* is any BDSM activity that involves the use of high-voltage, low amperage, low-frequency devices that deliver stimulation to the skin, typically in a fashion that *looks* much more intimidating than it actually merits. The most common of these types of devices are *TENS units* and *violet wands*. Electricity play can be dangerous for certain individuals, and these devices should never be used by anyone with a pacemaker, insulin pump, or any other kind of implanted electrically operated medical device or metallic joint replacements. Otherwise, they are safe for use almost anywhere on the body, except around the eyes. As is the case with *any* electrical device, they should not be used in or around liquids, particularly flammable liquids, which could be ignited by the electrical discharge. *(See also: TENS Unit, Purple Wand, Violet Wand.)*

Eloctrostimulation. *(See Electricity play, EMS Unit, TENS unit, Violet Wand)*

EMS Unit. *EMS* stands for *Electrical Muscle Stimulation.* EMS units are typically used in medicine, sports training, cosmetic treatments, and in therapy to produce repeated muscle contractions through electrical stimulation. EMS devices range in quality and complexity from the very intricate and expensive machines used by medical and sports professionals to the simpler, less expensive devices marketed to the flabby masses via late-night infomercials. The odd experience of having your muscles stimulated electrically to *involuntarily* contract and release in rapid succession makes the EMS unit an interesting option for BDSM sensation play. *(See also: Electricity play, TENS unit, Violet wand)*

Enema. Refers to the introduction of fluids into a person's rectum and colon, which results in an uncomfortable expansion of the lower intestinal tract. This procedure, which is done medically to treat conditions like constipation and encopresis, or to administer certain drugs, is sometimes done for recreational purposes by some in the BDSM lifestyle as part of control scenes, humiliation play, medical play, bathroom use restrictions, or punishment. *(See also: Bathroom Use Restrictions, Brown showers, Medical Play, Humiliation)*

Enforced Chastity. The practice of preventing one's submissive from engaging in any kind of sexual activity or stimulation involving the genitals. This may involve wearing a device such as a chastity belt or some other secure appliance around the groin area, or even bulky mitts or sleeves on the hands and arms to prevent masturbation. *(See also: Arm Sleeves, Chastity Belt, Mitts, Orgasm Control)*

Everyday Collar. *(See: Day collar)*

Eye Contact Restriction. This refers to the practice of forbidding or restricting direct eye contact between a submissive and his or her Dominant, and in some cases, other individuals. Eye contact restrictions are more common in the *Gorean* tradition, where slaves are traditionally taught to lower their gaze in the presence of Masters, but they may be practiced in a variety of other kinds of relationships and situations, as well. *(See also: Gor, Protocol.)*

Face-sitting. *Face sitting,* also sometimes referred to as *queening,* is typically a form of humiliation play that involves sitting on another person's face in such a way as to force the Dominant's genitals or anus into the submissive's mouth. The submissive may be held in position by the body weight of the Dominant, by restraints, or by a simple command to remain in position. Those who engage in this practice regularly may employ specialized equipment or furnishings, such a *queening stool, or smotherbox. (See also: Pussy worship, Queening,*

Queening stool, Smotherbox)

Felching. The act of sucking or licking semen from another person's anus; sometimes the term is also applied to the same activity performed on a woman's vagina. Felching is usually an act of humiliation forced upon a submissive by a Sadistic Dom or FemDom Mistress. It's typically far more common to hear it discussed for its shock value, the most common reaction being, *"There's a word for that?"* than it is to actually see it done. *(See also: FemDom, Humiliation, Sadistic Dom)*

Figging. *Figging* refers to the practice of inserting a piece of *freshly peeled ginger* into the anus, which causes a strong burning sensation which lasts twenty to thirty minutes without causing any permanent damage. *(See also: Sensation play, Torture)*

Fire Play. Any BDSM activity that typically involves flame or high heat. Two of the most common forms of fire play are *branding* and *cupping*. *(See also Branding, Cupping, Edge play, Scarification, Sensation Play.)*

Fist Fucking. *(See: Fisting)*

Fisting. *Fisting* refers to the insertion of the entire hand into the vagina or rectum, usually with the help of lubricants. Fisting is sometimes referred to as *handballing, or fist fucking*. Fisting may be done as part of masturbation, or performed on another person. Once the hand is inserted, the hand may be clenched or flexed to intensify the sensations.

Flame Play. *(See: Fire Play.)*

Flip-Flopper. *(See: Switch.)*

Fluid Bonding. *Fluid bonding (sometime referred to as body fluid monogamy)* generally refers to relationships between people who have agreed to engage in unprotected sex which involves the exchange of bodily fluids. A fluid bond can also sometimes refer to a BDSM toy or piece of equipment that should be reserved for the sole use of its owner because it comes into contact with bodily fluids such as semen, secretions, or blood. *(See also: Barebacking)*

Flogger. A small hand-held whip with multiple tails or strips of leather, which are called *falls*. Floggers are sometimes referred to as a *cats-o'-nine-tails.* Most modern floggers used by those in the lifestyle are specially constructed for specific purposes, such as appearance, force of impact or type of sensation *(high or low)*, durability, grip, and weight. Contrary to popular belief, floggings are seldom very painful. The sensations involved, when getting a flogging, are often compared by recipients to getting a "thuddy massage," and for many, the psychological effects of a flogging far outweigh the physical. Generally speaking, the heavier the flogger, the *"thuddier"* the flogging. The lighter and more wiry the flogger, the more it will sting. Either way, the longer the flogging continues the more sensitive the areas of the body being flogged will become. *(See also: Whip, Cat o' Nine Tails.)*

Flogging Horse. A *flogging horse* is typically a custom-built, padded piece of dungeon furniture which often resembles a bench or saw-horse used to secure and position a submissive in restraints while he or she is being flogged. *(See also: Flogger, Racks, St. Andrew's Cross, Table play, Whip)*

Food Control. Refers to any activity where the Dominant controls the type or quantity of food consumed by the submissive or the circumstances under which it may be consumed. Sometimes food control also includes the intake of fluids. Food control is often done for *dietary reasons* in an effort by a Dominant to reshape or modify a submissive's physical characteristics or weight, or to provide a submissive with the purpose, discipline, or willpower which he or she lacks. Other times, food control is done purely for disciplinary or punitive purposes. *(See also: Discipline)*

Foot Partialism. *(See: Foot Worship.)*

Foot Worship. *Foot worship* refers to foot fetishism, also sometimes called *foot partialism, or podophilia.* In *foot worship,* the feet are considered to be objects of adoration by the submissive, and they figure prominently into activities such as humiliation play, boot licking, and masturbation. *(See also: Body Worship, Boot Worship, Humiliation, Paraphilia.)*

Formal Collar. Also sometimes referred to as a *slave collar, full collar, or true collar.* The formal collar is often said to be analogous to a *wedding ring.* It is symbolic of what is usually intended to be a lifelong committed and loving relationship between a Dominant and his submissive. Formal collaring ceremonies, similar to weddings, are often performed to commemorate and consecrate the beginning of the relationship. The symbolism of a formal collar obviously means different things to different couples, but it is often referred to as the ultimate gift of one's submission and self to another; a manifestation of complete and total *power exchange.* *(See also: Collar, Collar of consideration, Collar of Protection, Day collar, Play collar, Training collar)*

Forced Bed Wetting. The practice of forcing submissives to urinate in the bed they must lie in, or to wet themselves in general, in order to emphasize the Dominant's control over the submissive, or as part of bathroom access control. *(See also: AB/DL, Age Play, Bathroom access control, Diaper play, Humiliation, Tickling, Urine Play)*

Forced Collaring. Forced collaring is a uniquely *online phenomenon* practiced almost entirely by pretenders to the D/s lifestyle. The notion that a person can be forced into a *collared relationship* against his or her will is ludicrous, but the mythology that surrounds it continues to be perpetuated by those who are ignorant of the lifestyle and the true symbolism of a collar. Many of the would-be submissives who encounter forced collaring for the first time in online chat rooms and similar venues have *no idea* that it's a farce, and so they play along, thinking that perhaps it's some sort of requirement for entry into the mysterious sisterhood of submissives. Invariably, the victim soon learns that the supposed Dominant *doesn't have a clue,* the entire situation was a *joke*, and that she's been made to look like a complete idiot. For more information on this topic, see Chapter 5: Online BDSM Relationships. *(See also: Collar)*

Forced Dressing. *Forced dressing* refers to any scene or activity where the Dominant requires the submissive to wear specific types or articles of clothing. Typically, forced dressing is used as a part of forced feminization or humiliation play; i.e. when a FemDom forces a submissive male to wear effeminate clothing or lingerie. *(See also: FemDom, Forced Feminization, Humiliation)*

Forced Feminization. *Forced Feminization* is the practice, commonly imposed by FemDom Mistresses upon submissive males, of forcing them to assume traditionally female roles, positions, and traits as part of a humiliation regimen. *(See also: FemDom, Forced Dressing, Humiliation)*

Forced Heterosexuality. *Forced heterosexuality* is the practice of compelling a submissive who typically self-identifies as homosexual to engage in sexual activity with a person of the opposite sex, generally as part of humiliation play. *(See also: FemDom, Humiliation.)*

Forced Homosexuality. *Forced homosexuality* is the practice of compelling a submissive who typically self-identifies as heterosexual to engage in sexual activity with a person of the same sex, generally as part of humiliation play. *(See also: FemDom, Humiliation.)*

Forced Masturbation. *Forced Masturbation* is the practice of forcing a submissive to engage in masturbation while the Dominant, and/or others observe. It is often utilized as part of humiliation play or age play. *(See also: Age Play, Humiliation.)*

Forced Nudity. *Forced Nudity* refers to the practice of denying a submissive the right or opportunity to wear clothing. Forced nudity may be for the duration of a single scene or event, or may be enforced 24/7 in a Dominant's household.

Forced Orgasm. *Forced Orgasm* is the practice of causing a person to experience an orgasm, *ostensibly* against their will. Since this is, in reality, *highly unlikely* for fairly obvious reasons, forced orgasm is generally associated with *role play* involving rape, abduction, bondage, and humiliation. While both men *and* women sometimes fantasize about being forced to have unwilling orgasms by a Dominant, men have the unique challenge of being unable to convincingly simulate an erection or orgasm. A question that frequently arises on this topic is: *Why wouldn't anyone want to have an orgasm?* The answer is quite simple: *Guilt.* Society teaches many of us from birth that we shouldn't be turned on by many of the things that we do find stimulating. There can also be religious, relationship-related, and psychological reasons for repressing the urge to orgasm. One fairly common example is the woman who, as the result of a rape or sexual abuse in her past, now associates sex with the abuse and finds it difficult, if not impossible, to have an orgasm the "normal" way. Role play that involves being "forced" to have an orgasm against her will allows her to enjoy the benefits of an orgasm without experiencing the associated guilt for having done so.

Forced Servitude. *Forced Servitude* is the practice of compelling a person, typically a submissive, to perform service-related tasks for a Dominant and/or other members of his or her household.

Forced Smoking. *Forced smoking* refers to the practice of compelling a bottom to inhale the Top's exhaled cigarette smoke. It is practiced perhaps most commonly by FemDoms as part of humiliation, sissification, asphyxiation, or torture play. This can be done in a variety of ways, ranging from simply blowing smoke into a bound bottom's face to pumping smoke into the bottom's hood or *gas mask.* The discomfort felt by the bottom, naturally, is significantly increased if he or she is a *non-smoker.* *(See also: Breath Play, FemDom, Humiliation, Sissification, Torture)*

Forniphilia. The derivation of pleasure from being considered and used as if you were a piece of furniture. This may include humiliation, bondage, blindfolds, gags or other forms of BDSM play, but may also be as simple as having a person kneel and be used as a footstool. Unlike most other forms of bondage, forniphilia play may involve remaining bound for extended periods of time, and in those cases, should be practiced with caution. *(See also: Human Furniture, Bondage, Humiliation, FemDom)*

Furry. This term refers to someone who engages in a particular form of animal *role play* characterized by adopting, to the greatest extent possible, the *appearance and some mannerisms* of a chosen animal. Furries envision themselves and role play the part of *humans in animal bodies* unlike *primals*, who typically imagine themselves as *animals in human bodies*. Many furry role players have an assortment of animal personas, avatars, or costumes to choose from and will switch between them frequently. The most common furry animal roles chosen are cats, dogs ponies, skunks, foxes, rabbits, wolves, and ferrets. Growth in the furry phenomenon has sprung mostly out of *cosplay fandom;* it is immensely popular among teens and young adults. It is, for that reason, sometimes viewed as a *gateway or introduction* to more traditional D/s relationships and BDSM activities. *Furry role play* is *not* the same thing as *pet role play*, even though there may sometimes be significant overlap. *(See also: Pet play, Pony play, Ponygirl/Ponyboy, Primal, Role play)*

Gag. A gag refers to just about anything placed in or over the mouth (OTM) or even over the nose (OTN) to prevent speech, outcries, biting, or the like. Gags can include such things as an unpretentious strip of cloth, a wide strip of duct tape, a wooden rod, a ball-gag, open-mouth bracing, or even a pony bit.

Gang Rape Fantasy. Refers to fantasies and/or role play involving being forced to submit to sex with multiple partners, usually in conjunction with abduction play, bondage, torture, or humiliation play. Expressing a gang rape fantasy or any kind of rape fantasy does *not* mean that someone desires to be raped in *real life.* When engaging in any form of rape-related role play, *particularly with new play partners*, it is *highly* recommended that you *thoroughly document* the consensual nature of the planned activity prior to the scene. *(See also: Consent, Consensual non-consent, Prison fantasy, Rape fantasy)*

Gas Mask. Gas masks are typically military surplus protective masks and/or hoods originally designed to filter chemical or biological toxins out of the wearer's breathing air. Usually, the original filters have been removed, so as not to restrict or affect the wearer's breathing. Gas masks are used for the same purposes as any other BDSM hood, which is commonly to create discomfort, restrict the wearer's vision, hearing, or ability to speak, produce feelings of claustrophobia, or to humiliate. Gas masks are also sometimes worn by bottoms in asphyxiation play or forced smoking play and by Tops in abduction or rape fantasy play to conceal their identities. *(See also: Abduction play, Asphyxiation play, Forced Smoking, Hoods, Humiliation, Smoking play)*

Gates of Hell. Refers to a device worn around the penis and testicles typically consisting of a connected series of rings that encircle the penis with a ring or strap that is secured around the testicles to keep the device in place. The gates of hell may or may not be locked into place with a lock or securing mechanism. The device is used primarily for cock and ball torture (CBT) or for aesthetic purposes. *(See also: CBT)*

Girlfag. A person who was born and remains assigned female, yet feels a strong sexual attraction to gay and bisexual men. A *girlfag* differs from a *fag hag* because while a *fag hag* has a strong affinity for gay and bisexual men, her relationships with them are strictly platonic; she is sexually attracted to heterosexual men.

Given Away. Being *"given away"* is typically an activity enjoyed by *some* Master/slave couples which consists of a Master bestowing a third party with the temporary use of his slave for purely sexual purposes. *(See also: Auction, Master, Slave)*

Golden Shower. *Golden showers* is a euphemistic term for one form of *urine play,* which is also called *urolagnia, urophilia, or water sports.* It is generally an activity enjoyed by people who are sexually aroused by the thought or sight of urine or urination. This sort of play may take various forms, to include infantilism, diaper play, bathroom access control play, humiliation play, urine consumption, clothes or bed wetting, or voyeurism. Contrary to popular belief, people are told to wash their hands after urination not because urine is unsanitary, but because *genitals* are. Uncontaminated urine is actually *sterile. (See also: Bathroom Access Control, Brown showers, Humiliation, Scat, Urine play, Water sports)*

Gor. Gor is the name of a fictional planet whose people were the subject of a series of pulp fiction novels by John Frederick Lange Jr. writing under the pen name *John Norman.* Devotees of the *"Gorean"* subculture of the D/s lifestyle pattern their relationship and social dynamics, language, customs, protocols, and even their sexual activities after the manner of the people of this fictional planet, which is also sometimes referred to by the series publishers as *"Counter-Earth."* The planet, as envisioned by John Norman, is ruled by a technologically advanced insect-like race of Priest-Kings who have, over the course of eons, transported large numbers of humans from earth to populate the planet, many of whom are made slaves, if they happen to be female. *(See also: Master, Kajira)*

Group Marriage. Generally refers to any marriage or relationship resembling a marriage that has more than two partners, typically without regard to the legal standing of the relationship in the eyes of the law. Group marriage is also sometimes referred to as *plural marriage. (See also: Polyamory, Polyandry, Polygyny.)*

Gun Play. *Gun play* is a form of BDSM *edge-play* which consists of using a firearm or simulated firearm to create sensations of fear and/or arousal in the bottom. This sort of play can be *extremely* dangerous if anyone involved in the scene is unfamiliar with basic weapons safety procedures. Even overly curious bystanders can put themselves or others at risk if proper precautions are not meticulously observed. Gun play is sometimes combined with abduction or rape fantasy play. *(See* *also: Abduction play, Edge play, Gang rape fantasy, Humiliation, Interrogation play, Rape fantasy)*

Guydyke. A person who was born and remains assigned male, yet his primary sexual attraction is to gay and bisexual females, usually to the complete exclusion of heterosexual females.

Hairbrush Spanking. Paddling or spanking with the flat back-side of a hairbrush. *(See also: Paraphilia, Paddling, Spanking)*

Hair Pulling. Refers to being sexually aroused by the grasping, pulling, binding, yanking or dragging by the hair in a scene or during sex play.

Handballing. *(See: Fisting)*

Handcuffs. *(See: Restraints)*

Harness. Refers to anything that is worn about the torso, and to which you attach *other things.* A simple example would be a *dildo harness,* which is usually *(but not always)* worn around the hips and groin and is designed to hold a dildo in place for *pegging.* Other common types of harnesses include cock and ball torture harnesses, chastity harnesses, purely decorative body harnesses, and specialty bondage harnesses. Some harnesses are designed to be used *only* with other types of equipment, fetish furniture, frames, hoists, swings or devices. *(See also: Bondage, Dildo harness, Pegging)*

Hoods. *Hoods*, unlike *blindfolds*, are typically fitted over the *entire head.* They are commonly constructed from cotton, silk, spandex, leather, rubber, PVC, nylon or other synthetic fabrics. Some hoods come with straps, flaps, and holes; others *may not*. Some are designed to keep people from seeing out; others are designed to keep people from seeing in. Most hoods function to limit a person's *vision;* others may be uniquely constructed to limit a person's ability to speak, hear, breathe, *or all of the above.* Hoods may be simple or devious, sensual or cruel, loose-fitting or elastic, and they may be secured in place by laces, zippers, snaps, buttons, straps, or Velcro. *(See also: Blindfold,*

Sensory deprivation, Masks)

Hot Wax Play. *Hot wax play* generally consists of dripping or pouring molten candle wax onto someone's skin to produce erotic *sensations*, for *aesthetic* purposes, or *both*. The types of candle wax used for erotic wax play *typically* fall into two categories: *paraffin* (a man-made, petroleum-based compound) and *beeswax* (which is secreted by the wax glands of worker bees). There are many other varieties of wax that can be used, but they all generally fall into these two categories, differing only in the various additives that are combined with the waxes to change its properties, such as its burn characteristics, melting point, plasticity, or effects upon the skin. *(See also: Sensation play)*

Human Furniture. *(See: Forniphilia)*

Humbler. A *humbler* is a device which consists of a testicle cuff mounted at the center of a bar or board that is mounted behind the legs. The cuff forces the wearer to keep his legs pulled forward, since straightening the legs causes discomfort by stretching the scrotum. *(See also: Ball crusher, Ball Stretching, CBT)*

Hypnotism. *Hypnotism* generally refers to a form of BDSM play which involves the *actual or simulated* placement of a person into a hypnotic or highly suggestible trance-like state, during which he or she may be instructed to act out imagined sexual or erotic scenarios. *(See also: Age Play, Infantilism, Kidnapping Fantasy, Knife Play, Rape Fantasy, etc.)*

Ice Play. *Ice play* refers to any BDSM play activity that utilizes ice to enhance erotic sensations, produce discomfort or pain, or even to startle a play partner. Ice play can range from the very simple act of running an ice cube over a person's erogenous zones, to very complex and potentially dangerous activities, such as the use of ice dildos. *(See also: Sensation Play)*

Immobilization. *Immobilization* refers to any BDSM activity that involves rendering a person immobile. This usually accomplished through various forms of bondage, but can also include other means, such as mental bondage, forniphilia, queening/smothering, or forcibly being held down. *(See also: Bondage, Face Sitting, Forniphilia, Kinbaku, Mummification, Queening, Restraints, Rope Play, Shibari, Smotherbox)*

Impact Play. Impact play is a generic term which refers to virtually any BDSM activity that involves striking, such as *spanking, slapping, caning, paddling, whipping, or cropping*. *(See also: Caning, Crops, Flogging, OTK spanking, Paddling, Slapping, Spanking, Whipping)*

Infantilism. Infantilism is sometimes referred to as Adult Baby/Diaper Lover (AB/DL) play. Infantilism in BDSM usually refers to the derivation of pleasure from fantasies and role play involving a return to infancy. This typically involves exhibiting baby-like behavior, such as wearing (and soiling) diapers, drinking from baby bottles, sucking on pacifiers, sleeping in cribs, and similar activities. Scenes involving infantilism generally requires another person, in addition to the *"baby,"* who assumes the role of a parent, caretaker, babysitter, and on rare occasions, another infant. The infantilism play *may or may not be sexual* in nature, as is the case with most kinds of *age play*. *(See also: AB/DL, Age Play, Babygirls, Diaper play, Littles, Role Play, Urine play)*

Injection Play. *Injection play* refers to the use of *hypodermics* in BDSM needle play. Hypodermic needles are *hollow*, and designed to inject or sample fluids from the body; that means the needle has to be *thicker* and will usually produce a slightly more painful poke. Some studies have shown that roughly 10% of the population suffers from *trypanophobia*, which is the fear of hypodermic needles. Hypodermic needle play occurs most often in BDSM *medical role-play scenes. (See also: Edge play, Needle play, Medical play)*

Interrogation Play. *Interrogation play* refers to role play that simulates the aggressive questioning of a suspect or prisoner, often under duress, the threat of harm, or torture. Interrogation play is most commonly engaged in as part of abduction play, humiliation play, medical play or hypnotism play. *(See also: Abduction play, Humiliation play, Hypnotism play, Injection play, Medical play, Prison fantasy, Straitjacket)*

Kajira. The term kajira *(plural: kajirae)* refers to the female slaves featured in the sci-fi erotic pulp fiction series of books about the planet Gor by John Norman. There are *male* slaves on Gor, as well, however they are far fewer in number and, unlike the women who are either bred for slavery or kidnapped from Earth, the male slaves of Gor typically become slaves as the result of war, criminality, or indebtedness. Male slaves are individually called *kajirus*, and *kajiri* in the plural. *(See also: Gor, Master, Slave)*

Kidnapping Fantasy. *(See: Abduction play)*

Kinbaku. *(See: Shibari.)*

Kitten Play. *(See: Pet play)*

Kneeling. *Kneeling* is sometimes used as a euphemism for *submitting* to a Dominant but is, more often than not, a reference to assuming a submissive posture by sitting on the floor on your knees. Various fetish culture sub-groups may place more or less emphasis on the significance of kneeling. Goreans, for example, teach slaves to assume a series of positions on command from their Masters, many of which are kneeling positions. *(See also: Gor, Kajira, Protocol, Master, Slave, Submissive)*

Knife Play. *Knife play* refers to any BDSM activity that involves knives, blades or other sharp objects. Knife play can be exceedingly dangerous when performed by inexperienced or reckless individuals. The blades used in knife play may or may not be terribly sharp, depending on the circumstances. In some cases, the mere thought of a blade – *sharp or not* – is enough to conjure up the requisite fear that makes knife play interesting for so many people. Regardless, *before* engaging in knife play with *anyone*, one should always learn something about the experience level of the person wielding the blades, learn how sharp and clean the blades are, and clarify whether or not there should be any *blood* involved. *(See also: Abduction play, Edge play, Fluid bonding, Interrogation play, Role play, Wet play)*

Lady-boy. Typically refers to an effeminate gay Southeast Asian male, usually in his teens or twenties, who appears in almost every respect, except for having male *sex organs*, to be a female. They often work as models, escorts, and prostitutes in the tourist regions of Thailand and the Philippines and have become well-known outside of Asia thanks to the internet.

Latex. *(See: Rubber)*

Lesser God Dominant. The Lesser God Dominant, *sometimes referred to as Lord, Prophet, Pharoah, or Pharoanic Lord,* is a Dominant who thrives on the worship of his submissives. This adoration and worship, which can sometimes take the form of highly ritualistic activities and behaviors, has but one purpose, which is the ego gratification of the Lesser God. It is relatively common for the real-life households of Lesser God Doms to forsake all traditional forms of religion in order to practice their own *home-grown* religion, with the Dominant at its head and submissives as adoring acolytes. In such cases, the Dominant is usually either regarded as a demi-god or prophet. *(See also: Dominant, Religious fantasy)*

Limits. Limits refer to qualifications or limitations that are placed on a BDSM scene or relationship that specify what the participants will or will not tolerate. Limits are typically discussed prior to participating in a scene, or at the beginning of a relationship. Dominants *and* submissives, Tops *and* bottoms can have limits. There are several different kinds of *limits*, including:

- **Hard Limits:** Activities that will not be tolerated, under any circumstances. Hard limits are, by *definition*, non-negotiable and not subject to debate or persuasion. Violating a person's hard limits is considered an extremely serious offense in the BDSM culture.
- **Soft Limits:** Activities that a person may be generally inclined to refuse, subject to circumstances, persuasion, or the right partner. Violating a soft limit without prior consent is still considered a serious breach of trust.

- **Must Limits:** An activity that is a requirement or a requisite condition of a scene. One example might be a bottom's requirement that aftercare be provided following a scene, or a Top's requirement that his play partners sign a declaration of good health prior to any scene.
- **Time Limits:** A limitation on how long a scene can last, or a set time where it must end.
- **No Limits:** The term is sometimes used as a synonym for Total Power Exchange (TPE), but most often refers to a consensual agreement between a Top and bottom that there will be no limits of any kind in an ensuing scene or relationship. This is generally considered to be an extremely unwise thing to do, since even the most experienced and hardened BDSM practitioners have *some limits.*

Little. *A Little,* sometimes referred to as a *Baby, Babygirl, Lolita, Loli, Lolly, Little Girl, Little One, or Tot,* is a submissive who finds great joy in embracing her inner child. This sort of *age play* often involves behaving, speaking and/or dressing in a child-like manner, and may or may not involve sex or other adult-appropriate themes. While the great majority of Littles and their Daddy Doms find age play to be sexually stimulating, there are also those who simply find comfort in the simulated adult-child dynamic, and do not associate it in any way with sex. *(See also: Age play, AB/DL, Daddy Dom, Diaper play, Infantilism)*

Lolita. *(See: Little.)*

Masochism. *Masochism,* which is sometimes referred to as *sadomasochism, S&M, or S/M,* refers to the derivation of arousal, pleasure, or sexual gratification from inflicting or receiving pain or humiliation. Aside from its association with *sadism* and *BDSM*, there are clinical psychological classifications of sexual masochism are sometimes the subject of debate. They are:

- Class I Sexual Masochist: Bothered by, but not seeking out, fantasies. May be preponderantly sadists with minimal masochistic tendencies and/or non-sadomasochistic with minimal masochistic tendencies

- Class II Sexual Masochist: Equal mix of sadistic and masochistic tendencies. Like to receive pain but also like to be dominant partner (in this case, sadists). Sexual orgasm is achieved without pain or humiliation.
- Class III Sexual Masochist: Masochists with minimal to no sadistic tendencies. Preference for pain and/or humiliation (which facilitates orgasm), but not necessary to orgasm. Capable of romantic attachment.
- Class IV Sexual Masochist: Exclusive masochists (i.e. Cannot form typical romantic relationships, cannot achieve orgasm without pain or humiliation).

Master. *Master* is an appellation, title, or even a term of endearment which may be used by a slave or submissive for his or her Dominant. Some Dominants consider *Master* to be a generic *synonym* for Dominant, although that practice is generally most prevalent in the Gorean subculture. Other Dominants reserve the use of the title of *Master* only to those whom they have collared. *(See also: Collar, Dominant, Gor, Slave, Submissive)*

Masturbation Restrictions. Refers to any activity or scene that prevents or limits a bottom's ability to masturbate, either in the short term (i.e. for a scene) or for the long term (i.e. days, weeks, or months). Masturbation restrictions may take the form of a command by the Dominant to avoid masturbation for a specific period of time or under specific circumstances, or can consist of restrictions enforced by devices or clothing. It is also sometimes used for amusement, teasing, or torture by having a bottom masturbate to the point where he or she is at the point of orgasm, and then is commanded to stop. Once the impending orgasm has been deferred, the cycle is repeated again and again, growing more frustrating for the bottom with each interrupted orgasm. *(See also: Chastity belt, Humiliation, Mitts)*

Medical Fantasy. Medical fantasy and role play refers to assuming the roles of a medical professional (doctor or nurse, for example) and patient for purposes of BDSM play or sexual arousal and gratification. Medical play typically consists of simulated examinations, treatments, procedures, injections, operations or torture. It is sometimes combined with age play, abduction and interrogation play, CBT, or even *pet play* in the form of *veterinary role play. (See also: Age play, Abduction play, CBT, Infantilism, Injection play, Interrogation play, Pet play)*

Mentoring. *Mentoring* refers to the practice of guiding, teaching and advising another on aspects of the D/s or BDSM lifestyles. Typically a Dominant will mentor another Dominant, or a submissive will mentor another submissive, and the relationship is a casual, friendly one rather than a formal one.

Misandry. Hatred or dislike of men as a class; not necessarily targeting men as individuals. Often used as a significant part of the FemDom's sadistic role-reversal repertoire. *(See also: CBT, FemDom, Humiliation, Sadism)*

Mitts. *BDSM mitts* are typically made of leather or other heavy-duty materials, and are used to prevent a bottom from using his or her hands and, most commonly, *to prevent masturbation.* Other common uses include immobilizing the wrists and hands by attaching them to other bondage gear, hobbling someone to make an assigned task near-impossible to accomplish, or for disciplinary or humiliation purposes. *(See also: Bondage, Humiliation, Masturbation restrictions)*

Mouth Bit. A *mouth bit* is a type of *gag* which consists of a cylindrical bar placed between the teeth of the wearer, and held in place by straps or a bridle. Actual horse bits are generally made of metal, but the mouth bits used in BDSM play are usually made from rubber or a rigid material (plastic/metal) with a pliable coating to provide more protection for the teeth and lips. Mouth bits are most commonly used in pony play, but are also used in other types of scenes and play. A mouth bit will not prevent speech, but will make it more difficult. *(See also: Bondage, Gags, Pet play, Pony Play)*

Mummification. *Mummification* refers to bondage play consisting of *wrapping* parts or all of a person's body with fabric, bandages, plastic wrap, rubber, duct tape, tarps, or similar materials. Mummification is often combined with abduction play, bondage play, humiliation play, breath play, torture, and many other forms of BDSM play. Mummification can create a risk of postural asphyxiation. When mummification includes the subject's head and face, great care must be taken to avoid suffocation. A reliable pair of heavy-duty emergency shears should always be kept nearby in the event that an emergency requires the rapid release of the wrapped subject. *(See also: Bondage, Breath play, Humiliation, Postural asphyxiation)*

Munch. A *munch* typically refers to a regular gathering of a D/s lifestyle group for socializing, meeting new people and, often, a meal. Munches are almost always conducted in public places, in an entirely *vanilla* fashion. This allows first-time visitors, who may be curious or hesitant, to attend the event and enjoy themselves without feeling any unnecessary pressure. Munches also allow the group to learn a little something about new or unfamiliar individuals before inviting them to other more sensitive events. *(See also: Protocol)*

Needle Play. Needle play typically consist of placing acupuncture needles into various fleshy parts of the body to induce or reduce fear, create aesthetically pleasing patterns or designs, stimulate the nervous system, cause or reduce pain, and for other therapeutic reasons. Acupuncture needles may be inserted into the flesh *perpendicular* to the skin or at a *secant*, where the needle is pushed through a fold of skin in such a way that the tip emerges again, leaving only the center part of the needle shaft below the skin. This aesthetic mode of needle play has recently become quite popular as a way to anchor *decorative corset lacing* to a person's back or chest. *(See also: Edge play, Injection play, Medical play)*

Novice Submissive. A *novice submissive* is typically a person who has very recently discovered and become excited about the D/s or BDSM lifestyle, and has decided that she badly wants to be a part of it as quickly as possible. This is sometimes referred to as *sub frenzy.* This often involves a frenzied quest to find a Master, *any Master*, as quickly as possible.

Odaxelagnia. *Odaxelagnia* refers to a fetish or *paraphilia* which involves becoming sexually aroused by biting. *(See also: Paraphilia.)*

Orgasm Control/Denial. The practice of denying or delaying a submissive's orgasm, which can be done for a multitude of reasons, to include heightening arousal, demonstrating a Dominant's power over a submissive, or to punish. Orgasm denial can be long term, meaning the subject may be denied permission to have an orgasm for days or weeks, or short term, where the orgasm is deferred for just seconds or minutes. Orgasm denial may or may not involve the submissive requesting from the Dominant permission to have an orgasm. (See also: Masturbation restrictions)

OTK. Acronym for *Over The Knee*. OTK refers to a specific style of spanking, generally (but not necessarily) practiced by those who are into *Age Play*. The submissive lies face down across the lap of the Dominant, who administers a spanking. The spanking may be characterized as punishment *or* reward, depending on the relationship dynamic, and may or may not involve genital fondling or other sexual activities. *(See also: Age play, Humiliation, Impact play, Spanking)*

Painslut. The *painslut* is typically an *extreme masochist*, or someone who enjoys the sensations of pain to an extreme or dangerous degree. The painslut's *primary* interest, attraction, and fetish is *pain.* The use of the suffix *slut* is not incidental, as Painsluts are often known almost as much for their promiscuity as they are for their extreme brand of masochism. *(See also: Masochism)*

Parachute. A small conical leather ring or collar with four or more small chains attached, which makes it resemble a tiny parachute. Parachutes are affixed around the scrotum, and weights are attached to the parachute's chains in order to stretch the scrotum as part of *cock and* *ball torture (CBT). Ball stretching* is a potentially dangerous activity. *(See also: Ball crusher, Ball stretching, CBT, Weights)*

Paraphilia. *Paraphilia* is a rather generic term which refers to being sexually aroused by objects, body parts, situations, or individuals not typically associated with eroticism or sex by members of the general population. *Paraphilia* is often used synonymously with *fetishism* though, technically, they differ in the sense that a fetish is a *requirement* for sexual gratification. Paraphilia may be more appropriate as a technical synonym for *kink.*

Pegging. *Pegging* typically and correctly refers to the sexual practice in which a woman penetrates a man's anus with a strap-on dildo, though it is also sometimes used to refer any penetrative sex involving a strap-on dildo, without regard to gender or orifice. *(See also: FemDom, Forced feminization, Strap-on)*

Pet Play. Pet play *(sometimes referred to as kitten play, puppy play, pony play, ponyism, or animal role play)* consists of two or more role players, one of whom takes on the characteristics of a cherished pet while the other typically plays the role of an owner, caretaker, trainer or rider. Pet play can be sexual or asexual, and in the case of sexual pet play, may include role play scenarios involving discipline, humiliation and sado-masochism, as might be applied by an owner to his naughty puppy, for example. *(See also: Furry, Pony play, Ponygirl/Ponyboy, Primal)*

Pharoanic Lord. *(See: Lesser God Dom.)*

Piercing. *(See: Needle play)*

Pillory. *(See: Stocks)*

Pinwheel. A *pinwheel* is a small device, also known as a Wartenburg Neurowheel. It is named after its inventor, Robert Wartenberg, who invented it to test nerve sensitivity as it was rolled across a patient's skin. It was commonly used in in the past in many kinds of BDSM scenes, but less so today due to health concerns, since it breaks the skin with its tiny sharp spikes, which are arranged like a child's pinwheel toy. *(See also: Sensation play)*

Play Collar. A *play collar* refers to any collar that is worn primarily for *utilitarian purposes* during a BDSM play session. Typically, play collars are constructed of leather or metal, but they can literally be made of any material that is appropriate for the type of play that is going to take place. The most common type of play collar used in *bondage* scenes are constructed of durable leather and heavy-duty steel D-rings which facilitate the attachment of chains, straps, rope, or other restraints to the collar. Other types of play collars may include posture collars, neck corsets, steel lockable collars, rubber or PVC collars, medical (cervical) collars, ball gag collars, bit gag collars, or hooded collars. *(See also: Collar, Collar of consideration, Collar of protection, Day collar)*

Plural Marriage. *(See also: Polyamory, Group marriage)*

Podophilia. *(See: Foot Worship)*

Polyamory. The practice or ability to love more than one person at a time; from the Latin *poly* (many) and *amor* (love). Just because polyamory is relatively common in the D/s lifestyle doesn't mean that people in the lifestyle are any better at it than anyone else. It is a profoundly difficult thing to be successfully polyamorous in *any* relationship, D/s or otherwise. For more on Polyamory, see Chapter 12: Polyamory,

Polyandry. Refers to a polyamorous relationship in which a woman has more than one male partner. It is typically used to describe a polygamous or plural *marriage* consisting of a wife with two or more husbands. *(See also: Group marriage, Polyamory)*

Polyfidelous. The practice of being faithful to more than one partner, usually in a polyamorous relationship, is called *polyfidelity*. For example, a polyamorous Dominant with two submissives may choose to be *polyfidelous* to his two partners, not engaging in intimate relations with anyone else. This may or may not include BDSM fetish-play, as many people in the BDSM lifestyle do not consider such activity as "intimate." Ultimately, the meaning of polyfidelity should be mutually agreed upon by the individuals in the relationship. *(See also: Group marriage, Polyamory)*

Polygyny. Refers to a polyamorous relationship in which a man has more than one female partner. It is typically used to describe a polygamous or plural *marriage* consisting of a husband with two or more wives. *(See also: Group marriage, Polyamory)*

Polyvinyl Chloride (PVC). *Polyvinyl Chloride or PVC,* as it is commonly referred to, is a synthetic polymer plastic that can be produced in rigid or flexible form. In its pure form, PVC resembles the hard white plastic generally associated with plastic piping and conduits. When PVC is combined with certain other substances, it becomes pliable and a less expensive substitute for leather, natural rubber, or other materials used in fetish-wear. PVC can be produced to be glossy or matte, flexible or rigid. It is often confused for leather, rubber, latex, or other types of plastic. *(See also: Latex, Rubber)*

Pony Play. Pony Play refers to a form of pet play that involves assuming the role of a pet pony. Ponies typically fall into three categories: cart ponies, riding ponies, and show ponies. Cart ponies pull a small cart called a sulky, which carries her owner or other riders. Riding ponies prefer to be ridden directly, either while on all fours, or standing, with the rider on her back or shoulders. Since this can be problematic due to the rider's weight, it is often simulated. Show ponies are all about the *dressage*, and often wear very elaborate plumes, braids, harnesses, bridles, and other decorative items. *(See also: Pet play, Ponygirl, Ponyboy, Pony Slave)*

Ponygirl / Ponyboy / Pony Slave. Refers to a person who enjoys or gets sexually aroused by assuming the role of a pony for pony play. *(See also: Pet play, Pony play.)*

Poppers. Typically refers to small glass ampules encased in a pouch made of absorbent material. The ampules, when crushed, release a liquid that soaks the absorbent material and becomes an inhalant that produces a momentary feeling of heart-pounding euphoria or inebriation. Poppers usually contain amyl nitrate, butyl nitrate or other similar compounds and are sold over-the-counter in adult retail establishments under various brand names as liquid incense. The same inhalants are also often sold in liquid form in small bottles as solvents, cleaners, or air fresheners. Inhaling the fumes during sex often results in intense orgasm, increased heart rate and respiration, and relaxation of the anal sphincter. Overuse of poppers and similar inhalants can lead to serious medical problems, including death.

Postural Asphyxiation. *Postural asphyxiation* occurs when a person's *body position* makes it difficult or impossible for that person to breathe. Different people may be susceptible to postural asphyxiation as a result of different positions, which makes it extremely difficult to anticipate or take preventative measures for. The best strategy for mitigating the effects of postural asphyxiation is *continuous monitoring* of the bottom's physical, emotional, and cognitive condition. *(See also: Asphyxiation, Autoerotic asphyxiation)*

Predicament Bondage. *Predicament bondage* typically refers to a scene that features either a bondage position that is untenable or difficult to maintain for very long, or the dilemma of having to choose between two equally uncomfortable or painful options. An example of the former would be a bondage position that requires a bottom to stand on his or her tiptoes in order to reduce the discomfort of a partial suspension. As the tiptoe stance becomes untenable and the bottom stands *flat-footed*, the discomfort of the partial suspension becomes significantly more intense. An example of the latter would be a bottom who is given a choice between having her ass spanked and having her pussy spanked. When she gives a signal that one has become unbearable, the Top will switch to the other, alternating back and forth as appropriate. Predicament bondage is generally considered to be a form of *edge play*, meaning that it carries a higher than average risk of injury. *(See also: Bondage, Kinbaku, Restraints, Shibari)*

Primal. A person who embraces his or her *animalistic or primal instincts*. Primals are often neither inherently dominant nor submissive by nature. Primals tend to prefer nontraditional poly relationships patterned on the *pack or pride dynamic*, similar to that of wolves and lions. Primals *do* treat dominance and submission as a significant part of their interactions with others, but it is something that is fluid and spontaneous, and often established in an ad-hoc, spur of the moment fashion upon meeting someone for the first time. This process of establishing dominance or submission may involve stare-downs, sniffing, verbal sparring, or even physical aggression. On a hypothetical spectrum with *role play* at one end and *real life* at the other, primalism tends to be a core personality trait, while furryism is more a matter of role play. A primal considers himself an *animal in a human body*, while a furry *envisions* himself and role plays as a human in an *animal body. (See also: Furry, Pet play, Role play)*

Prison Fantasy. *Prison fantasies and role play* typical involve simulations of being held captive in a jail cell, prison, or cage and being humiliated, punished or coerced to engage in sexual acts. This type of role play is often combined with abduction play, medical play, humiliation and bondage. *(See also: Abduction play, Bondage, Caging, Humiliation, Medical play)*

Protocol: The customs, courtesies and practices of a group which have become semi-formalized over time, and are generally expected to be observed by members of the group. There are certain protocols common to almost all aspects of the D/s lifestyle, as well as certain protocols that are specific only to subcultures within the lifestyle. One example of a protocol that is common to the BDSM lifestyle in general is the customary use of honorifics, such as *Master, Mistress, Sir, or Ma'am*. An example of a custom or protocol common to the *Littles subculture* might be the practice of addressing a Dominant as *Mister, Mistress, Daddy, or Mommy.* For more information about typical BDSM munch group customs and protocols, see Chapter 10 - BDSM Groups and Activities.

Puppy Play. *(See: Pet play)*

Pussy Spanking. *Pussy spanking* consists of strikes to a woman's genitalia with a bare, open hand. The strikes may be soft or hard, singular or multiple strikes, slow or fast-paced, or any combination of the above. Pussy spanking is often done in conjunction with other types of impact play, to include traditional OTK spankings, and bondage play. *(See also: Impact play, OTK spanking, Spanking)*

Pussy Whipping. *Pussy whipping* generally refers to any activity that consists of striking a female bottom's genitals with an implement such as a whip, crop, slapper, flogger, or cane. Pussy whipping is often done while a bottom is immobilized by restraints or as a part of humiliation play. *(See also: Bondage, Crops, Humiliation, Impact play, Pussy spanking)*

Pussy Worship. *Pussy worship* consists of an intense, demonstrated adoration of female genitalia. While it is technically a *fetish*, pussy worship is not a *paraphilia*, since the genitalia *is normally* associated with sexual arousal. *(See also: FemDom, Humiliation, Paraphilia, Queening, Queening Stool, Smotherbox)*

Quad. A *quad* is a polyamorous relationship consisting of four people. *(See also: Polyamory.)*

Queening. *(See: Face Sitting)*

Queening Stool. A *queening stool* is a specialized stool that allows access to the seated person's bare genitals to a person lying on his or her back below. It is used primarily for *forced cunnilingus, or face sitting. (See also: Face Sitting, Humiliation, Queening, Smotherbox)*

Rack. *Racks* are sometimes referred to as *torture* or *stretching racks* and were used for torture, and sometimes even *execution,* for over two thousand years. A traditional rack consisted of a wooden frame or table-like device which sat horizontally or at a slight incline, with *ratcheting rollers or cylinders* at each end. Attached to the ratcheting rollers were ropes, chains or cables which were, in turn, attached to wrist or ankle cuffs. A subject would be placed on the rack and restrained by the wrist and ankle cuffs before his torturer would begin ratcheting the rollers tight to put excruciating tension on the arms and legs. Often, the person would be held immobile on the rack by the tension while other forms of torture, such as whipping, burning, or cutting were applied. Eventually, the tension would be increased and the subject's cartilage, ligaments, and bones would begin to pop, tear, and dislocate. Modern-day racks used in BDSM play apply the same general mechanism to stretch a person out lengthwise by his wrists and ankles, typically to immobilize the subject while *other* things are done to him. *(See also: St. Andrews Cross, Table play, Torture)*

R.A.C.K. Acronym for Risk Aware Consensual Kink. Refers to the practice of knowing and evaluating the *realistic risks* of what you are doing, and whom you are doing it with, before engaging in any BDSM activity. *(See also: S.S.C.)*

Rape Fantasy. Sexual arousal or gratification from thinking about or acting out a fantasy or simulated rape scene is relatively common, yet rarely discussed openly in polite society for a number of good reasons. In the BDSM lifestyle, rape role play is generally referred to as a form of *"consensual non-consent"*, meaning that a bottom gives actual consent to the activity *prior to a scene*, with the understanding that *any non-consent that is expressed during a scene is not to be taken seriously.* Obviously, this can be a very risky activity for everyone involved, since even the simplest misunderstanding can have serious ramifications. This sort of play is also highly controversial in the sense that there are people who feel that it glorifies or legitimizes violence against women and that *even discussing* it can needlessly traumatize those who have been victimized in the past. *(See also: Abduction play, Bondage, Consent, Consensual non-consent, Prison fantasy, R.A.C.K., and S.S.C.)*

Religious Fantasy. *Religious fantasy and role play* typically relies on iconic religious symbols, rituals, or authority figures such as priests and nuns for sexual arousal or gratification. The fantasies often rely heavily upon the societal taboo of mixing sex and religion which, for many people, makes it feel all the more sacrilegious and naughty. For some, particularly people who may have been raised in a religious home, a religious authority figure may be viewed as the *ultimate Dominant,* acting with the *authority of God.* Still others may have no religious background at all, but take great joy in skewering society's *sacred cows* in a variety of kinky ways. Religious fantasy and role play should *not* be confused with the relationship dynamic that exists between a *Lesser God Dominant* and his or her *acolytes. (See also: Acolyte, Lesser God Dominant, Role play)*

Restraints. *Restraints* refer to virtually anything that can be used to immobilize or limit the movement of a bottom in a bondage scene. The most common forms of BDSM restraints are wrist and ankle cuffs, handcuffs, thigh cuffs, arm cuffs, collars, arm sleeves, bondage harnesses, spreader bars, and similar types of bondage gear. *(See also: Arm/Leg sleeves, Bondage, Collars, Harness, Kinbaku, Shibari, Spreader bar)*

Role Play. *Role playing* refers to any activity that involves *acting out roles* in a hypothetical or fantasy scenario. Role play in the BDSM lifestyle is typically erotic in nature and usually involves a power exchange dynamic of some sort. The most common forms of BDSM role play are Topping, bottoming, and switching. A person need not necessarily be a Dominant to Top, nor a submissive to bottom. Sexual role play is also often associated with various types of *paraphilia*, or sexual arousal from things not typically associated with sex. *(See also: AB/DL, Abandonment, Abduction play, Age play, Auctions, Bottom, Diaper play, Forniphilia, Gor, Infantilism, Injection play, Interrogation play, Kiajira, Medical Play, Paraphilia, Pet play, Pony play, Ponygirl/ponyboy, Prison Fantasy, Religious fantasy, Switch, Top, Veterinary play)*

Rope Play. Any BDSM activity that involves *rope bondage* or *suspension*. *(See also: Bondage, Kinbaku, Restraints, Shibari, Suspension).*

Rubber. *Rubber* comes in two varieties - natural and synthetic. *Latex,* which is sometimes erroneously considered to be something different from rubber, is actually the sap that is a natural *component* of rubber. Synthetic rubber, on the other hand, is produced from petroleum compounds and does *not* contain latex. This distinction is relatively unimportant to most people, unless you happen to suffer allergic reactions to latex products. *Rubber* is a term that is often generically applied to just about any material which demonstrates a high degree of *elasticity,* to include some types of PVC which are technically *not* a form of rubber. Rubber is popular and commonly used in the BDSM culture for sex toys, impact toys, restraints, and high-end specialty fetish-wear. *(See also: Polyvinyl chloride/PVC)*

Sadism. *Sadism* is the enjoyment, satisfaction, or sexual arousal from inflicting *physical or emotion pain*, suffering, humiliation, or discomfort upon another person. It can manifest itself as a personality trait that has no connection whatsoever to the fetish culture, or as an intense sexual kink, or anything in-between. In extreme cases, it can even be classified as a mental disorder. The *psychological* classifications of sexual sadists fall into four categories:

- The Class I Sexual Sadist has sadistic thoughts and fantasies of inflicting pain and suffering on his or her sex partners, but *does not act* on those sadistic sexual fantasies.
- The Class II Sexual Sadist has sadistic thoughts and fantasies of inflicting pain and suffering on his or her sex partners and acts out those sadistic urges, but *only with consenting adult partners.*
- The Class III Sexual Sadist commits criminal acts by acting on his or her sadistic compulsions with *non-consenting victims,* but doesn't go so far as to seriously injure or kill his victims.

- Class IV Sexual Sadist commits criminal acts by acting on his or her sadistic compulsions with *non-consenting victims* and *does* seriously injure or kill them.

In short, Class I sexual sadists are *in the closet*. Class II sexual sadists fit right in with your typical BDSM lifestyle kinksters. Class III sexual sadists are *criminal predators*, and Class IV sexual sadists are *pathologically dangerous criminals*. *(See also: BDSM, Masochism, Sadistic Dominant)*

Sadistic Dominant. A Sadistic Dominant is one who enjoys or is sexually aroused by inflicting physical or emotional pain, suffering or humiliation upon his partners. Whether or not the Sadistic Dom's partner is a masochist is usually *not relevant* to the pleasure he derives from it. *(See also: Dominant, Masochism, Sadism)*

Sadomasochism. *(See: Masochism, Sadism, Sadistic Dominant)*

Safe Word. A *safe word* is a pre-arranged, mutually understood and agreed-upon code-word that can be used by a bottom during a BDSM scene to signal to the Top and/or anyone else present that all activity must stop immediately. The use of a safe-word is typically the result of one or more of the bottom's soft or hard limits being exceeded; however, for all practical purposes, it can be used *anytime* a bottom cannot continue with a scene, since one of the defining characteristics of a safe word is that no explanation is required, nor should one be demanded when it is used. A safe word should be *unusual* enough that it is not uttered inadvertently or misunderstood when it is used deliberately, however it should not be *so* unusual that it can't be recalled or is difficult to say when in pain or under stress.

Saint Andrews Cross. The *St Andrew's cross*, which is also sometimes referred to as an *X-frame* or *saltire cross*, consists essentially of two cross-beams in the form of a large letter "X", with hardware at the ends of the beams to facilitate the attachment of wrist and ankle restraints. It may or may not be padded, may be completely vertical or canted, and can be constructed from practically any sturdy material. Bottoms may be attached facing the cross or facing outward, depending on the type of play being contemplated. *(See also: Bondage, Racks, Restraints)*

S.A.M./Sammy. Acronym for *Smart-ass Masochist.* A *Sammy* is a submissive who intentionally misbehaves, lacks discipline, and/or refuses to observe generally accepted customs and protocol. *(See also: Brat, Masochist, Protocol, Service Top, Submissive, Topping from the Bottom)*

Saran Wrap. *(See: Bondage, Breath play, Mummification, Immobilization, Postural asphyxiation)*

Scene. A BDSM *scene* may refer to any BDSM activity and setting; however it more accurately refers to a BDSM activity that is done in front of an *audience.* A scene should be considered a *performance*, and not be interrupted or interfered with in any way. Scenes do not usually involve explicitly *sexual* activity, but there are always exceptions, and it is not uncommon for participants (or even observers) to experience a *sexual reaction* to what might be considered by most to be a *non-sexual* activity. Before participating in any kind of BDSM scene, always be sure that all participants are clear on exactly what will be involved, whether it will involve sex, and what safety measures will be in effect. *(See also: Bondage, Bottom, Impact play, Fluid bonding, Role play, Safe word, Top)*

Sensation Play. *Sensation play* refers to any activity that involves a sharp focus on the physical sensations of touch, temperature, taste, smell, hearing, and sight. Some types of sensation play may be very subtle and others not quite so subtle. Sensation play may also include sensory deprivation activities, such as the use of blindfolds. Other examples of sensation play are: tickle play, temperature play (i.e. ice or hot wax), electrical play (i.e. violet wands or TENS units), abrasion, and cupping. *(See also: Abrasion play, Blindfolds, Cupping, Electrical play, EMS units, Hot wax play, TENS units, Tickle play, Violet wand)*

Service Sub/Slave. *(See also: Domestic)*

Service Top. A *Service Top* is a person who is *topping*, or acting in a dominant role, at the request or direction of their partner, who is a *bottom, submissive, or switch*. This type of direction or guidance by the bottom is sometimes called *topping from the bottom. (See also: Top, Switch, Bottom, Topping from the bottom.)*

Shibari. A form of Japanese rope bondage that involves highly intricate and visually appealing patterns and knots. In the BDSM lifestyle, there is a robust sub-culture devoted almost entirely to rope bondage in general, and Japanese rope bondage in particular. Some devotees of shibari make the distinction between shibari, which is technically the art of tying and knotting, and *kinbaku*, which is the application of that art in an erotic or sexual way. *(See also: Bondage, Kinbaku, Restraints, Rope play, Suspension)*

Slapping. Striking the face with an open hand; usually done to heighten a submissive's emotional state. Face slapping is often an activity enjoyed by those who seek *humiliation* as part of their BDSM play. As a general rule, it is usually a good idea to *ensure* that your partner wants to have this done before engaging in it, since this is an activity that can be an instant source of misunderstanding, and can turn ugly *really fast. (See also: Humiliation, Impact play, Spanking)*

Slave. A submissive who cultivates and enjoys the illusion that he or she has no free will. The fact that this is an illusion should surprise no one, since the foundation of any D/s relationship is always *consent*. Many in the lifestyle consider this a form of consensual non-consent. The many different types of slaves could literally fill an entire book, but it should suffice to say that the word *slave* can mean very different things to different people. Anyone considering becoming a slave should define exactly what that means to everyone involved, especially when one considers the fact that the law takes a dim view of anything that resembles *actual* slavery. *(See also: Consent, Consensual non-consent, Gor, Master)*

Slave Contract. A *slave contract* is an agreement which requires the slave to relinquish all personal rights, property, finances and decision making powers to the slave-owner or Master. Even though they are quite popular, especially in the online BDSM community, there are numerous reasons why slave contracts are illegal and unenforceable. *(See also: Consent, Consensual non-consent, Gor, Master)*

Sleep Sack. A *sleep sack* is simply a cloth bag similar to a *sleeping bag* which can be used to enclose a person either entirely or with the head protruding. It is used most commonly as a unique form of bondage and often in conjunction with other forms of BDSM play such as age play and abduction play. *(See also: Bondage, Restraints)*

Smotherbox. A *smother box is a* device used in activities involving *queening or face sitting*. It is a box with two openings - one on the vertical face of the box to allow the head entry into the box, and the other in the top of the box to expose the face to the Dominant's genitals, above. The inside of a smotherbox is sometimes padded to prevent the head from moving. *(See also: Face sitting, Humiliation, Queening, Queening stool.)*

Spanking. Any striking activity that involves an open hand, unless it is to the face or breasts, in which case it is usually considered *slapping.* While spanking is generally associated with strikes to the buttocks, it is also fairly common for spankings to target the inner thighs, backs of the legs, and the groin area. Depending on the D/s dynamic, spankings can be delivered as either reward or punishment, or even a combination of the two. Some people like to differentiate an *erotic spanking* (which usually involves sexual fondling or other sex acts) from a simple spanking, which does not. A spanking can be an end in itself, or used as a type of foreplay that is used to heighten psychological or physical arousal. Spankings are often combined with bondage, age play, and other types of scenes. *(See also: Impact play, Pussy spanking, Slapping)*

Speculum. A *speculum (plural: specula)* is a hand-held medical device which facilitates looking into body cavities. It is used most commonly by a gynecologist to examine a woman's vagina, obtain a Pap test sample, or to conduct a biopsy. Specula may come in a variety of designs, to include vaginal, anal, dilating, and even some with mechanisms to inflate the body cavity with air. In the BDSM culture, specula are used primarily in medical role play. *(See also: Medical play)*

Spreader Bar. A *spreader bar* is a device designed to keep a person's legs spread wide apart in order to provide easy access to his or her genitalia. It is essentially just a stick, two to four feet in length, with rings at each end, to which *ankle (or sometimes, wrist) cuff*s may be attached. Some spreader bar designs incorporate additional features such as center-mounted shackles for wrists or collars, adjustable length, extra rings or clips, or suspension gear. *(See also: Bondage, Restraints)*

Squick. *Squick* is a recently coined word which means to be viscerally turned-off by something. It is often used synonymously for *repulsed or disgusted,* as in, *"Scat play really squicks me out."* It is generally believed that the word is a combination of *squeamish and icky,* though the actual etymology is unclear. There has been some controversy regarding whether or not *repulsion* and/or *disgust* carry connotations of *judgment and moralizing.* This is a particularly sensitive topic in a culture where judging and moralizing are generally considered the ultimate taboo. Being *disguste*d by a BDSM scene *may imply to some* that you consider what the participants are doing to be *morally wrong.* On the other hand, certain foods can disgust you without there being any implication of moral judgment. This controversy is not likely to be settled anytime soon.

S.S.C. Acronym for *Safe, Sane, and Consensual.* For many years, SSC was a popular mantra of the BDSM culture; however recently it has come under a great deal of scrutiny and criticism for being far too subjective to be useful. Obviously, one person's notion of what is "safe" can differ greatly from another's, and *sanity* can be hard to define in *any* context. *(See also: Consent, Consensual non-consent, R.A.C.K.)*

Stocks. Stocks and pillories were popular in medieval times as a form of public humiliation and punishment. The two terms are often used interchangeably, but they are technically two very *different* devices.

Both typically consist of hinged or sliding planks of wood with cut-outs used for restraining certain parts of the human body. A *pillory,* however, is used to restrain the *hands and neck only,* and is supported in such a way that the person in it *must stand. Stocks* are set *vertically* and used to immobilize only the subject's *arms and legs* while he typically *sits.* Some variations immobilize *all three* appendages - the neck, arms, *and* legs. Stocks, pillories, and similar devices are usually generically referred to as *stocks. (See also: Bondage, Discipline, Humiliation)*

Strait Jacket. A *straitjacket* is typically a canvas garment top that closes in the back and has overly long sleeves which, when worn, are crossed over the chest and then tied or buckled in the back, which prevents the wearer from using his arms and hands. Some newer designs are made with leather, latex rubber, PVC or a combination of those materials. Minor variations can include arms that cross in the back instead of across the chest, the addition of wrist or crotch straps, breast-access zippers, built-in toy harnesses, built-in chastity belts, and sturdy closures or fasteners that will accommodate padlocks. *(See also: Abduction play, Bondage, Interrogation play, Medical play, Prison fantasy)*

Strap-on. A *strap-on dildo* is a phallic sex toy designed to be worn with a harness. They exist in a variety of different configurations and styles which are usually worn over the groin area, but are also sometimes worn on other parts of the body and even the face. Strap-ons can be worn by either sex, and are used for vaginal sex, anal sex, oral sex, and even masturbation. *(See also: Bottom, Pegging, Top)*

Strapping. *Strapping* is a generic term for using a length of leather, such as a belt, in impact play. The term may also sometimes also refer to *restraints,* as in, *"strapping someone to the equipment." (See also: Impact play, Whipping)*

Submissive. A submissive is someone who acts in a compliant or submissive role in life, and especially in *relationships.* A submissive may be a *"true submissive"* in the sense that this trait is firmly hard-wired into his or her psyche and the submissive simply doesn't know any other way to be, or he or she may be *acting out a role,* consciously or unconsciously. A submissive is defined primarily by his or her deep-seated desire to *serve* and *please* another, while feeling loved, cherished and cared for by a Dominant partner. A submissive may or may not have any knowledge or connection to the BDSM lifestyle. A submissive may or may not be a bottom, and vice versa. A bottom is someone who temporarily or situationally assumes the *role* of a submissive specifically for BDSM play. *(See also: Bottom, Dominant, Role play, Scene)*

Subspace. *Subspace* refers to an altered state of consciousness that *may* occur when a submissive or bottom experiences intense levels of pain, pleasure, or emotion either during or after a BDSM scene or activity. It is, in many ways, similar to a mild hypnotic state, to which each individual reacts differently. Subspace may manifest itself as a euphoric feeling, detachment from reality, confusion, incoherence, inability to speak, and/or unusual or inappropriate behaviors. There has been some controversy regarding whether it is a real phenomenon with broad application *at all*, with some experts claiming that subspace may simply be a matter of *individual physiology* and body chemistry. Some people, when in pain or under a great deal of stress or highly aroused, release a flood of *endorphins, serotonin or dopamine* into their bloodstreams, which are natural painkillers and can produce a *euphoric state.* Regardless of whether it is something that can happen to *anyone*, or is reserved for the lucky few who have the right body chemistry, it happens often enough that precautions should be taken, and after-care provided following a scene. *(See also: Aftercare, Bottom, Masochism, Topspace)*

Suspension. Refers to a sub-category of *rope play* that involves suspending the subject from the ceiling or frames by rope, harness, or other device. Suspensions may be highly elaborate, as in the case of certain *shibari* practices, or very simple, involving not much more than a store-bought leather harness or swing. *(See also: Bondage, Kinbaku, Restraints, Rope play, Shibari)*

Switch. A Switch is a person in the D/s lifestyle who, on the *"dominance scale,"* falls somewhere between *Dominant* on one end of the scale and *submissive* on the other end. The switch has characteristics of *both* and is generally able to assume either role as appropriate for role play and sometimes, in real life as well. It is a commonly held misconception that Switches make the best Dominants (or submissives), just as it is a myth that one must *first* learn to be a good submissive, *before* becoming a Dominant. Switches fall into two general categories. *BDSM Switches* are individuals who enjoy *performing* in either the role of a *Top* or a *Bottom,* depending upon the circumstances, their moods, or their partners. D/s Switches are people who *feel and relate* to their partners as *Dominants* or *submissives,* for essentially the same reasons.

Swolly. *Swolly* refers to a person who is both polyamorous and a swinger. Specifically, one who has multiple simultaneous loving relationships, yet also enjoys recreational sex in a swinging context. *(See also: Polyamory)*

Table Play. *Table play* refers to BDSM activities that occur on a table, typically a table that has been specially outfitted for play with padding, securing rings, or other devices. Tables may be outfitted for use as bondage platforms, torture racks, or even medical examination tables. *(See also: Medical play, Racks)*

Tampon Training. *Tampon play* is any scene related activity that involves tampons. The tampons themselves may not necessarily be the object of a paraphilia (sexual arousal from objects not typically associated with sex) but may be used to create a sense of embarrassment or humiliation. Tampons may be used in tampon play in a variety of ways, to include vaginally, anally, orally, and for public humiliation purposes. *(See also: FemDom, Forced feminization, Humiliation, Paraphilia)*

TENS Unit. Acronym which stands for Transcutaneous Electrical Nerve Stimulation. A device that uses electrical current to stimulate nerves by attaching two or more electrodes to the skin and passing a current through them. Not to be confused with a purple wand, or violet wand. *(See also: Electricity play, EMS unit, Violet Wand)*

Temperature Play. *(See: Sensation play)*

Thigh Cuffs. *(See: Restraints)*

Thumb Cuffs. *(See: Restraints)*

Third. Common term for an additional or third person who is invited into a primary couple's relationship for intimacy, love, sex, or fetish play purposes. *(See also: Polyamory)*

Ticklers. A *tickler* is usually a sort of *mini-crop or novelty flogger* with an elongated (15"-24") slender rod used for a handle. The falls, or strips of material at the business end of the tickler, may be comprised of leather, rubber, plastic, beads, delicate chains, rope, cloth, or even feathers. *(See also: Crop, Flogger)*

Tickling. *Tickling or tickle play* refers to a scene or activity that incorporates *tickling* as a reward, a punishment, as part of age play, or as a form of humiliation. Tickle play is often combined with various forms of bondage to prevent the bottom from avoiding or preventing the tickling. It is also a very common component of age play, since tickling is an archetypal adult-child interaction that universally occurs in most cultures. One example of how tickling may be incorporated into a humiliation scene is when it is used to cause a bottom to lose control of his bladder and wet himself. Not everyone is ticklish, but for those who are, the possibilities are endless. *(See also: Age play, Forced Bed Wetting, Humiliation, Sensation play, Torture, Urine play)*

Top. A *Top* is someone who *situationally or temporarily* assumes the dominant, leading, or aggressive role as part of an *activity* which is *usually*, but not necessarily limited to, a BDSM scene. A Top *may or* *may not* be a Dominant. Conversely and less commonly, a Dominant is not always a Top. *(See also: Bottom, Dominant, Master, Scene, Submissive)*

Topping from the Bottom. A submissive's practice of manipulating or influencing the decisions or behavior of a Dominant. This behavior by the submissive can be overt, purposeful, and conscious, or it can be covert, subtle, and unconscious. It is sometimes accomplished with the full knowledge and approval of the Dominant. Other times, the Dominant may be oblivious to it, even if everyone else can see it. The brat sub is the type of submissive that is most commonly associated with this sort of behavior, but in reality, it is practiced by *all* kinds of submissives, in every category of D/s relationship. A would-be Dominant who is topped from the bottom is sometimes referred to as a *Service Top. (See also: Bottom, Dominant, Service top, Submissive, Top)*

Topspace. *Topspace* refers to an altered state of consciousness which is sometimes experienced by a Top during or following a BDSM scene or activity. It is sometimes (and probably erroneously) equated with *subspace,* a mental state which may occur when a bottom experiences intense pain, pleasure or emotions. Topspace is more likely to be the product of a Top's hyper-focus, adrenaline, physical exertion, and intense emotions. Regardless of the causes, it is a real phenomenon which occurs infrequently, but often enough that precautions (such as monitoring) should be taken and aftercare provided, as needed. *(See also: Aftercare, Bottom, Scene, Subspace, Top)*

Torture. *Torture* refers to any *sustained activity over time* that consists of the intentional infliction of physical or emotional pain upon another person. One of the key elements of torture is the fact that it is sustained over a period of time; a single poke or squeeze may not qualify as torture, but a hundred of them over the course of an hour might. The most common forms of BDSM torture play are CBT, breast and nipple torture, predicament bondage, orgasm denial, and bathroom restrictions; however the list is literally endless. Torture play is also typically combined with other forms of role play or BDSM scenes, such as abduction play, interrogation play and medical play. *(See also: Abduction play, Bathroom use restrictions, Ball crushing, Ball stretching, Castration play, CBT, Interrogation play, Medical play)*

Training Collar. A training collar is, for *many* submissives, the logical second step that follows a short period of consideration and decision to move forward into a more serious and committed relationship. It is a recognition that, while a more intense and formal relationship is *desired* by both parties, there is still much to be learned by the submissive before a formal collar can be offered. During training, every action by a submissive in a training collar reflects *directly* upon the Dominant, telegraphing to all his competence - *or lack thereof* – as a trainer of submissives. This can also be a period of great stress and contention as the Dominant and submissive adjust to their new roles in the relationship, and learn to reconcile their expectations and preconceptions with reality. *(See also: Collar, Collar of consideration, Collar of protection, Day collar, Play collar)*

Triad. A *triad* is any polyamorous relationship consisting of three people. Triad relationships exist worldwide in many cultures, not just in the Poly or D/s lifestyles. *(See also: Polyamory)*

Uniform Play. *Uniform play* refers to activities which utilize a *uniform paraphilia*, or sexual arousal from either wearing or seeing others in a uniform. The uniforms are typically those worn by military service members, police officers, doctors, nurses, priests, schoolgirls, or the costumes worn by fictional superheroes. Uniforms are frequently perceived as symbolic of authority, integrity, discipline or power. Other times, as in the case of nurses, schoolgirls, and priests, they may represent chastity, purity, innocence, or caring. The arousal or emotions evoked by uniform play are sometimes used to add intensity to abduction play, age play, interrogation play, medical play, or religious fantasies. *(See also: Abduction play, Age play, Interrogation play, Littles, Medical play, Paraphilia, Religious fantasy)*

Urethra Play. *Urethra play* refers to any activity that stimulates or focuses on the urethra which, for males is the tube through which urine and semen pass and exit from the head of the penis, and for females is the tube through which urine passes and exits between the clitoris and the vagina. Urethra play typically focuses on the *male* urethra, and generally consists of inserting objects into the urethra to stimulate, arouse, or torture the subject. It is considered by some to be a form of *edge play* due to its high potential for pain or damage. *(See also: CBT, Torture)*

Urine Play. *Urine play* (sometimes referred to as *water sports*) is simply any activity that involves the fascination with, adoration of, or sexual arousal from *urine.* Urine play can take many forms, to include voyeurism (i.e. being aroused by watching others urinate), diaper play (i.e. being aroused by the sensations of a wet diaper), bathroom use restrictions (i.e. being aroused by being forced to wet oneself), golden showers (arousal from urinating on others, or from being urinated upon), and even *drinking it* which is, contrary to popular belief, actually sterile and relatively safe in small amounts. *(See also: AB/DL, Bathroom use restrictions, Diaper play, Golden showers, Paraphilia)*

Vanilla. Term used by those in the D/s, BDSM or fetish lifestyles to describe those who are outside of the lifestyle. It is generally used in the sense that anything that is *vanilla flavored* (i.e. ice cream) is considered to be unexciting or bland. The term *vanilla* is *rarely* used as a serious pejorative or insult, though some people will occasionally choose to interpret it as such. More commonly, it is simply used as a playful way of saying *"normal."*

Velcro Collar. A generally derisive term referring to the practice of *casual frequent collaring*, usually the collaring of inexperienced submissives by inexperienced Dominants, neither of whom fully grasp the symbolism of the collar, or the commitment to a relationship that it implies. "Velcro", which is a registered trademark of Velcro Industries B.V., is a reference to the *easy on, easy off* nature of this sort of collar. *(See also: Collar, Collar of consideration, Collar of protection, Play collar, Training collar)*

Versatile. *(See Switch)*

Veterinary Play. Refers to *Medical role play* that is associated with *pet play.* Instead of role playing the parts of a patient and doctor, veterinary play involves role playing as *pet and veterinarian*. *(See also: Medical play, Pet play)*

Violet Ray. *(See Violet wand)*

Violet Wand. An electrical device similar to decorative *lightning plasma globes,* but with an elongated wand-like shape, that is specifically produced for BDSM *sensation and electrical play*. As is the case with many BDSM-related toys, the violet wand *looks* a lot scarier than it really *is*, and therein lies its attraction. The artificial lightning electrical display delivers a tingling or ticklish sensation to the skin or any erogenous zone it touches, and the intensity can usually be adjusted from a mild tickle to intense pain. Most violet wands allow for a wide selection of interchangeable electrode attachments which are designed for specific purposes or sensations. At the highest settings and if left in place long enough a violet wand can actually burn or brand the skin. When first popularized in the 1920s as quack medical devices, they were called *violet rays. (See also: Branding, Electrical play, Sensation play)*

Water Sports. *(See: Urine play)*

Water Torture. *Water torture* refers to any activity that *utilizes* water to create discomfort or pain over time. Various forms of water torture may include the use of high-pressure hoses in combination with prison play, the use of extremely *hot or cold* water for sensation play, or the use of highly focused needle-like streams of water from a device like a Waterpik for stimulation or torture of sensitive areas. *(See also: Prison fantasy, Sensation play, Torture)*

Wax Play. *Wax play* generally consists of dripping or pouring molten candle wax onto someone's skin to produce erotic *sensations*, for *aesthetic* purposes, or *both*. The types of candle wax used for erotic wax play *typically* fall into two categories: *paraffin* (a man-made, petroleum-based compound) and *beeswax* (which is secreted by the wax glands of worker bees). There are many other varieties of wax that can be used, but they all generally fall into these two categories, differing only in the various additives that are combined with the waxes to change its properties, such as its burn characteristics, melting point, plasticity, or effects upon the skin. *(See also: Chapter 9 - BDSM Toys and Safety)*

Weights. *Weights* are sometimes used in various types of BDSM scenes or play to add stress, discomfort or pain as needed. Weights are most commonly used in *CBT ball stretching*, but may also be used in breast and nipple torture, labia torture, predicament bondage, mummification, and humiliation play. *(See also: Ball crushing, Ball stretching, CBT, Predicament bondage, Torture)*

Whip. A *whip* can refer to a wide range of BDSM toys, including floggers, lashes, cats-o'-nine-tails, and crops. Usually, when the word *whip* is used, it is a reference to *single-tail whips*. Single-tail whips come in three basic styles: *stock whips, bullwhips, and snake whips.* See Chapter 9 - BDSM Toys and Safety for more information on whips. *(See also: Canes, Crops, Floggers, Impact play)*

Whipping Post. A *whipping post* is a sturdy pole, frame or device used primarily for the purpose of restraining a bottom in a *standing position* to facilitate being whipped, cropped, caned, paddled, or spanked. *(See also: St. Andrews cross, Caning, Crop, Flogger, Impact play, Paddle, Rack, Torture, Whip)*

Appendix B:

Silly Shit Mike Makai Says

Have you ever uttered a sentence aloud and immediately, upon hearing it come out of your own mouth, think to yourself, "I really should *write that down.* I'm *sure* it will come in handy someday?" But of course, it never does. And so you end up with a crazy hodgepodge of quips and quotes - some funny, some profound, some just plain dopey, and you have no idea what you should *do* with them, but you're unwilling to just throw them away.

I'm a lover of words; I can't just toss them out. I have a hard enough time just lending out a book. Perhaps that makes me a little like those whack-jobs on *Hoarders* who sit around watching TV while sharing a ratty couch with a big stinking pile of dead cats. Okay, that was a really *bad* analogy. I'm *nothing* like that.

Some of these quips consist of brief commentaries on life and personal witticisms that I've *tweeted* to my followers on Twitter. On days when I'm feeling a little *cocky*, I'll sometimes ask a friend, "So, did you see what I tweeted today?" to which the typical response is, "No, unlike you, *I have a life."* That's when I hit them with my *"I-may-be-a-Dom-but-I-can-do-sad-puppy-dog-eyes-as-good-as-any-subbie"* look, and they fold like a dollar-store card table under a fat kid twerking on You Tube.

They beg me to show them what they've been missing.

And so, here it is.

# # #

If only it were as easy as going to the pharmacy, purchasing a test kit, and taking it home to pee on a little plastic stick. Red for Dominant, blue for submissive, purple for switch, and yellow for everyone else. Life would be *so* much simpler.

There's nothing sexier than confidence, and nothing dumber than over-confidence. Life is all about where you *draw the line* between the two.

I always bring a pig-slapper to a flogger fight. I don't even know what that means. I honestly just love the sound of it.

"Pussy spanking" sounds so *severe*. Try to think of it as an open-handed, rapid-fire, impact massage for your clitoris.

Saran Wrap is the Bondage Gods' way of telling you not to take your BDSM toys - *or yourself* - too seriously. Always buy an extra roll. Or ten.

People are like M&Ms. They come in a variety of colors, they're hard on the outside, and full of obscene yumminess on the inside.

I love redheads. It's not the hair color, it's the crazy.

I need a little sign in my car that says, "For your own safety, please buckle your seat belt, ankle cuffs, wrist restraints and ball gag."

Questions real people actually ask me: "So, do you know a lot about sex?" No, I just *write books* about it.

I wouldn't say I'm terribly religious, but I *am* looking for someone who's really into cock worship.

Some days, I ponder the mysteries of the universe. Other days, about the best I can do is wonder why *"now"* and *"snow"* don't rhyme.

Some people are a complete waste of our time. Others are a complete waste of our oxygen.

I prefer my version: "Abstinence makes the hard-on seek fondlers."

If this day gets any slower, I'll be moving backward in time. Can we stop at age 21 please? *That* would be *really cool.*

Entering into or even considering a D/s relationship knowing that you *cannot trust* is a little like skydiving without a parachute. It may start out great, but it *never ends well.*

Sure, I'd *love* to meet your mom. That way I can see what your boobs will look like in 20 years. Did I just say that out loud?

I don't care about your excuses. I don't care about *anyone's* excuses; not even my own. Either we accomplish what we have set out to do, *or we don't.* Not much else matters. No one asks why Jefferson Davis lost the civil war. They just know that he *did.*

Some women just make you want to know what makes them tick. Others make you wonder what happens when the ticking *stops.*

A dirty mind is a terrible thing to waste.

I think the employees at my local ranch supply store are beginning to wonder why I'm always in the tack section checking out their leather pig-slappers. I don't own a ranch. *Or* pigs.

[After seeing a photograph of a pretty redhead wearing glasses and reading a book] Did I mention I love redheads? And glasses? And short skirts? And girls who read? And... Oh fuck it, just take my 401(k) already.

Dear people who try to call me at 5:30am: *Knock that shit off.* And have a nice day.

It's easy to fall in love online with someone you'd slide away from on a bus stop bench. A little *too* damn easy.

A cage stokes our emotions and imaginations, regardless of whether you are inside looking out, or outside looking in.

I actually got asked this: *"What's your favorite safe word?"* I replied, *"More!"*

No one should ever have to get out of bed before McDonalds switches to burgers.

How we relate to our partners in relationships is a microcosm of how we relate to the world. On a completely unrelated note, have I ever mentioned that I've always wanted to conquer the world?

Relationships are something that women go into hoping that their men will change, and men go into hoping that their women won't.

How do you make someone do crazy, kinky, pervy things? You don't. At best, you can make them *want* to. Are we there yet?

Bottoming doesn't make you a submissive, any more than standing in my kitchen makes you a cook. By the way, while you're there, please make me a sandwich.

You can't *fake* being a Dominant. You *can* fake being a top. The same goes for Subs.

When I was an Army Ranger, sometimes other soldiers would tell me, *"I* could do that, if I wanted to." I'd always reply: Maybe so, but then *no one* ever really *wants* to go hungry for a week, sleep in a swamp, or parachute out of a perfectly good airplane into pitch darkness, do they? *That's* the difference between me and you. *Neither* of us wants to do that, but I do it anyway.

For $425 you can buy pills containing real gold that make your poop sparkle. How have I lived this long without sparkly poop?

Emotional whiplash: Being irresistibly attracted to a beautiful young woman while simultaneously coming to the realization that I probably have food in my refrigerator older than she is.

If you're looking for a *real* partner, then *you* need to be real. This is doubly so online. If you want a *phony partner,* then go ahead and misrepresent yourself.

A submissive who says she *trusts* you, but doesn't *believe* you, *doesn't* trust you.

A highway patrol officer pulled me over the other day and told me, "Contrary to popular belief, we don't have a *frequent flyer program* along this stretch of freeway." He wrote me a ticket, and then said, "This ain't *Cheers.* It's *not* a good thing when *we all know your name."*

There's a time and a place for everything. Like, right now, your panties belong in your panty drawer.

I have to see a doctor every few years about my ADHD medications. Today, when I saw him, he asked me if I was OCD. I said, "I don't think so. Why do you ask?" He replied, "Most people just fill out our questionnaires. You *redesigned* them."

My new and improved Golden Rule: Dom unto others and you would have God Dom unto you.

Appendix C:

About the Author

Michael Makai is an unapologetically atypical White Knight Dominant with over thirty-five years of experience in both D/s relationships and the BDSM lifestyle. He was born in Japan and raised in Hawaii and California, where he worked as a waiter and bartender to pay his own way at the University of California, Riverside. He has lived all over the United States, and spent ten years living in Europe in the Rheinland-Pfalz region of Germany, near the Franco-German border. He currently resides near Wichita Falls, Texas.

Mike spent twenty years on active duty in the United States Army, serving in a wide variety of positions, to include paratrooper, Ranger forward observer, NATO liaison officer, research development test & evaluation NCO, military doctrine instructor, and NCO academy school chief.

In addition to being an author, Mike's civilian vocations have included bartender, freelance writer, magazine publisher, web site designer, internet service provider, small business consultant, banker, stock market day trader, marketing director, graphics designer, and online retailer.

Mike's hobbies and preferred pastimes include koi ponds, music, alpine skiing, beaches, travel, foreign languages, and Scrabble.

His *kinks* are eclectic.

Printed in Great Britain
by Amazon